ce

OPEN

OPEN

An Autobiography

ANDRE AGASSI

HARPER

HARPER

An Imprint of HarperCollins*Publishers*
77–85 Fulham Palace Road,
Hammersmith, London W6 8JB

www.harpercollins.co.uk

First published in the USA in 2009 by Alfred A. Knopf
This edition published in 2010 by HarperCollins*Publishers*

9

Andre Agassi asserts the moral right to be
identified as the author of this work

A catalogue record of this book is
available from the British Library

ISBN 978-0-00-728143-5

Printed and bound in Great Britain by
Clays Ltd, St Ives plc

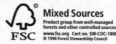

Mixed Sources
Product group from well-managed
forests and other controlled sources
www.fsc.org   Cert no. SW-COC-1806
© 1996 Forest Stewardship Council

FSC is a non-profit international organisation established to promote the
responsible management of the world's forests. Products carrying the FSC
label are independently certified to assure consumers that they come
from forests that are managed to meet the social, economic and
ecological needs of present and future generations.

Find out more about HarperCollins and the environment at
www.harpercollins.co.uk/green

For Stefanie, Jaden, and Jaz

One cannot always tell what it is that keeps us shut in, confines us, seems to bury us, but still one feels certain barriers, certain gates, certain walls. Is all this imagination, fantasy? I do not think so. And then one asks: My God! Is it for long, is it for ever, is it for eternity? Do you know what frees one from this captivity? It is very deep serious affection. Being friends, being brothers, love, that is what opens the prison by supreme power, by some magic force.

—Vincent van Gogh, *letter to his brother, July 1880*

OPEN

THE END

I OPEN MY EYES and don't know where I am or who I am. Not all that unusual—I've spent half my life not knowing. Still, this feels different. This confusion is more frightening. More total.

I look up. I'm lying on the floor beside the bed. I remember now. I moved from the bed to the floor in the middle of the night. I do that most nights. Better for my back. Too many hours on a soft mattress causes agony. I count to three, then start the long, difficult process of standing. With a cough, a groan, I roll onto my side, then curl into the fetal position, then flip over onto my stomach. Now I wait, and wait, for the blood to start pumping.

I'm a young man, relatively speaking. Thirty-six. But I wake as if ninety-six. After three decades of sprinting, stopping on a dime, jumping high and landing hard, my body no longer feels like my body, especially in the morning. Consequently my mind doesn't feel like my mind. Upon opening my eyes I'm a stranger to myself, and while, again, this isn't new, in the mornings it's more pronounced. I run quickly through the basic facts. My name is Andre Agassi. My wife's name is Stefanie Graf. We have two children, a son and daughter, five and three. We live in Las Vegas, Nevada, but currently reside in a suite at the Four Seasons hotel in New York City, because I'm playing in the 2006 U.S. Open. My last U.S. Open. In fact my last tournament ever. I play tennis for a living, even though I hate tennis, hate it with a dark and secret passion, and always have.

As this last piece of identity falls into place, I slide to my knees and in a whisper I say: Please let this be over.

Then: I'm not ready for it to be over.

Now, from the next room, I hear Stefanie and the children. They're eating breakfast, talking, laughing. My overwhelming desire to see and touch them, plus a powerful craving for caffeine, gives me the inspiration

I need to hoist myself up, to go vertical. Hate brings me to my knees, love gets me on my feet.

I glance at the bedside clock. Seven thirty. Stefanie let me sleep in. The fatigue of these final days has been severe. Apart from the physical strain, there is the exhausting torrent of emotions set loose by my pending retirement. Now, rising from the center of the fatigue comes the first wave of pain. I grab my back. It grabs me. I feel as if someone snuck in during the night and attached one of those anti-theft steering wheel locks to my spine. How can I play in the U.S. Open with the Club on my spine? Will the last match of my career be a forfeit?

I was born with spondylolisthesis, meaning a bottom vertebra that parted from the other vertebrae, struck out on its own, rebelled. (It's the main reason for my pigeon-toed walk.) With this one vertebra out of sync, there's less room for the nerves inside the column of my spine, and with the slightest movement the nerves feel that much more crowded. Throw in two herniated discs and a bone that won't stop growing in a futile effort to protect the damaged area, and those nerves start to feel downright claustrophobic. When the nerves protest their cramped quarters, when they send out distress signals, a pain runs up and down my leg that makes me suck in my breath and speak in tongues. At such moments the only relief is to lie down and wait. Sometimes, however, the moment arrives in the middle of a match. Then the only remedy is to alter my game—swing differently, run differently, do everything differently. That's when my muscles spasm. Everyone avoids change; muscles can't abide it. Told to change, my muscles join the spinal rebellion, and soon my whole body is at war with itself.

Gil, my trainer, my friend, my surrogate father, explains it this way: Your body is saying it doesn't want to do this anymore.

My body has been saying that for a long time, I tell Gil. Almost as long as I've been saying it.

Since January, however, my body has been shouting it. My body doesn't want to retire—my body has already retired. My body has moved to Florida and bought a condo and white Sansabelts. So I've been negotiating with my body, asking it to come out of retirement for a few hours here, a few hours there. Much of this negotiation revolves around a cortisone shot that temporarily dulls the pain. Before the shot works, however, it causes its own torments.

I got one yesterday, so I could play tonight. It was the third shot this year, the thirteenth of my career, and by far the most alarming. The doctor, not my regular doctor, told me brusquely to assume the position.

I stretched out on his table, face down, and his nurse yanked down my shorts. The doctor said he needed to get his seven-inch needle as close to the inflamed nerves as possible. But he couldn't enter directly, because my herniated discs and bone spur were blocking the path. His attempts to circumvent them, to break the Club, sent me through the roof. First he inserted the needle. Then he positioned a big machine over my back to see how close the needle was to the nerves. He needed to get that needle almost flush against the nerves, he said, without actually touching. If it were to touch the nerves, even if it were to only nick the nerves, the pain would ruin me for the tournament. It could also be life-changing. In and out and around, he maneuvered the needle, until my eyes filled with water.

Finally he hit the spot. Bull's-eye, he said.

In went the cortisone. The burning sensation made me bite my lip. Then came the pressure. I felt infused, embalmed. The tiny space in my spine where the nerves are housed began to feel vacuum packed. The pressure built until I thought my back would burst.

Pressure is how you know everything's working, the doctor said.

Words to live by, Doc.

Soon the pain felt wonderful, almost sweet, because it was the kind that you can tell precedes relief. But maybe all pain is like that.

MY FAMILY IS GROWING LOUDER. I limp out to the living room of our suite. My son, Jaden, and my daughter, Jaz, see me and scream. Daddy, Daddy! They jump up and down and want to leap on me. I stop and brace myself, stand before them like a mime imitating a tree in winter. They stop just before leaping, because they know Daddy is delicate these days, Daddy will shatter if they touch him too hard. I pat their faces and kiss their cheeks and join them at the breakfast table.

Jaden asks if today is the day.

Yes.

You're playing?

Yes.

And then after today are you *retire*?

A new word he and his younger sister have learned. *Retired*. When they say it, they always leave off the last letter. For them it's *retire*, forever ongoing, permanently in the present tense. Maybe they know something I don't.

Not if I win, son. If I win tonight, I keep playing.

But if you lose—we can have a dog?

To the children, retire equals puppy. Stefanie and I have promised them that when I stop training, when we stop traveling the world, we can buy a puppy. Maybe we'll name him Cortisone.

Yes, buddy, when I lose, we will buy a dog.

He smiles. He hopes Daddy loses, hopes Daddy experiences the disappointment that surpasses all others. He doesn't understand—and how will I ever be able to explain it to him?—the pain of losing, the pain of playing. It's taken me nearly thirty years to understand it myself, to solve the calculus of my own psyche.

I ask Jaden what he's doing today.

Going to see the bones.

I look at Stefanie. She reminds me she's taking them to the Museum of Natural History. Dinosaurs. I think of my twisted vertebrae. I think of my skeleton on display at the museum with all the other dinosaurs. Tennis-aurus Rex.

Jaz interrupts my thoughts. She hands me her muffin. She needs me to pick out the blueberries before she eats it. Our morning ritual. Each blueberry must be surgically removed, which requires precision, concentration. Stick the knife in, move it around, get it right up to the blueberry without touching. I focus on her muffin and it's a relief to think about something other than tennis. But as I hand her the muffin, I can't pretend that it doesn't feel like a tennis ball, which makes the muscles in my back twitch with anticipation. The time is drawing near.

AFTER BREAKFAST, after Stefanie and the kids have kissed me goodbye and run off to the museum, I sit quietly at the table, looking around the suite. It's like every hotel suite I've ever had, only more so. Clean, chic, comfortable—it's the Four Seasons, so it's lovely, but it's still just another version of what I call Not Home. The non-place we exist as athletes. I close my eyes, try to think about tonight, but my mind drifts backward. My mind these days has a natural backspin. Given half a chance it wants to return to the beginning, because I'm so close to the end. But I can't let it. Not yet. I can't afford to dwell too long on the past. I get up and walk around the table, test my balance. When I feel fairly steady I walk gingerly to the shower.

Under the hot water I groan and scream. I bend slowly, touch my quads, start to come alive. My muscles loosen. My skin sings. My pores fly open. Warm blood goes sluicing through my veins. I feel something begin to stir. Life. Hope. The last drops of youth. Still, I make no sudden movements. I don't want to do anything to startle my spine. I let my spine sleep in.

Standing at the bathroom mirror, toweling off, I stare at my face. Red eyes, gray stubble—a face totally different from the one with which I started. But also different from the one I saw last year in this same mirror. Whoever I might be, I'm not the boy who started this odyssey, and I'm not even the man who announced three months ago that the odyssey was coming to an end. I'm like a tennis racket on which I've replaced the grip four times and the strings seven times—is it accurate to call it the same racket? Somewhere in those eyes, however, I can still vaguely see the boy who didn't want to play tennis in the first place, the boy who wanted to quit, the boy who *did* quit many times. I see that golden-haired boy who hated tennis, and I wonder how he would view this bald man, who still hates tennis and yet still plays. Would he be shocked? Amused? Proud? The question makes me weary, lethargic, and it's only noon.

Please let this be over.

I'm not ready for it to be over.

The finish line at the end of a career is no different from the finish line at the end of a match. The objective is to get within reach of that finish line, because then it gives off a magnetic force. When you're close, you can feel that force pulling you, and you can use that force to get across. But just before you come within range, or just after, you feel another force, equally strong, pushing you away. It's inexplicable, mystical, these twin forces, these contradictory energies, but they both exist. I know, because I've spent much of my life seeking the one, fighting the other, and sometimes I've been stuck, suspended, bounced like a tennis ball between the two.

Tonight: I remind myself that it will require iron discipline to cope with these forces, and whatever else comes my way. Back pain, bad shots, foul weather, self-loathing. It's a form of worry, this reminder, but also a meditation. One thing I've learned in twenty-nine years of playing tennis: Life will throw everything but the kitchen sink in your path, and then it will throw the kitchen sink. It's your job to avoid the obstacles. If you let them stop you or distract you, you're not doing your job, and failing to do your job will cause regrets that paralyze you more than a bad back.

I lie on the bed with a glass of water and read. When my eyes get tired I click on the TV. *Tonight, Round Two of the U.S. Open! Will this be Andre Agassi's farewell?* My face flashes on the screen. A different face than the one in the mirror. My game face. I study this new reflection of me in the distorted mirror that is TV and my anxiety rises another click or two. Was that the final commercial? The final time CBS will ever promote one of my matches?

I can't escape the feeling that I'm about to die.

It's no accident, I think, that tennis uses the language of life. Advantage, service, fault, break, love, the basic elements of tennis are those of everyday existence, because every match is a life in miniature. Even the structure of tennis, the way the pieces fit inside one another like Russian nesting dolls, mimics the structure of our days. Points become games become sets become tournaments, and it's all so tightly connected that any point can become the turning point. It reminds me of the way seconds become minutes become hours, and any hour can be our finest. Or darkest. It's our choice.

But if tennis is life, then what follows tennis must be the unknowable void. The thought makes me cold.

Stefanie bursts through the door with the kids. They flop on the bed, and my son asks how I'm feeling.

Fine, fine. How were the bones?

Fun!

Stefanie gives them sandwiches and juice and hustles them out the door again.

They have a playdate, she says.

Don't we all.

Now I can take a nap. At thirty-six, the only way I can play a late match, which could go past midnight, is if I get a nap beforehand. Also, now that I know roughly who I am, I want to close my eyes and hide from it. When I open my eyes, one hour has passed. I say aloud, It's time. No more hiding. I step into the shower again, but this shower is different from the morning shower. The afternoon shower is always longer—twenty-two minutes, give or take—and it's not for waking up or getting clean. The afternoon shower is for encouraging myself, coaching myself.

Tennis is the sport in which you talk to yourself. No athletes talk to themselves like tennis players. Pitchers, golfers, goalkeepers, they mutter to themselves, of course, but tennis players *talk* to themselves—and *answer*. In the heat of a match, tennis players look like lunatics in a public square, ranting and swearing and conducting Lincoln-Douglas debates with their alter egos. Why? Because tennis is so damned lonely. Only boxers can understand the loneliness of tennis players—and yet boxers have their corner men and managers. Even a boxer's opponent provides a kind of companionship, someone he can grapple with and grunt at. In tennis you stand face-to-face with the enemy, trade blows with him, but never touch him or talk to him, or anyone else. The rules forbid a tennis player from even talking to his coach while on the court. People sometimes mention the track-and-field runner as a comparably lonely figure, but I have to laugh. At least the runner can feel and smell his opponents. They're inches away. In tennis you're on an island. Of all the games men and women play, tennis is the closest to solitary confinement, which inevitably leads to self-talk, and for me the self-talk starts here in the afternoon shower. This is when I begin to say things to myself, crazy things, over and over, until I believe them. For instance, that a quasi-cripple can compete at the U.S. Open. That a thirty-six-year-old man can beat an opponent just entering his prime. I've won 869 matches in my career, fifth on the all-time list, and many were won during the afternoon shower.

With the water roaring in my ears—a sound not unlike twenty thousand fans—I recall particular wins. Not wins the fans would remember, but wins that still wake me at night. Squillari in Paris. Blake in New York. Pete in Australia. Then I recall a few losses. I shake my head at the disappointments. I tell myself that tonight will be an exam for which I've been studying twenty-nine years. Whatever happens tonight, I've already been through it at least once before. If it's a physical test, if it's mental, it's nothing new.

Please let this be over.

I don't want it to be over.

I start to cry. I lean against the wall of the shower and let go.

I GIVE MYSELF STRICT ORDERS as I shave: Take it one point at a time. Make him work for everything. No matter what happens, hold your head up. And for God's sake enjoy it, or at least try to enjoy moments of it, even the pain, even the losing, if that's what's in store.

I think about my opponent, Marcos Baghdatis, and wonder what he's doing at this moment. He's new to the tour, but not your typical newcomer. He's ranked number eight in the world. He's a big strong Greek kid from Cyprus, in the middle of a superb year. He's reached the final of the Australian Open and the semis of Wimbledon. I know him fairly well. During last year's U.S. Open we played a practice set. Typically I don't play practice sets with other players during a Grand Slam, but Baghdatis asked with disarming grace. A TV show from Cyprus was doing a piece about him, and he asked if it would be all right if they filmed us practicing. Sure, I said. Why not? I won the practice set, 6–2, and afterward he was all smiles. I saw that he's the type who smiles when he's happy or nervous, and you can't tell which. It reminded me of someone, but I couldn't think who.

I told Baghdatis that he played a little like me, and he said it was no accident. He grew up with pictures of me on his bedroom wall, patterned his game after mine. In other words, tonight I'll be playing my mirror image. He'll play from the back of the court, take the ball early, swing for the fences, just like me. It's going to be toe-to-toe tennis, each of us trying to impose our will, each of us looking for chances to smoke a backhand up the line. He doesn't have an overwhelming serve, nor do I, which means long points, long rallies, lots of energy and time expended. I brace myself for flurries, combinations, a tennis of attrition, the most brutal form of the sport.

Of course the one stark difference between me and Baghdatis is physical. We have different bodies. He has my former body. He's nimble, fast, spry. I'll have to beat the younger version of myself if I am to keep the older version going. I close my eyes and say: Control what you can control.

I say it again, aloud. Saying it aloud makes me feel brave.

I shut off the water and stand, shivering. How much easier it is to be brave under a stream of piping hot water. I remind myself, however, that hot-water bravery isn't true bravery. What you feel doesn't matter in the end; it's what you do that makes you brave.

STEFANIE AND THE KIDS RETURN. Time to make the Gil Water.

I sweat a lot, more than most players, so I need to begin hydrating many hours before a match. I down quarts of a magic elixir invented for me by Gil, my trainer for the last seventeen years. Gil Water is a blend of carbs, electrolytes, salt, vitamins, and a few other ingredients Gil keeps a closely guarded secret. (He's been tinkering with his recipe for two decades.) He usually starts force-feeding me Gil Water the night before a match, and keeps forcing me right up to match time. Then I sip it as the match wears on. At different stages I sip different versions, each a different color. Pink for energy, red for recovery, brown for replenishment.

The kids love helping me mix Gil Water. They fight over who gets to scoop out the powders, who gets to hold the funnel, who gets to pour it all into plastic water bottles. No one but me, however, can pack the bottles into my bag, along with my clothes and towels and books and shades and wristbands. (My rackets, as always, go in later.) No one but me touches my tennis bag, and when it's finally packed, it stands by the door, like an assassin's kit, a sign that the day has lurched that much closer to the witching hour.

At five, Gil rings from the lobby.

He says, You ready? Time to throw down. It's on, Andre. It's on.

Nowadays everyone says *It's on,* but Gil has been saying it for years, and no one says it the way he does. When Gil says *It's on,* I feel my booster rockets fire, my adrenaline glands pump like geysers. I feel as if I can lift a car over my head.

Stefanie gathers the children at the door and tells them it's time for Daddy to leave. What do you say, guys?

Jaden shouts, Kick butt, Daddy!

Kick butt, Jaz says, copying her brother.

Stefanie kisses me and says nothing, because there's nothing to say.

IN THE TOWN CAR Gil sits in the front seat, dressed sharp. Black shirt, black tie, black jacket. He dresses for every match as if it's a blind date or a mob hit. Now and then he checks his long black hair in the side mirror or rearview. I sit in the backseat with Darren, my coach, an Aussie who always rocks a Hollywood tan and the smile of a guy who just hit the Powerball. For a few minutes no one says anything. Then Gil speaks the lyrics of one of our favorites, an old Roy Clark ballad, and his deep basso fills the car:

> Just going through the motions and pretending
> we have something left to gain—

He looks to me, waits.

I say, We Can't Build a Fire in the Rain.

He laughs. I laugh. For a second I forget my nervous butterflies.

Butterflies are funny. Some days they make you run to the toilet. Other days they make you horny. Other days they make you laugh, and long for the fight. Deciding which type of butterflies you've got going (monarchs or moths) is the first order of business when you're driving to the arena. Figuring out your butterflies, deciphering what they say about the status of your mind and body, is the first step to making them work for you. One of the thousand lessons I've learned from Gil.

I ask Darren for his thoughts on Baghdatis. How aggressive do I want to be tonight? Tennis is about degrees of aggression. You want to be aggressive enough to control a point, not so aggressive that you sacrifice control and expose yourself to unnecessary risk. My questions about Baghdatis are these: How will he try to hurt me? If I hit a backhand cross-court to start a point, some players will be patient, others will make a statement right away, crush the ball up the line or come hard to the net. Since I've never played Baghdatis outside of our one practice set, I want to know how he'll react to conservative play. Will he step up and jack that routine crosscourt, or lie back, bide his time?

Darren says, Mate, I think if you get too conservative on your rally shot, you can expect this guy to move around it and hurt you with his forehand.

I see.

As far as his backhand goes, he can't hit it easily up the line. He won't be quick to pull that trigger. So if you find he *is* hitting backhands up the line, that definitely means you're not putting enough steam on your rally shot.

Does he move well?

Yes, he's a good mover. But he's not comfortable being on the defensive. He's a better mover offensively than defensively.

Hm.

We pull up to the stadium. Fans are milling about. I sign a few autographs, then duck through a small door. I walk down a long tunnel and into the locker room. Gil goes off to consult with security. He always wants them to know exactly when we're going out to the court to practice, and when we're coming back. Darren and I drop our bags and walk straight to the training room. I lie on a table and beg the first trainer who comes near me to knead my back. Darren ducks out and returns five minutes later, carrying eight freshly strung rackets. He sets them atop my bag. He knows I want to place them in the bag myself.

I obsess about my bag. I keep it meticulously organized, and I make no apologies for this anal retentiveness. The bag is my briefcase, suitcase, toolbox, lunchbox, and palette. I need it just right, always. The bag is what I carry onto the court, and what I carry off, two moments when all my senses are extra acute, so I can feel every ounce of its weight. If someone were to slip a pair of argyle socks into my tennis bag, I'd feel it. The tennis bag is a lot like your heart—you have to know what's in it at all times.

It's also a question of functionality. I need my eight rackets stacked chronologically in the tennis bag, the most recently strung racket on the bottom and the least recently strung on the top, because the longer a racket sits, the more tension it loses. I always start a match with the racket strung least recently, because I know that's the racket with the loosest tension.

My racket stringer is old school, Old World, a Czech artiste named Roman. He's the best, and he needs to be: a string job can mean the difference in a match, and a match can mean the difference in a career, and a career can mean the difference in countless lives. When I pull a fresh racket from my bag and try to serve out a match, the string tension can be worth hundreds of thousands of dollars. Because I'm playing for my family, my charitable foundation, my school, every string is like a wire in an airplane engine. Given all that lies beyond my control, I obsess about the few things I can control, and racket tension is one such thing.

So vital is Roman to my game that I take him on the road. He's officially a resident of New York, but when I'm playing in Wimbledon, he lives in London, and when I'm playing in the French Open, he's a Parisian. Occasionally, feeling lost and lonely in some foreign city, I'll sit with Roman and watch him string a few rackets. It's not that I don't trust him. Just the opposite: I'm calmed, grounded, inspired by watching a craftsman. It reminds me of the singular importance in this world of a job done well.

The raw rackets come to Roman in a great big box from the factory, and they're always a mess. To the naked eye they look identical; to Roman they're as different as faces in a crowd. He spins them, back and forth, furrows his brow, then makes his calculations. At last he begins. He starts by removing the factory grip and putting on my grip, the custom grip I've had since I was fourteen. My grip is as personal as my thumbprint, a by-product not just of my hand shape and finger length but the size of my calluses and the force of my squeeze. Roman has a mold of my grip, which he applies to the racket. Then he wraps the mold with calfskin, which he pounds thinner and thinner until it's the width he wants. A millimeter difference, near the end of a four-hour match, can feel as irritating and distracting as a pebble in my shoe.

With the grip just so, Roman laces in the synthetic strings. He tightens them, loosens them, tightens them, tunes them as carefully as strings on a viola. Then he stencils them and vigorously waves them through the air, to let the stenciling dry. Some stringers stencil the rackets right before match time, which I find wildly inconsiderate and unprofessional. The stencil rubs off on the balls, and there's nothing worse than playing a guy who gets red and black paint on the balls. I like order and cleanliness, and that means no stencil-specked balls. Disorder is distraction, and every distraction on the court is a potential turning point.

Darren opens two cans of balls and shoves two balls in his pocket. I take a gulp of Gil Water, then a last leak before warm-ups. James, the security guard, leads us into the tunnel. As usual he's squeezed into a tight yellow security shirt, and he gives me a wink, as if to say, *We security guards are supposed to be impartial, but I'm rooting for you.*

James has been at the U.S. Open almost as long as I have. He's led me down this tunnel before and after glorious wins and excruciating losses. Large, kind, with tough-guy scars that he wears with pride, James is a bit like Gil. It's almost as though he takes over for Gil during those few hours on the court, when I'm outside Gil's sphere of influence. There are people you count on seeing at the U.S. Open—office staffers, ball boys, trainers—and their presence is always reassuring. They help you remember where and who you are. James is at the top of that list. He's one of the first people I look for when I walk into Arthur Ashe Stadium. Seeing him, I know I'm back in New York, and I'm in good hands.

Ever since 1993, when a spectator in Hamburg rushed onto the court and stabbed Monica Seles during a match, the U.S. Open has positioned one security guard behind each player's chair during all breaks and changeovers. James always makes sure to be the one behind my chair. His inability to remain impartial is endlessly charming. During a grueling match, I'll often catch James looking concerned, and I'll whisper, Don't worry, James, I've got this chump today. It always makes him chuckle.

Now, walking me out to the practice courts, he's not chuckling. He looks sad. He knows that this could be our last night together. Still, he doesn't deviate from our pre-match ritual. He says the same thing he always says:

Let me help you with that bag.

No, James, no one carries my bag but me.

I've told James that when I was seven years old I saw Jimmy Connors make someone carry his bag, as though he were Julius Caesar. I vowed then and there that I would always carry my own.

OK, James says, smiling. I know, I know. I remember. Just wanted to help.

Then I say: James, you got my back today?

I got your back, baby. I got it. Don't worry about nothing. Just take care of business.

We emerge into a dusky September night, the sky a smear of violet and orange and smog. I walk to the stands, shake hands with a few fans, sign a few more autographs before practicing. There are four practice courts, and James knows I want the one farthest from the crowd, so Darren and I can have a little privacy as we hit and talk strategy.

I groan as I guide the first backhand up the line to Darren's forehand.

Don't hit that shot tonight, he says. Baghdatis will hurt you with that.

Really?

Trust me, mate.

And you say he moves well?

Yes, quite well.

We hit for twenty-eight minutes. I don't know why I notice these details—the length of an afternoon shower, the duration of a practice session, the color of James's shirt. I don't want to notice, but I do, all the time, and then I remember forever. My memory isn't like my tennis bag; I have no say over its contents. Everything goes in, and nothing ever seems to come out.

My back feels OK. Normal stiffness, but the excruciating pain is gone. The cortisone is working. I feel good—though, of course, the definition of good has evolved in recent years. Still, I feel better than I did when I opened my eyes this morning, when I thought of forfeiting. I might be able to do this. Of course tomorrow there will be severe physical consequences, but I can't dwell on tomorrow any more than I can dwell on yesterday.

Back inside the locker room I pull off my sweaty clothes and jump in the shower. My third shower of the day is short, utilitarian. No time for coaching or crying. I slip on dry shorts, a T-shirt, put my feet up in the training room. I drink more Gil Water, as much as I can hold, because it's six thirty, and the match is nearly one hour off.

There is a TV above the training table, and I try to watch the news. I can't. I walk down to the offices and look in on the secretaries and officials of the U.S. Open. They're busy. They don't have time to talk. I step through a small door. Stefanie and the children have arrived. They're in a little playground outside the locker room. Jaden and Jaz are taking turns on the plastic slide. Stefanie is grateful, I can tell, to have the children here for distraction. She's more keyed up than I. She looks almost irritated. Her frown says, *This thing should have started already! Come on!* I love the way my wife spoils for a fight.

I talk to her and the children for a few minutes, but I can't hear a word they're saying. My mind is far away. Stefanie sees. She feels. You don't win twenty-two Grand Slams without a highly developed intuition. Besides, she was the same way before her matches. She sends me back into the locker room: Go. We'll be here. Do what you need to do.

She won't watch the match from ground level. It's too close for her. She'll stay in a skybox with the children, alternately pacing, praying, and covering her eyes.

PERE, ONE OF the senior trainers, walks in. I can tell which of his trays is for me: the one with the two giant foam donuts and two dozen precut strips of tape. I lie on one of six training tables, and Pere sits at my feet. A messy business, getting these dogs ready for war, so he puts a trash can under them. I like that Pere is tidy, meticulous, the Roman of calluses. First he takes a long Q-tip and applies an inky goo that makes my skin sticky, my instep purple. There's no washing off that ink. My instep hasn't been ink-free since Reagan was president. Now Pere sprays on skin toughener. He lets that dry, then taps a foam donut onto each callus. Next come the strips of tape, which are like rice paper. They instantly become part of my skin. He wraps each big toe until it's the size of a sparkplug. Finally he tapes the bottoms of my feet. He knows my pressure points, where I land, where I need extra layers of padding.

I thank him, put on my match shirt, socks, shoes, unlaced. Now, as everything begins to slow down, the volume goes up. Moments ago the stadium was quiet, now it's beyond loud. The air is filled with a buzzing, a humming, the sound of fans rushing to their seats, hurrying to get settled, because they don't want to miss a minute of what's coming.

I stand, shake out my legs.

I won't sit again.

I try a jog down the hall. Not bad. The back is holding. All systems go.

Across the locker room I see Baghdatis. He's suited up, fussing with his hair in front of a mirror. He's flicking it, combing it, pulling it back. Wow, he has a lot of hair. Now he's positioning his headband, a white Cochise wrap. He gets it perfect, then gives one last tug on his ponytail. A decidedly more glamorous pre-match ritual than cushioning your toe calluses. I remember my hair issues early in my career. For a moment I feel jealous. I miss my hair. Then I run a hand over my bare scalp and feel grateful that, with all the things I'm worried about right now, hair isn't one of them.

Baghdatis begins stretching, bending at the waist. He stands on one leg and pulls one knee to his chest. Nothing is quite so unsettling as watching your opponent do pilates, yoga, and tai chi when you can't so much as curtsy. He now maneuvers his hips in ways I haven't dared since I was seven.

And yet he's doing too much. He's antsy. I can almost hear his central nervous system, a sound like the buzz of the stadium. I watch the interaction between him and his coaches, and they're antsy too. Their faces, their body language, their coloring, everything tells me they know they're in for a street fight, and they're not sure they want it. I always like my opponent and his team to show nervous energy. A good omen, but also a sign of respect.

Baghdatis sees me and smiles. I remember that he smiles when he's happy or nervous, and you can never tell which. Again, it reminds me of someone, and I can't think who.

I raise a hand. Good luck.

He raises a hand. We who are about to die . . .

I duck into the tunnel for one last word with Gil, who's staked out a corner where he can be alone but still keep an eye on everything. He puts his arms around me, tells me he loves me, he's proud of me. I find Stefanie and give her one last kiss. She's bobbing, weaving, stomping her feet. She'd give anything to slip on a skirt, grab a racket, and join me out there. My pugnacious bride. She tries a smile but it ends up a wince. I see in her face everything she wants to say but will not let herself say. I hear every word she refuses to utter: Enjoy, savor, take it all in, notice each fleeting detail, because this could be it, and even though you hate tennis, you might just miss it after tonight.

This is what she wants to say, but instead she kisses me and says what she always says before I go out there, the thing I've come to count on like air and sleep and Gil Water.

Go kick some butt.

AN OFFICIAL OF THE U.S. OPEN, wearing a suit and carrying a walkie-talkie as long as my forearm, approaches. He seems to be in charge of network coverage and on-court security. He seems to be in charge of everything, including arrivals and departures at LaGuardia. Five minutes, he says.

I turn to someone and ask, What time is it?

Go time, they say.

No. I mean, what time? Is it seven thirty? Seven twenty? I don't know, and it suddenly feels important. But there are no clocks.

Darren and I turn to each other. His Adam's apple goes up and down.

Mate, he says, your homework is done. You're ready.

I nod.

He holds out his fist for a bump. Just one bump, because that's what we did before my first-round win earlier this week. We're both superstitious, so however we start a tournament, that's how we finish. I stare at Darren's fist, give it one decisive bump, but don't dare lift my gaze and make eye contact. I know Darren is tearing up, and I know what that sight will do to me.

Last things: I lace up my shoes. I tape my wrist. I always tape my own wrist, ever since my injury in 1993. I tie my shoes.

Please let this be over.

I'm not ready for it to be over.

Mr. Agassi, it's time.

I'm ready.

I walk into the tunnel, three steps behind Baghdatis, James again leading the way. We stop, wait for a signal. The buzzing sound all around us becomes louder. The tunnel is meat-locker cold. I know this tunnel as well as I know the front foyer of my house, and yet tonight it feels about fifty degrees colder than usual and a football field longer. I look to the side. There along the walls are the familiar photos of former champions. Navratilova. Lendl. McEnroe. Stefanie. Me. The portraits are three feet tall and spaced evenly—too evenly. They're like trees in a new suburban development. I tell myself: *Stop noticing such things.* Time to narrow your mind, the way the tunnel narrows your vision.

The head of security yells, OK, everyone, it's showtime!

We walk.

By careful prearrangement, Baghdatis stays three paces ahead as we move toward the light. Suddenly a second light, a blinding ethereal light, is in our faces. A TV camera. A reporter asks Baghdatis how he feels. He says something I can't hear.

Now the camera is closer to my face and the reporter is asking the same question.

Could be your last match ever, the reporter says. How does that make you feel?

I answer, no idea what I'm saying. But after years of practice I have a sense that I'm saying what he wants me to say, what I'm expected to say. Then I resume walking, on legs that don't feel like my own.

The temperature rises dramatically as we near the door to the court. The buzzing is now deafening. Baghdatis bursts through first. He knows how much attention my retirement has been getting. He reads the papers. He expects to play the villain tonight. He thinks he's prepared. I let him go, let him hear the buzzing turn to cheers. I let him think the crowd is cheering for both of us. *Then* I walk out. Now the cheers triple. Baghdatis turns and realizes the first cheer was for him, but this cheer is mine, all mine, which forces him to revise his expectations and reconsider what's in store. Without hitting a single ball I've caused a major swing in his sense of well-being. A trick of the trade. An old-timer's trick.

The crowd gets louder as we find our way to our chairs. It's louder than I thought it would be, louder than I've ever heard it in New York. I keep my eyes lowered, let the noise wash over me. They love this moment; they love tennis. I wonder how they would feel if they knew my secret. I stare at the court. Always the most abnormal part of my life, the court is now the only space of normalcy in all this turmoil. The court, where I've felt so lonely and exposed, is where I now hope to find refuge from this emotional moment.

I CRUISE THROUGH THE FIRST SET, winning 6–4. The ball obeys my every command. So does my back. My body feels warm, liquid. Cortisone and adrenaline, working together. I win the second set, 6–4. I see the finish line.

In the third set I start to tire. I lose focus and control. Baghdatis, meanwhile, changes his game plan. He plays with desperation, a more powerful drug than cortisone. He starts to live in the now. He takes risks, and every risk pays off. The ball now disobeys me and conspires with him. It consistently bounces his way, which gives him confidence. I see the confidence shining from his eyes. His initial despair has turned to hope. No, anger. He doesn't admire me anymore. He hates me, and I hate him, and now we're sneering and snarling and trying to wrest this thing from each other. The crowd feeds on our anger, shrieking, pounding their feet after every point. They're not clapping their hands as much as slapping them, and it all sounds primitive and tribal.

He wins the third set, 6–3.

I can do nothing to slow the Baghdatis onslaught. On the contrary, it's getting worse. He's twenty-one, after all, just warming up. He's found his rhythm, his reason for being out here, his right to be here, whereas I've burned through my second wind and I'm painfully aware of the clock inside my body. I don't want a fifth set. I can't handle a fifth set. My mortality now a factor, I start to take my own risks. I grab a 4–0 lead. I'm up two service breaks, and again the finish line is within sight, within reach. I feel the magnetic force, pulling me.

Then I feel the other force pushing. Baghdatis starts to play his best tennis of the year. He just remembered he's number eight in the world. He pulls triggers on shots I didn't know he had in his repertoire. I've set a perilously high standard, but now he meets me there, and exceeds me. He breaks me to go 4–1. He holds serve to go 4–2.

Here comes the biggest game of the match. If I win this game, I retake command of this set and reestablish in his mind—and mine—that he was fortunate to get one break back. If I lose, it's 4–3, and everything resets. Our night will begin again. Though we've bludgeoned each other for ten rounds, if I lose this game the fight will start over. We play at a furious pace. He goes for broke, holds nothing back—wins the game.

He's going to take this set. He'll die before he loses this set. I know it and he knows it and everyone in this stadium knows it. Twenty minutes ago I was two games from winning and advancing. I'm now on the brink of collapse.

He wins the set, 7–5.

The fifth set begins. I'm serving, shaking, unsure my body can hold out for another ten minutes, facing a kid who seems to be getting younger and stronger with every point. I tell myself, Do *not* let it end this way. Of all ways, not this way, not giving up a two-set lead. Baghdatis is talking to himself also, urging himself on. We ride a seesaw, a pendulum of high-energy points. He makes a mistake. I give it back. He digs in. I dig in deeper. I'm serving at deuce, and we play a frantic point that ends when he hits a backhand drop shot that I wing into the net. I scream at myself. Advantage Baghdatis. The first time I've trailed him all night.

Shake it off. Control what you can control, Andre.

I win the next point. Deuce again. Elation.

I give him the next point. Backhand into the net. Advantage Baghdatis. Depression.

He wins the next point also, wins the game, breaks to go up 1–0.

We walk to our chairs. I hear the crowd murmuring the first Agassi eulogies. I take a sip of Gil Water, feeling sorry for myself, feeling old. I look over at Baghdatis, wondering if he's feeling cocky. Instead he's asking a trainer to rub his legs. He's asking for a medical time-out. His left quad is strained. He did that to me on a strained quad?

The crowd uses the lull in the action to chant. *Let's go, Andre! Let's go, Andre!* They start a wave. They hold up signs with my name.

Thanks for the memories, Andre!

This is Andre's House.

At last Baghdatis is ready to go. His serve. Having just broken me to take the lead in the match, he should have a full head of steam. But instead the lull seems to have disrupted his rhythm. I break him. We're back on serve.

For the next six games we each hold. Then, knotted at four–all, with me serving, we play a game that seems to last a week, one of the most taxing and unreal games of my career. We grunt like animals, hit like gladiators, his forehand, my backhand. Everyone in the stadium stops breathing. Even the wind stops. Flags go limp against the poles. At 40–30, Baghdatis hits a swift forehand that sweeps me out of position. I barely get there in time to put my racket on it. I sling the ball over the net— screaming in agony—and he hits another scorcher to my backhand. I scurry in the opposite direction—oh, my back!—and reach the ball just in time. But I've wrenched my spine. The spinal column is locked up and the nerves inside are keening. Goodbye, cortisone. Baghdatis hits a winner to the open court and as I watch it sail by I know that for the rest of this night my best effort is behind me. Whatever I do from this point on will be limited, compromised, borrowed against my future health and mobility.

I look across the net to see if Baghdatis has noticed my pain, but he's hobbling. Hobbling? *He's cramping.* He falls to the ground, grabbing his legs. He's in more pain than I. I'll take a congenital back condition over sudden leg cramps any day. As he writhes on the ground I realize: All I have to do is stay upright, move this goddamned ball around a little while longer, and let his cramps do their work.

I abandon all thought of subtlety and strategy. I say to myself, Fundamentals. When you play someone wounded, it's about instinct and reaction. This will no longer be tennis, but a raw test of wills. No more jabs, no more feints, no more footwork. Nothing but roundhouses and haymakers.

Back on his feet, Baghdatis too has stopped strategizing, stopped thinking, which makes him more dangerous. I can no longer predict what he'll do. He's crazed with pain, and no one can predict crazy, least of all on a tennis court. At deuce, I miss my first serve, then give him a fat, juicy second serve, seventy-something miles an hour, on which he unloads. Winner. Advantage Baghdatis.

Shit. I slump forward. The guy can't move, but he still crushes my serve?

Now, yet again, I'm one slender, skittish point away from falling behind 4–5, which will set up Baghdatis to serve for the match. I close my eyes. I miss my first serve again. I hit another tentative second serve just to get the point going and somehow he flubs an easy forehand. Deuce again.

When your mind and body teeter on the verge of all-out collapse, one easy point like that feels like a pardon from the governor. And yet, I nearly squander my pardon. I miss my first serve. I make my second and he returns it wide. Another gift. Advantage Agassi.

I'm one point from a commanding 5–4 lead. Baghdatis grimaces, bears down. He won't yield. He wins the point. Deuce number three.

I promise myself that if I gain the advantage again, I won't lose it.

By now Baghdatis isn't merely cramping, he's a cripple. Awaiting my serve, he's fully bent over. I can't believe he's managing to stay on the court, let alone give me such a game. The guy has as much heart as he has hair. I feel for him, and at the same time tell myself to show him no mercy. I serve, he returns, and in my eagerness to hit to the open court, I hit far wide. Out. A choke. Clearly, a choke. Advantage Baghdatis.

He can't capitalize, however. On the next point he hits a forehand several feet beyond the baseline. Deuce number four.

We have a long rally, ending when I drive a deep shot to his forehand that he misplays. Advantage Agassi. Again. I promised myself I wouldn't waste this opportunity if it came around again, and here it is. But Baghdatis won't let me keep the promise. He quickly wins the next point. Deuce number five.

We play an absurdly long point. Every ball he hits, moaning, catches a piece of the line. Every ball I hit, screaming, somehow clears the net. Forehand, backhand, trick shot, diving shot—then he hits a ball that nicks the baseline and takes a skittish sideways hop. I catch it on the rise and hit it twenty feet over him and the baseline. Advantage Baghdatis.

Stick to basics, Andre. Run him, run him. He's gimpy, just make him move. I serve, he hits a vanilla return, I send him side to side until he yowls in pain and hits the ball into the net. Deuce number six.

While waiting for my next serve, Baghdatis is leaning on his racket, using it as an old man uses a walking stick. When I miss a first serve, however, he creeps forward, crablike, and with his walking stick he whacks my serve well beyond the reach of my forehand. Advantage Baghdatis.

His fourth break point of this game. I hit a timid first serve, so paltry, so meek, my seven-year-old self would have been ashamed, and yet Baghdatis hits a defensive return. I hit to his forehand. He nets. Deuce number seven.

I make another first serve. He gets a racket on it but can't get it over the net. Advantage Agassi.

I'm serving again for the game. I recall my twice-broken promise. Here, one last chance. My back, however, is spasming. I can barely turn, let alone toss the ball and hit it 120 miles an hour. I miss my first serve, of course. I want to crush a second serve, be aggressive, but I can't. Physically I cannot. I tell myself, Three-quarter kick, put the ball above his shoulder, make him go side to side until he pukes blood. Just don't double-fault.

Easier said than done. The box is shrinking. I watch it gradually diminish in size. Can everyone else see what I'm seeing? The box is now the size of a playing card, so small that I'm not sure this ball would fit if I walked it over there and set it down. I toss the ball, hit an alligator-armed serve. Out. Of course. Double fault. Deuce number eight.

The crowd screams in disbelief.

I manage to make a first serve. Baghdatis hits a workmanlike return. With three-quarters of his court wide open, I punch the ball deep to his backhand, ten feet from him. He scampers toward it, waves his racket limply, can't get there. Advantage Agassi.

On the twenty-second point of the game, after a brief rally, Baghdatis finally whips a backhand into the net. Game, Agassi.

During the changeover I watch Baghdatis sit. Big mistake. A young man's mistake. Never sit when cramping. Never tell your body that it's time to rest, then tell it, Just kidding! Your body is like the federal government. It says, Do anything you like, but when you get caught, don't lie to me. So he's not going to be able to serve. He's not going to be able to get out of that chair.

And then he gets out and holds serve.

What's keeping this man up?

Oh. Yes. Youth.

At 5–all, we play a stilted game. He makes a mistake, goes for the knockout. I counterpunch and win. I lead, 6–5.

His serve. He goes up 40–15. He's one point from pushing this match to a tiebreaker.

I fight him to deuce.

Then I win the next point, and now I have match point.

A quick, vicious exchange. He hits a wild forehand, and as it leaves his strings I know it's out. I know I've won this match, and at the same moment I know that I wouldn't have had energy for one more swing.

I meet Baghdatis at the net, take his hand, which is trembling, and hurry off the court. I don't dare stop. *Must keep moving.* I stagger through the tunnel, my bag slung over my left shoulder, feeling as if it's slung over my right shoulder, because my whole body is twisted. By the time I reach the locker room I'm unable to walk. I'm unable to stand. I'm sinking to the floor. I'm on the ground. Darren and Gil arrive, slip my bag off my shoulder and lift me onto a table. Baghdatis's people deposit him on the table next to me.

Darren, what's wrong with me?

Lie down, mate. Stretch out.

I can't, I can't—

Where does it hurt? Is it a cramp?

No, it's a constriction. I can't *breathe.*

What?

I can't—Darren, I can't—*breathe.*

Darren is helping someone put ice on my body, raising my arms, calling for doctors. He's begging me to reach, reach, stretch.

Just release, mate. Unclench. Your body is clenched. Just let go, mate, let go.

But I can't. And that's the whole problem, isn't it? I can't let go.

A KALEIDOSCOPE OF FACES appears above me. Gil, squeezing my arm, handing me a recovery drink. I love you, Gil. Stefanie, kissing me on the forehead and smiling—happy or nervous, I can't tell. *Oh, yes, of course, that's where I've seen that smile before.* A trainer, telling me the doctors are on the way. He turns on the TV above the table. Something to do while you wait, he says.

I try to watch. I hear moans to my left. I turn my head slowly and see Baghdatis on the next table. His team is working on him. They stretch his quad, his hamstring cramps. They stretch his hamstring, his quad cramps. He tries to lie flat, his groin cramps. He curls into a ball and begs them to leave him be. Everyone clears out of the locker room. It's just the two of us. I turn back to the TV.

Moments later something makes me turn back to Baghdatis. He's smiling at me. Happy or nervous? Maybe both. I smile back.

I hear my name coming from the TV. I turn my head. Highlights from the match. The first two sets, so misleadingly easy. The third, Baghdatis starting to believe. The fourth, a knife fight. The fifth, the never-ending ninth game. Some of the best tennis I've ever played. Some of the best I've ever seen. The commentator calls it a classic.

In my peripheral vision I detect slight movement. I turn to see Baghdatis extending his hand. His face says, We *did* that. I reach out, take his hand, and we remain this way, holding hands, as the TV flickers with scenes of our savage battle.

At last I let my mind go where it's wanted to go. I can't stop it anymore. No longer asking politely, my mind is now forcibly spinning me into the past. And because my mind notes and records the slightest details, I see everything with bright, startling clarity, every setback, victory, rivalry, tantrum, paycheck, girlfriend, betrayal, reporter, wife, child, outfit, fan letter, grudge match, and crying jag. As if a second TV above me were showing highlights from the last twenty-nine years, it all flies past in a high-def whirl.

People often ask what it's like, this tennis life, and I can never think how to describe it. But that word comes closest. More than anything else, it's a wrenching, thrilling, horrible, astonishing *whirl*. It even exerts a faint centrifugal force, which I've spent three decades fighting. Now, lying on my back under Arthur Ashe Stadium, holding hands with a vanquished opponent and waiting for someone to come help us, I do the only thing I can do. I stop fighting it. I just close my eyes and watch.

1

I'M SEVEN YEARS OLD, talking to myself, because I'm scared, and because I'm the only person who listens to me. Under my breath I whisper: Just quit, Andre, just give up. Put down your racket and walk off this court, right now. Go into the house and get something good to eat. Play with Rita, Philly, or Tami. Sit with Mom while she knits or does her jigsaw puzzle. Doesn't that sound nice? Wouldn't that feel like heaven, Andre? To just quit? To never play tennis again?

But I can't. Not only would my father chase me around the house with my racket, but something in my gut, some deep unseen muscle, won't let me. I hate tennis, hate it with all my heart, and still I keep playing, keep hitting all morning, and all afternoon, because I have no choice. No matter how much I want to stop, I don't. I keep begging myself to stop, and I keep playing, and this gap, this contradiction between what I want to do and what I actually do, feels like the core of my life.

At the moment my hatred for tennis is focused on the dragon, a ball machine modified by my fire-belching father. Midnight black, set on big rubber wheels, the word PRINCE painted in white block letters along its base, the dragon looks at first glance like the ball machine at every country club in America, but it's actually a living, breathing creature straight out of my comic books. The dragon has a brain, a will, a black heart—and a horrifying voice. Sucking another ball into its belly, the dragon makes a series of sickening sounds. As pressure builds inside its throat, it groans. As the ball rises slowly to its mouth, it shrieks. For a moment the dragon sounds almost silly, like the fudge machine swallowing Augustus Gloop in *Willy Wonka & the Chocolate Factory*. But when the dragon takes dead aim at me and fires a ball 110 miles an hour, the sound it makes is a bloodcurdling roar. I flinch every time.

My father has deliberately made the dragon fearsome. He's given it an extra-long neck of aluminum tubing, and a narrow aluminum head, which recoils like a whip every time the dragon fires. He's also set the dragon on a base several feet high, and moved it flush against the net, so the dragon towers above me. At seven years old I'm small for my age. (I look smaller because of my constant wince and the bimonthly bowl haircuts my father gives me.) But when standing before the dragon, I look tiny. Feel tiny. Helpless.

My father wants the dragon to tower over me not simply because it commands my attention and respect. He wants the balls that shoot from the dragon's mouth to land at my feet as if dropped from an airplane. The trajectory makes the balls nearly impossible to return in a conventional way: I need to hit every ball on the rise, or else it will bounce over my head. But even that's not enough for my father. Hit earlier, he yells. Hit *earlier.*

My father yells everything twice, sometimes three times, sometimes ten. Harder, he says, *harder.* But what's the use? No matter how hard I hit a ball, no matter how early, the ball comes back. Every ball I send across the net joins the thousands that already cover the court. Not hundreds. Thousands. They roll toward me in perpetual waves. I have no room to turn, to step, to pivot. I can't move without stepping on a ball—and yet I can't step on a ball, because my father won't bear it. Step on one of my father's tennis balls and he'll howl as if you stepped on his eyeball.

Every third ball fired by the dragon hits a ball already on the ground, causing a crazy sideways hop. I adjust at the last second, catch the ball early, and hit it smartly across the net. I know this is no ordinary reflex. I know there are few children in the world who could have seen that ball, let alone hit it. But I take no pride in my reflexes, and I get no credit. It's what I'm supposed to do. Every hit is expected, every miss a crisis.

My father says that if I hit 2,500 balls each day, I'll hit 17,500 balls each week, and at the end of one year I'll have hit nearly one million balls. He believes in math. Numbers, he says, don't lie. A child who hits one million balls each year will be unbeatable.

Hit *earlier,* my father yells. Damn it, Andre, hit *earlier.* Crowd the ball, crowd the ball.

Now he's crowding me. He's yelling directly into my ear. It's not enough to hit everything the dragon fires at me; my father wants me to hit it *harder* and *faster* than the dragon. He wants me to beat the dragon. The thought makes me panicky. I tell myself: You can't beat the dragon. How can you beat something that never stops? Come to think of it, the dragon is a lot like my father. Except my father is worse. At least the dragon stands before me, where I can see it. My father stays behind me. I rarely see him, only hear him, day and night, yelling in my ear.

More topspin! Hit harder. Hit *harder.* Not in the net! Damn it, Andre! *Never in the net!*

Nothing sends my father into a rage like hitting a ball into the net. He dislikes when I hit the ball wide, he yells when I hit a ball long, but when I muff a ball into the net, he foams at the mouth. Errors are one thing, the net is something else. Over and over my father says: The net is your biggest enemy.

My father has raised the enemy six inches higher than regulation, to make it that much harder to avoid. If I can clear my father's high net, he figures I'll have no trouble clearing the net one day at Wimbledon. Never mind that I don't want to play Wimbledon. What I want isn't relevant. Sometimes I watch Wimbledon on TV with my father, and we both root for Björn Borg, because he's the best, he never stops, he's the nearest thing to the dragon—but I don't want to be Borg. I admire his talent, his energy, his style, his ability to lose himself in his game, but if I ever develop those qualities, I'd rather apply them to something other than Wimbledon. Something of my own choosing.

Hit harder, my father yells. Hit *harder.* Now backhands. *Backhands.*

My arm feels like it's going to fall off. I want to ask, How much longer, Pops? But I don't ask. I do as I'm told. I hit as hard as I can, then slightly harder. On one swing I surprise myself by how hard I hit, how cleanly. Though I hate tennis, I like the feeling of hitting a ball dead perfect. It's the only peace. When I do something perfect, I enjoy a split second of sanity and calm.

The dragon responds to perfection, however, by firing the next ball faster.

Short backswing, my father says. Short back—that's it. Brush the ball, brush the ball.

At the dinner table my father will sometimes demonstrate. Drop your racket under the ball, he says, and brush, brush. He makes a motion like a painter, gently wafting a brush. This might be the only thing I've ever seen my father do gently.

Work your volleys, he yells—or tries to. An Armenian, born in Iran, my father speaks five languages, none of them well, and his English is heavily accented. He mixes his Vs and Ws, so it sounds like this: *Vork your wolleys.* Of all his instructions, this is his favorite. He yells this until I hear it in my dreams. *Vork your wolleys, vork your wolleys.*

I've vorked so many wolleys I can no longer see the court. Not one patch of green cement is visible beneath the yellow balls. I slidestep, shuffling like an old man. Finally, even my father has to admit there are too many balls. It's counterproductive. If I can't move we won't make our daily quota of 2,500. He revs up the blower, the giant machine for drying the court after it rains. Of course it never rains where we live—Las Vegas, Nevada—so my father uses the blower to corral tennis balls. Just as he did with the ball machine, my father has modified a standard blower, made it into another demonic creature. It's one of my earliest memories: five years old, getting pulled out of kindergarten, going with my father to the welding shop and watching him build this insane lawnmower-like machine that can move hundreds of tennis balls at once.

Now I watch him push the blower, watch the tennis balls scurry from him, and feel sympathy for the balls. If the dragon and the blower are living things, maybe the balls are too. Maybe they're doing what I would if I could—running from my father. After blowing all the balls into one corner, my father takes a snow shovel and scoops the balls into a row of metal garbage cans, slop buckets with which he feeds the dragon.

He turns, sees me watching. What the hell are you looking at? Keep hitting! Keep hitting!

My shoulder aches. I can't hit another ball.

I hit another three.

I can't go on another minute.

I go another ten.

I get an idea. Accidentally on purpose, I hit a ball high over the fence. I manage to catch it on the wooden rim of the racket, so it sounds like a misfire. I do this when I need a break, and it crosses my mind that I must be pretty good if I can hit a ball wrong at will.

My father hears the ball hit wood and looks up. He sees the ball leave the court. He curses. But he heard the ball hit wood, so he knows it was an accident. Besides, at least I didn't hit the net. He stomps out of the yard, out to the desert. I now have four and a half minutes to catch my breath and watch the hawks circling lazily overhead.

My father likes to shoot the hawks with his rifle. Our house is blanketed with his victims, dead birds that cover the roof as thickly as tennis balls cover the court. My father says he doesn't like hawks because they swoop down on mice and other defenseless desert creatures. He can't stand the thought of something strong preying on something weak. (This also holds true when he goes fishing: whatever he catches, he kisses its scaly head and throws it back.) Of course he has no qualms about preying on me, no trouble watching me gasp for air on his hook. He

31

doesn't see the contradiction. He doesn't care about contradictions. He doesn't realize that I'm the most defenseless creature in this godforsaken desert. If he did realize, I wonder, would he treat me differently?

Now he stomps back onto the court, slams the ball into a garbage can, and sees me staring at the hawks. He glares. What the fuck are you *doing*? Stop thinking. No fucking thinking!

The net is the biggest enemy, but thinking is the cardinal sin. Thinking, my father believes, is the source of all bad things, because thinking is the opposite of doing. When my father catches me thinking, daydreaming, on the tennis court, he reacts as if he caught me taking money from his wallet. I often think about how I can stop thinking. I wonder if my father yells at me to stop thinking because he knows I'm a thinker by nature. Or, with all his yelling, has he turned me into a thinker? Is my thinking about things other than tennis an act of defiance?

I like to think so.

OUR HOUSE IS AN OVERGROWN SHACK, built in the 1970s, white stucco with peeling dark trim around its edges. The windows have bars. The roof, under all the dead hawks, has wood shingles, many of which are loose or missing. The door has a cowbell that rings every time someone comes or goes, like the opening bell of a boxing match.

My father has painted the high cement wall around the house a bright forest green. Why? Because green is the color of a tennis court. Also, my father likes the convenience of directing someone to the house like this: Turn left, go down half a block, then look for the bright green wall.

Not that we ever have any visitors.

Surrounding the house on all sides is desert, and more desert, which to me is another word for death. Dotted with sticker bushes, tumbleweed, and coiled rattlers, the desert around our house seems to have no reason for existence, other than providing a place for people to dump things they no longer want. Mattresses, tires, other people. Vegas—the casinos, the hotels, the Strip—stands off in the distance, a glittering illusion. My father commutes to the illusion every day. He's a captain at one of the casinos, but he refuses to live closer. We moved out here to the middle of nowhere, the heart of nothingness, because it's only here that my father could afford a house with a yard big enough for his ideal tennis court.

It's another early memory: driving around Vegas with my father and the real estate agent. It would have been funny if it hadn't been scary. At house after house, even before the agent's car came to a full stop my father would jump out and march up the front walk. The agent, close on my father's heels, would be yakking about local schools, crime rates, interest rates, but my father wouldn't be listening. Staring straight ahead, my father would storm into the house, through the living room, through the kitchen, into the backyard, where he'd whip out his tape measure and count off thirty-six feet by seventy-eight feet, the dimensions of a tennis court. Time after time he'd yell, Doesn't fit! Come on! Let's go! My father would then march back through the kitchen, through the living room, down the front walk, the real estate agent struggling to keep pace.

We saw one house my older sister Tami desperately wanted. She begged my father to buy it, because it was shaped like a T, and T stood for Tami. My father almost bought it, probably because T also stood for Tennis. I liked the house. So did my mother. The backyard, however, was inches too short.

Doesn't fit! Let's go!

Finally we saw this house, its backyard so big that my father didn't need to measure. He just stood in the middle of the yard, turning slowly, gazing, grinning, seeing the future.

Sold, he said quietly.

We hadn't carried in the last cardboard box before my father began to build his dream court. I still don't know how he did it. He never worked a day in construction. He knew nothing about concrete, asphalt, water drainage. He read no books, consulted no experts. He just got a picture in his head and set about making that picture a reality. As with so many things, he willed the court into being through sheer orneriness and energy. I think he might be doing something similar with me.

He needed help, of course. Pouring concrete is a big job. So each morning he'd drive me to Sambo's, a diner on the Strip, where we'd recruit a few old-timers from the gang that hung out in the parking lot. My favorite was Rudy. Battle-scarred, barrel-chested, Rudy always looked at me with a half smile, as if he understood that I didn't know who or where I was. Rudy and his gang would follow me and my father back to our house, and there my father would tell them what needed doing. After three hours my father and I would run down to McDonald's and buy huge sacks of Big Macs and French fries. When we returned, my father would let me ring the cowbell and call the men to lunch. I loved rewarding Rudy. I loved watching him eat like a wolf. I loved the concept of hard work leading to sweet rewards—except when hard work meant hitting tennis balls.

The days of Rudy and the Big Macs passed in a blur. Suddenly my father had his backyard tennis court, which meant I had my prison. I'd helped feed the chain gang that built my cell. I'd helped measure and paint the white lines that would confine me. Why did I do it? I had no choice. The reason I do everything.

No one ever asked me if I wanted to play tennis, let alone make it my life. In fact, my mother thought I was born to be a preacher. She tells me, however, that my father decided long before I was born that I would be a professional tennis player. When I was one year old, she adds, I proved my father right. Watching a ping-pong game, I moved only my eyes, never my head. My father called to my mother.

Look, he said. See how he moves only his eyes? A natural.

She tells me that when I was still in the crib, my father hung a mobile of tennis balls above my head and encouraged me to slap at them with a ping-pong paddle he'd taped to my hand. When I was three he gave me a sawed-off racket and told me to hit whatever I wanted. I specialized in salt shakers. I liked serving them through glass windows. I aced the dog. My father never got mad. He got mad about many things, but never about hitting something hard with a racket.

When I was four he had me hitting with tennis greats who passed through town, beginning with Jimmy Connors. My father told me that Connors was one of the finest to ever play. I was more impressed that Connors had a bowl haircut just like mine. When we finished hitting, Connors told my father that I was sure to become very good.

I already know that, my father said, annoyed. Very good? He's going to be number one in the world.

He wasn't seeking Connors's confirmation. He was seeking someone who could give me a game.

Whenever Connors comes to Vegas, my father strings his rackets. My father is a master stringer. (Who better than my old man to create and maintain tension?) It's always the same drill. In the morning Connors gives my father a box of rackets, and eight hours later my father and I meet Connors at a restaurant on the Strip. My father sends me in, cradling the restrung rackets. I ask the manager if he can point me to Mr. Connors's table. The manager sends me to a far corner, where Connors sits with his entourage. Connors is at the center, back to the wall. I hold his rackets toward him, carefully, not saying a word. The conversation at the table comes to a halt, and everyone looks down at me. Connors takes the rackets roughly and sets them on a chair. For a moment I feel important, as though I've delivered freshly sharpened swords to one of the Three Musketeers. Then Connors tousles my hair, says something sarcastic about me or my father, and everyone at the table guffaws.

THE BETTER I GET AT TENNIS, the worse I get at school, which pains me. I like books, but feel overmatched by them. I like my teachers, but don't understand much of what they say. I don't seem to learn or process facts the way other kids do. I have a steel-trap memory, but trouble concentrating. I need things explained twice, three times. (Maybe that's why my father yells everything twice?) Also, I know that my father resents every moment I spend in school; it comes at the cost of court time. Disliking school, therefore, doing poorly in school, feels like loyalty to Pops.

Some days, when he's driving me and my siblings to school, my father will smile and say: I'll make you guys a deal. Instead of taking you to school, how about I take you to Cambridge Racquet Club? You can hit balls all morning. How does that sound?

We know what he wants us to say. So we say it. *Hooray!*

Just don't tell your mother, my father says.

Cambridge Racquet Club is a long, low-roofed dump, just east of the Strip, with ten hard courts and a seedy smell—dust, sweat, liniment, plus something sour, something just past its expiration date, that I can never quite identify. My father treats Cambridge like an addition to our house. He stands with the owner, Mr. Fong, and they watch us closely, making sure we play, that we don't waste our time talking or laughing. Eventually my father lets out a short whistle, a sound I'd know anywhere. He puts his fingers in his mouth, gives one hard blast, and that means game, set, match, stop hitting and get in the car, now.

My siblings always stop before I do. Rita, the oldest, Philly, my older brother, and Tami—they all play tennis well. We're like the von Trapps of tennis. But me, the youngest, the baby, I'm the best. My father tells me so, tells my siblings, tells Mr. Fong. Andre is the chosen one. That's why my father gives me most of his attention. I'm the last best hope of the Agassi clan. Sometimes I like the extra attention from my father, sometimes I'd rather be invisible, because my father can be scary. My father does things.

For instance, he often reaches a thumb and forefinger inside his nostril and, bracing himself for the eye-watering pain, pulls out a thick bouquet of black nose hairs. This is how he grooms himself. In the same spirit, he shaves his face without soap or cream. He simply runs a disposable razor up and down his dry cheeks and jaw, shredding his skin, then letting the blood trickle down his face until it dries.

When stressed, when distracted, my father often stares off into space and mumbles: *I love you, Margaret.* I ask my mother one day: Who's Pops talking to? Who's Margaret?

My mother says that when my father was my age, he was skating on a pond and the ice cracked. He fell through and drowned—stopped breathing for a long time. He was pulled from the water and revived by a woman named Margaret. He'd never seen her before and never saw her again. But every so often he sees her in his mind, and speaks to her, and thanks her in his most tender voice. He says this vision of Margaret comes upon him like a seizure. He has no knowledge while it's happening, and only a dim memory afterward.

Violent by nature, my father is forever preparing for battle. He shadowboxes constantly. He keeps an ax handle in his car. He leaves the house with a handful of salt and pepper in each pocket, in case he's in a street fight and needs to blind someone. Of course some of his most vicious battles are with himself. He has chronic stiffness in his neck, and he's perpetually loosening the neck bones by angrily twisting and yanking his head. When this doesn't work he shakes himself like a dog, whipping his head from side to side until the neck makes a sound like popcorn popping. When even *this* doesn't work, he resorts to the heavy punching bag that hangs from a harness outside our house. My father stands on a chair, removes the punching bag, and places his neck in the harness. He then kicks away the chair and drops a foot through the air, his momentum abruptly halted by the harness. The first time I saw him do this, I was walking through the rooms of the house. I looked up and there was my father, kicking the chair, hanging by his neck, his shoes three feet off the ground. I had no doubt he'd killed himself. I ran to him, hysterical.

Seeing the stricken look on my face, he barked: What the fuck is the matter with you?

Most of his battles, however, are against others, and they typically begin without warning, at the most unexpected times. In his sleep, for instance. He boxes in his dreams, and frequently hauls off and punches my dozing mother. In the car too. My father enjoys few things more than driving his green diesel Oldsmobile, singing along to his eight-track of Laura Branigan. But if another driver crosses him, if another driver cuts him off or objects to being cut off by my father, everything goes dark.

I'm driving with my father one day, going to Cambridge, and he gets into a shouting match with another driver. My father stops his car, steps out, orders the man out of his. Because my father is wielding his ax handle, the man refuses. My father whips the ax handle into the man's headlights and taillights, sending sprays of glass everywhere.

Another time my father reaches across me and points his handgun at another driver. He holds the gun level with my nose. I stare straight ahead. I don't move. I don't know what the other driver has done wrong, only that it's the automotive equivalent of hitting into the net. I feel my father's finger tensing on the trigger. Then I hear the other driver speed away, followed by a sound I rarely hear—my father laughing. He's busting a gut. I tell myself that I'll remember this moment—my father laughing, holding a gun under my nose—if I live to be one hundred.

When he puts the gun back into the glove box and throws the car into drive, my father turns to me. Don't tell your mother, he says.

I can't imagine why he says this. What would my mother do if we told her? She never raises a word of protest. Does my father think there's a first time for everything?

On a rare rainy day in Vegas, my father is driving me to pick up my mother at her office. I'm standing on my end of the bench seat, horsing around, singing. My father gets in the left lane to make a turn. A trucker honks at my father. My father apparently forgot to signal. My father gives the trucker the finger. His hand flies up so fast, it nearly hits my face. The trucker yells something. My father lets fly a stream of curses. The trucker stops, opens his door. My father stops, jumps out.

I crawl into the backseat and watch through the back window. The rain is falling harder. My father approaches the trucker. The trucker throws a punch. My father ducks, deflects the punch with the top of his head, then throws a blazingly fast combination, ending with an uppercut. The trucker is lying on the pavement. He's dead—I'm sure of it. If he's not dead, he soon will be, because he's in the middle of the road and someone will run him over. My father gets back in the car and we peel away. I stay in the backseat, watching the trucker through the back window, rain pelting his unconscious face. I turn to see my father, mumbling, throwing combinations against the steering wheel. Just before we pick up my mother he looks down at his hands, clenches and unclenches his fists to make sure the knuckles aren't broken. Then he looks in the backseat, directly into my eyes, though it feels as if he's seeing Margaret. Somewhat tenderly he says, Don't tell your mother.

Such moments, and many more, come to mind whenever I think about telling my father that I don't want to play tennis. Besides loving my father, and wanting to please him, I don't want to upset him. I don't dare. Bad stuff happens when my father is upset. If he says I'm going to play tennis, if he says I'm going to be number one in the world, that it's my destiny, all I can do is nod and obey. I would advise Jimmy Connors or anyone else to do the same.

THE ROAD TO NUMBER ONE goes over Hoover Dam. When I'm almost eight years old my father says the time has come to move from backyard sessions with the dragon and hit-arounds at Cambridge to actual tournaments, against real live little boys, all over Nevada and Arizona and California. Every weekend the whole family piles into the car and drives, either north on U.S. 95, toward Reno, or south, through Henderson and over Hoover Dam, across the desert to Phoenix or Scottsdale or Tucson. The last place I want to be, other than a tennis court, is in a car with my father. But it's all settled. I'm condemned to divide my childhood between these two boxes.

I win my first seven tournaments in the ten-and-under bracket. My father has no reaction. I'm simply doing what I'm supposed to do. Driving back over Hoover Dam, I stare at all the water bottled up behind the massive wall. I look at the inscription on the base of the flagpole: *In honor of those men who, inspired by a vision of lonely lands made fruitful* . . . I turn this phrase over in my mind. Lonely lands. Is there a land lonelier than our house in the desert? I think about the rage bottled up in my father, like the Colorado River inside the Hoover Dam. Only a matter of time before it bursts. Nothing to do but scramble for high ground.

For me, that means winning. Always winning.

We go to San Diego. Morley Field. I play a kid named Jeff Tarango, who isn't nearly on my level. But he wins the first set, 6–4. I'm stunned. Scared. My father is going to kill me. I bear down, win the second set, 6–0. Early in the third set Tarango twists his ankle. I start drop-shotting him, trying to make him run on the bad ankle. But he's only faking. His ankle is fine. He comes bounding in and smashes my drop shots and wins every point.

My father screams from the stands: No more drop shots! No more drops!

But I can't help myself. I have a strategy, I'm sticking with it.

We go to a tiebreak. It's best-of-nine. Back and forth we trade points, until it's 4–all. Here it is. Sudden death. One point for the whole match. I've never lost and can't imagine what my father's reaction will be if I do.

38

I play as if my life hangs in the balance, which it does. Tarango must have a father like mine, because he's playing the same way.

I haul off and rope a fizzing backhand crosscourt. I hit it as a rally shot but it comes off my racket bigger and hotter than I intended. It's a screaming winner, three feet in but well beyond Tarango's reach. I howl in triumph. Tarango, standing in the center of the court, bows his head and seems to cry. Slowly he walks toward the net.

Now he stops. All of a sudden, he looks back at where the ball hit. He smiles.

Out, he says.

I stop.

The ball was out! Tarango yells.

This is the rule in juniors. Players act as their own linesmen. Players call balls in or out, and there is no appeal. Tarango has decided he'd rather do this than lose, and he knows there's nothing anyone can do about it. He raises his hands in victory.

Now I start to cry.

Bedlam breaks out in the stands, parents arguing, shouting, nearly coming to blows. It's not fair, it's not right, but it's reality. Tarango is the winner. I refuse to shake his hand. I run away into Balboa Park. When I return half an hour later, all cried out, my father is furious. Not because I disappeared, but because I didn't do what he said during the match.

Why didn't you listen to me? Why did you keep hitting drop shots?

For once I'm not afraid of my father. No matter how angry he is with me, I'm angrier. I'm furious with Tarango, with God, with myself. Even though I feel Tarango cheated me, I shouldn't have put him in a position to cheat me. I shouldn't have let the match get that close. Because I did, I'll now have a loss on my record—forever. Nothing can ever change it. I can't endure the thought, but it's inescapable: I'm fallible. Blemished. Imperfect. A million balls hit against the dragon—for what?

After years of hearing my father rant at my flaws, one loss has caused me to take up his rant. I've internalized my father—his impatience, his perfectionism, his rage—until his voice doesn't just feel like my own, it is my own. I no longer need my father to torture me. From this day on, I can do it all by myself.

2

My father's mother lives with us. She's a nasty old lady from Tehran with a wart the size of a walnut on the edge of her nose. Sometimes you can't hear a word she's saying because you can't take your eyes off that wart. But it doesn't matter, she's surely saying the same nasty things she said yesterday, and the day before, and probably saying them to my father. This seems to be the reason Grandma was put on earth, to harass my father. He says she nagged him when he was a boy and often beat him. When he was extra bad, she made him wear hand-me-down girl clothes to school. That's why he learned to fight.

If she's not pecking at my father, the old lady is squawking about the old country, sighing about the folks she left behind. My mother says Grandma is *homesick*. The first time I hear this word I ask myself, How can you be sick about not being home? Home is where the dragon lives. Home is the place where, when you go there, you have to play tennis.

If Grandma wants to go back home, I'm all for it. I'm only eight, but I'll drive her to the airport myself, because she causes more tension in a house that doesn't need one bit more. She makes my father miserable, she bosses me and my siblings around, and she engages in a strange competition with my mother. My mother tells me that when I was a baby, she walked into the kitchen and found Grandma breastfeeding me. Things have been awkward between the two women ever since.

Of course, there is one good thing about Grandma living with us. She tells stories about my father, about his childhood, and this sometimes gets my father reminiscing, causes him to open up. If not for Grandma we wouldn't know much about my father's past, which was sad and lonely and helps explain his odd behavior and boiling rage. Sort of.

Oh, Grandma says with a sigh, we were poor. You can't imagine how poor. And *hungry,* she says, rubbing her belly. We had no food—also, no running water, no electricity. And not a stick of furniture.

Where did you sleep?

We slept on the dirt floor! All of us in one tiny room! In an old apartment house built around a filthy courtyard. In one corner of the courtyard was a hole—that was the toilet for all the tenants.

My father chimes in.

Things got better after the war, he says. Overnight, the streets were filled with British and American soldiers. I liked them.

Why did you like the soldiers?

They gave me candy and shoes.

They also gave him English. The first word my father learned from the GIs was *victory*. That's all they talked about, he says. *Wictory*.

Whoa, were they big, he adds. And strong. I followed them everywhere, watching them, studying them, and one day I followed them to the place where they spent all their free time—a park in the woods with two clay tennis courts.

There were no fences around the courts, so the ball would go bouncing away every few seconds. My father would run after the ball and bring it back to the soldiers, like a puppy dog, until finally they made him their unofficial ball boy. Then they made him the official court custodian.

My father says: Every day I swept and watered and combed the courts with a heavy roller. I painted the lines white. What a job that was! I had to use chalk water.

How much did they pay you?

Pay? Nothing! They gave me a tennis racket. It was a piece of junk. An old wooden thing strung with steel wire. But I loved it. I spent hours with that racket, hitting a tennis ball against a brick wall, alone.

Why alone?

No one else in Iran played tennis.

The only sport that could offer my father a steady supply of opponents was boxing. His toughness was tested first in one street fight after another, and then as a teenager he strode into a gym and set to work learning formal boxing techniques. A natural, the trainers called him. Quick with his hands, light on his feet—and he had a grudge against the world. His rage, so hard for us to deal with, was an asset in the squared circle. He won a spot on the Iranian Olympic team, boxing in the bantamweight division, and went to the 1948 Games in London. Four years later he went to the Games in Helsinki. He didn't do well at either.

The judges, he grumbles. They were crooked. The whole thing was fixed, rigged. The world was very biased against Iran.

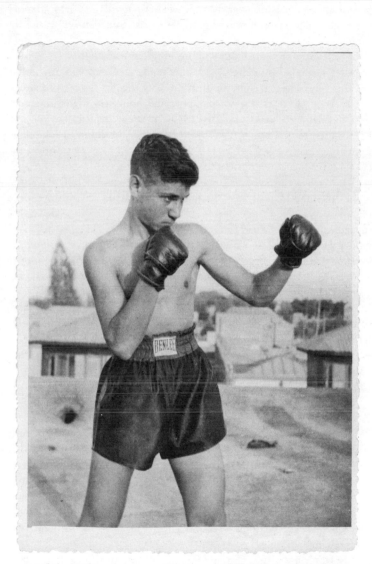

My father, Mike, as a scrappy eighteen-year-old bantamweight in Tehran

But my son, he adds—maybe they will make tennis an Olympic sport once again, and my son will win a gold medal, and that will make up for it.

A little extra pressure to go with my everyday pressure.

After seeing a bit of the world, after being an Olympian, my father couldn't return to that same single room with the dirt floor, so he snuck out of Iran. He doctored his passport and booked a flight under an assumed name to New York City, where he spent sixteen days on Ellis Island, then took a bus to Chicago, where he Americanized his name. Emmanuel became Mike Agassi. By day he worked as an elevator operator at one of the city's grand hotels. By night he boxed.

His coach in Chicago was Tony Zale, the fearless middleweight champ, often called the Man of Steel. Famous for his part in one of the sport's bloodiest rivalries, a three-bout saga with Rocky Graziano, Zale lauded my father, told him he had tons of raw talent, but pleaded with him to hit harder. Hit *harder*, Zale would scream at my father as he peppered the speed bag. Hit *harder*. Every punch you throw, throw it from the floor up.

With Zale in his corner my father won the Chicago Golden Gloves, then earned a prime-time fight at Madison Square Garden. His big break. But on fight night my father's opponent fell ill. The promoters scrambled, trying to find a substitute. They found one, all right—a much better boxer, and a welterweight. My father agreed to the fight, but moments before the opening bell he got the shakes. He ducked into a bathroom, crawled out the window above the toilet, then took the train back to Chicago.

Sneaking out of Iran, sneaking out of the Garden—my father is an escape artist, I think. But there's no escaping him.

My father says that when he boxed, he always wanted to take a guy's best punch. He tells me one day on the tennis court: When you know that you just took the other guy's best punch, and you're still standing, and the other guy knows it, you will rip the heart right out of him. In tennis, he says, same rule. Attack the other man's strength. If the man is a server, take away his serve. If he's a power player, overpower him. If he has a big forehand, takes pride in his forehand, go after his forehand until he hates his forehand.

My father has a special name for this contrarian strategy. He calls it putting a blister on the other guy's brain. With this strategy, this brutal philosophy, he stamps me for life. He turns me into a boxer with a tennis racket. More, since most tennis players pride themselves on their serve, my father turns me into a counterpuncher—a returner.

. . .

EVERY ONCE IN A WHILE my father gets homesick too. He especially misses his oldest brother, Isar. Someday, he vows, your uncle Isar will sneak out of Iran, like I did.

But first Isar needs to sneak out his money. Iran is falling apart, my father explains. Revolution is brewing. The government is teetering. That's why they're watching everyone, making sure people don't drain their bank accounts and flee. Uncle Isar, therefore, is slowly, secretly converting his cash to jewels, which he then hides in packages he sends us in Vegas. It feels like Christmas every time a brown-wrapped box from Uncle Isar arrives. We sit on the living-room floor and cut the string and tear the paper and shriek when we find, hidden under a tin of cookies or inside a fruitcake, diamonds and emeralds and rubies. Uncle Isar's packages arrive every few weeks, and then one day comes a much larger package. Uncle Isar. Himself. On the doorstep, smiling down.

You must be Andre.

Yes.

I'm your uncle.

He reaches out and touches my cheek.

He's the mirror image of my father, but his personality is the exact opposite. My father is shrill and stern and filled with rage. Uncle Isar is soft-spoken and patient and funny. He's also a genius—he was an engineer back in Iran—so he helps me every night with my homework. Such a relief from my father's tutoring sessions. My father's way of teaching is to tell you once, then tell you a second time, then shout at you and call you an idiot for not getting it the first time. Uncle Isar tells you, then smiles and waits. If you don't understand, no problem. He tells you again, more softly. He has all the time in the world.

I stare at Uncle Isar as he strolls through the rooms and hallways of our house. I follow him the way my father followed the British and American soldiers. As I grow familiar with Uncle Isar, as I get to know him better, I like to hang from his shoulders and swing from his arms. He likes it too. He likes to roughhouse, to be tackled and tickled by his nephews and nieces. Every night I hide behind the front door and jump out when Uncle Isar comes home, because it makes him laugh. His booming laughter is the opposite of the sounds that come from the dragon.

One day Uncle Isar goes to the store for a few things. I count the minutes. At last, the front gate clanks open, then clanks shut, meaning I have exactly twelve seconds until Uncle Isar walks through the front door. It always takes people twelve seconds to go from the gate to the door. I crouch, count to twelve, and as the door opens I leap out.

Boo!

It's not Uncle Isar. It's my father. Startled, he yells, steps back, then shoots out his fist. Even though he only puts a fraction of his weight into it, my father's left hook hits my jaw flush and sends me flying. One second I'm excited, joyful, the next I'm sprawled on the ground.

My father stands over me, scowling. What the fuck is the matter with you? Go to your room.

I run to my room and throw myself on my bed. I lie there, shaking, I don't know how long. An hour? Three? Eventually the door opens and I hear my father.

Grab your racket. Get on the court.

Time to face the dragon.

I hit for half an hour, my head throbbing, my eyes tearing.

Hit *harder,* my father says. Goddamn it, hit *harder.* Not in the fucking net!

I turn and face my father. The next ball from the dragon I hit as hard as I can, but high over the fence. I aim for the hawks and I don't bother pretending it's an accident. My father stares. He takes one menacing step toward me. He's going to hit *me* over the fence. But then he stops, calls me a bad name, and warns me to stay out of his sight.

I run into the house and find my mother lying on her bed, reading a romance novel, her dogs at her feet. She loves animals, and our house is like Dr. Dolittle's waiting room. Dogs, birds, cats, lizards, and one mangy rat named Lady Butt. I grab one of the dogs and hurl it across the room, ignoring its insulted yelp, and bury my head in my mother's arm.

Why is Pops so mean?

What happened?

I tell her.

She strokes my hair and says my father doesn't know any better. Pa has his own ways, she says. Strange ways. We have to remember that Pa wants what's best for us, right?

Part of me feels grateful for my mother's endless calm. Part of me, however, a part I don't like to acknowledge, feels betrayed by it. Calm sometimes means weak. She never steps in. She never fights back. She never throws herself between us kids and my father. She should tell him to back off, ease up, that tennis isn't life.

But it's not in her nature. My father disturbs the peace, my mother keeps it. Every morning she goes to the office—she works for the State of Nevada—in her sensible pantsuit, and every night she comes home at six, bone tired, not uttering one word of complaint. With her last speck of energy she cooks dinner. Then she lies down with her pets and a book, or her favorite: a jigsaw puzzle.

Only every great once in a while does she lose her temper, and when she does, it's epic. One time my father made a remark about the house being unclean. My mother walked to the cupboard, took out two boxes of cereal, and waved them around her head like flags, spraying Corn Flakes and Cheerios everywhere. She yelled: You want the house clean? Clean it yourself!

Moments later, she was calmly working on a jigsaw puzzle.

She particularly loves Norman Rockwell puzzles. There is always some half-assembled scene of idyllic family life spread across the kitchen table. I can't imagine the pleasure my mother takes in jigsaw puzzles. All that fractured disorder, all that chaos—how can that be relaxing? It makes me think my mother and I are complete opposites. And yet, anything soft in me, any love or compassion I have for people, must come from her.

Lying against her, letting her continue to stroke my hair, I think there is so much about her that I can't understand, and it all seems to flow from her choice of a husband. I ask how she ever ended up with a guy like my father in the first place. She gives a short, weary laugh.

It was a long time ago, she says. Back in Chicago. A friend of a friend told your father: You should meet Betty Dudley, she's just your type. And vice versa. So your father phoned me one night at the Girls Club where I was renting a furnished room. We talked a long, long time, and your father seemed sweet.

Sweet?

I know, I know. But he did. So I agreed to meet him. He showed up the next day in a spiffy new Volkswagen. He drove me around town, no place in particular, just round and round, telling me his story. Then we stopped to get something to eat and I told him my story.

My mother told my father about growing up in Danville, Illinois, 170 miles from Chicago, the same small town where Gene Hackman and Donald O'Connor and Dick Van Dyke grew up. She told him about being a twin. She told him about her father, a crotchety English teacher, a stickler for proper English. My father, with his broken English, must have cringed. More likely, he didn't hear. I imagine my father not capable of listening to my mother on their first date. He would have been too mes-merized by her flaming auburn hair and bright blue eyes. I've seen pic-tures. My mother was a rare beauty. I wonder if he liked her hair best because it was the color of a clay tennis court. Or was it her height? She's several inches taller than he. I can imagine him perceiving that as a chal-lenge.

My mother says it took eight blissful weeks for my father to convince her that they should combine their stories. They ran away from her crotchety father and her twin sister and eloped. Then they kept running. My father drove my mother clear out to Los Angeles, and when they had trouble finding jobs there, he drove her across the desert, to a new gam-bling boomtown. My mother landed her job with the state government, and my father caught on at the Tropicana Hotel, giving tennis lessons. It didn't pay much, so he got a second job waiting tables at the Landmark Hotel. Then he got a job as a captain at the MGM Grand casino, which kept him so busy he dropped the other two jobs.

Over their first ten years of marriage, my parents had three kids. Then, in 1969, my mother went to the hospital with ominous stomach

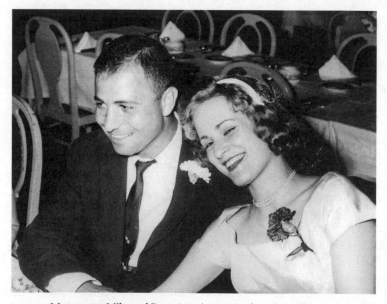

My parents, Mike and Betty Agassi, 1959, newlyweds in Chicago

pains. Need to do a hysterectomy, the doctor said. But a second round of tests showed she was pregnant. With me. I was born April 29, 1970, at Sunrise Hospital, two miles from the Strip. My father named me Andre Kirk Agassi, after his bosses at the casino. I ask my mother why my father named me after his bosses. Were they friends? Did he admire them? Did he owe them money? She doesn't know. And it's not the kind of question you can ask my father directly. You can't ask my father anything directly. So I file it away with all the other things I don't know about my parents— permanently missing pieces in the jigsaw puzzle that is me.

MY FATHER WORKS HARD, puts in long hours on the night shift at the casino, but tennis is his life, his reason for getting out of bed. No matter where you sit in the house, you see scattered evidence of his obsession. Aside from the backyard court, and the dragon, there is my father's laboratory, also known as the kitchen. My father's stringing machine and tools take up half the kitchen table. (My mother's latest Norman Rockwell takes up the other half—two obsessions vying for one busy room.) On the kitchen counter stand several stacks of rackets, many sawed in half so my father can study their guts. He wants to know *everything* about tennis, everything, which means dissecting its various parts. He's forever conducting experiments on this or that piece of equipment. Lately, for instance, he's been using old tennis balls to extend the lives of our shoes. When the rubber starts to wear down, my father cuts a tennis ball in half and puts one half on each toe.

I tell Philly: It's not bad enough that we live in a tennis laboratory— now we have to wear tennis balls on our feet?

I wonder why my father loves tennis. Yet another question I can't ask him directly. Still, he drops clues. He talks sometimes about the beauty of the game, its perfect balance of power and strategy. Despite his imperfect life—or maybe because of it—my father craves perfection. Geometry and mathematics are as close to perfection as human beings can get, he says, and tennis is all about angles and numbers. My father lies in bed and sees a court on the ceiling. He says he can actually see it there, and on that ceiling court he plays countless imaginary matches. It's a wonder he has any energy when he goes to work.

As a casino captain it's my father's job to seat people at the shows. Right this way, Mr. Johnson. Nice to see you again, Miss Jones. The MGM pays him a small salary, the rest he earns in tips. We live on tips, which makes life unpredictable. Some nights my father comes home with his pockets bulging with cash. Other nights his pockets are perfectly flat. Whatever he pulls from his pockets, no matter how little, gets carefully counted and stacked, then stashed in the family safe. It's nerve-wracking, never knowing how much Pops is going to be able to tuck in the safe.

My father loves money, makes no apologies for loving it, and he says there's good money to be made in tennis. Clearly this is one big part of his love for tennis. It's the shortest route he can see to the American dream. He takes me to the Alan King Tennis Classic and we watch a beautiful woman dressed as Cleopatra being carried onto center court by four half-naked musclemen in togas, followed by a man dressed as Caesar, pushing a wheelbarrow full of silver dollars. First prize for the winner of the tournament. My father stares at that silvery haze sparkling in the Vegas sun and looks drunk. He wants that. He wants me to have that.

Soon after that fateful day, when I'm almost nine years old, he finagles me a job as a ball boy for the Alan King tournament. But I don't give a damn about silver dollars—I want a mini Cleopatra. Her name is Wendi. She's one of the ball girls, about my age, a vision in her blue uniform. I love her instantly, with all my heart and part of my spleen. I lie awake at night, picturing her on the ceiling.

During matches, as Wendi and I dart past each other along the net, I shoot her a smile, try to get her to give me a smile in return. Between matches I buy her Cokes and sit with her, trying to impress her with my knowledge of tennis.

The Alan King tournament attracts big-time players, and my father cajoles most of them into hitting a few balls with me. Some are more willing than others. Borg acts as if there is nowhere else he'd rather be. Connors clearly wants to say no, but can't, because my father is his stringer. Ilie Nastase tries to say no, but my father pretends to be deaf. A champion of Wimbledon and the French Open, ranked number one in the world, Nastase has other places he'd rather be, but he quickly discovers that refusing my father is next to impossible. The man is relentless.

As Nastase and I hit, Wendi watches from the net post. I'm nervous, Nastase is visibly bored—until he spots Wendi.

Hey, he says. Is this your girlfriend, Snoopy? Is this pretty thing over here your sweetheart?

I stop. I glare at Nastase. I want to punch this big, stupid Romanian in the nose, even though he's got two feet and 100 pounds on me. Bad enough that he calls me Snoopy, but then he dares to mention Wendi in such a disrespectful way. A crowd has gathered, two hundred people at

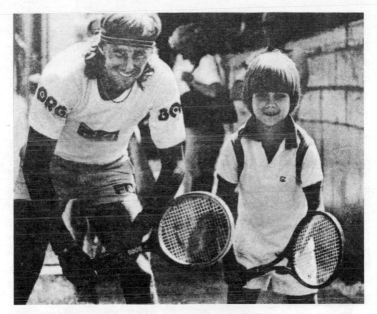

Eight years old, hitting a few balls
with my idol, Björn Borg

least. Nastase begins playing to the crowd, calling me Snoopy again and again, teasing me about Wendi. And I thought my father was relentless.

At the very least, I wish I had the courage to say: Mr. Nastase, you're embarrassing me, please stop. But all I can do is keep hitting harder. Hit *harder.* Then Nastase makes yet another wisecrack about Wendi, and that's it, I can't take any more. I drop my racket and walk off the court. Up yours, Nastase.

My father stares, openmouthed. He's not angry, he's not embarrassed—he's incapable of embarrassment, and he recognizes his own genes when he sees them in action. I don't know that I've ever seen him prouder.

BESIDES THE OCCASIONAL EXHIBITION with a top-ranked player, my public matches are mostly hustle jobs. I have a slick routine to lure in the suckers. First, I pick a highly visible court, where I play by myself, knocking the ball all over the place. Second, when some cocky teenager or drunken guest strolls by I invite them to play. Third, I let them beat me, soundly. Finally, in my most pitiful voice I ask if they'd like to play for a dollar. Maybe five? Before they know what's happening, I'm serving for match point and twenty bucks, enough to keep Wendi in Cokes for a month.

Philly taught me how to do it. He gives tennis lessons and often hustles his students, plays them for the price of the lesson, then double or nothing. But Andre, he says, with your size and youth, you should be raking in the dough. He helps me develop and rehearse the routine. Now and then it occurs to me that I only think I'm hustling, that people are happy to shell out for the show. Later they can brag to their friends that they saw a nine-year-old tennis freak who never misses.

I don't tell my father about my side business. Not that he'd think it was wrong. He loves a good hustle. I just don't feel like talking to my father about tennis any more than is absolutely necessary. Then my father stumbles into his own hustle. It happens at Cambridge. As we walk in one day, my father points to a man talking with Mr. Fong.

That's Jim Brown, my father whispers to me. Greatest football player of all time.

He's an enormous block of muscle wearing tennis whites and tube socks. I've seen him before at Cambridge. When he's not playing tennis for money, he's playing backgammon, or shooting craps—also for money. Like my father, Mr. Brown talks a lot about money. At this moment he's complaining to Mr. Fong about a money match that fell through. He was supposed to play a guy, and the guy didn't show. Mr. Brown is taking it out on Mr. Fong.

I came to play, Mr. Brown is saying, and I want to play.

My father steps forward.

You looking for a game?

Yeah.

My son Andre will play you.

Mr. Brown looks at me, then back at my father.

I ain't playing no eight-year-old boy!

Nine.

Nine? Oooh, well, I didn't realize.

Mr. Brown laughs. A few men within earshot laugh too.

I can tell that Mr. Brown doesn't take my father seriously. Big mistake. Just ask that trucker lying in the road. I close my eyes and see him, the rain pelting his face.

Look, Mr. Brown says, I don't play for fun, OK? I play for *money*.

My son will play you for money.

I feel a bead of sweat start down my armpit.

Yeah? How much?

My father laughs and says, I'll bet you my fucking house.

I don't need your house, Mr. Brown says. I got a house. Let's say ten grand.

Done, my father says.

I walk toward the court.

Slow down, Mr. Brown says. I need to see some money up front.

I'll go home and get it, my father says. I'll be right back.

My father hurries out the door. I sit in a chair and picture him opening the safe and pulling out stacks of money. All those tips I've seen him count through the years, all those nights of hard work. Now he's going to let it ride on me. I feel a heaviness in the center of my chest. I'm proud, of course, to think my father has such faith in me. But mainly I'm scared. What happens to me, to my father, to my mother and my siblings, not to mention Grandma and Uncle Isar, if I lose?

I've played under this kind of pressure before, when my father, without warning, has chosen an opponent and ordered me to beat him. But it's always been another kid, and there's never been money involved. It usually happens in the middle of the afternoon. My father will wake me from a nap and yell, Grab your racket! There's someone here you need to beat! It never occurs to him that I'm taking a nap because I'm exhausted from a morning playing the dragon, that nine-year-olds don't often take naps. Rubbing the sleep from my eyes I'll go outside and see some strange kid, some prodigy from Florida or California who happens to be in town. They're always older and bigger—like that punk who'd just moved to Vegas, and heard about me, and rang our doorbell. He had a white Rossignol and a head like a pumpkin. He was at least three years older than I, and he smirked as I walked out of the house, because I was so small. Even after I beat him, even after I wiped that smirk off his face, it took hours for me to calm down, to shed the feeling that I'd just run along a tightrope stretched across Hoover Dam.

This thing with Mr. Brown, however, is different, and not just because my family's life savings are riding on the outcome. Mr. Brown disrespected my father, and my father can't knock him out. He needs me to do it. So this match will be about more than money. It will be about respect and manhood and honor—against the greatest football player of all time. I'd rather play in the final of Wimbledon. Against Nastase. With Wendi as the ballgirl.

Slowly I become aware that Mr. Brown is watching me. Staring. He walks over and introduces himself, shakes my hand. His hand is one big callus. He asks how long I've been playing, how many matches I've won, how many I've lost.

I never lose, I say quietly.

His eyes narrow.

Mr. Fong pulls Mr. Brown aside and says: Don't do this, Jim.

Guy's asking for it, Mr. Brown whispers. Fool and his money.

You don't understand, Mr. Fong says. You are going to lose, Jim.

What the hell are you—? He's a kid.

That's not just any kid.

You must be crazy.

Look, Jim, I like having you come here. You're a friend, and it's good for business to have you at my club. But when you lose ten grand to this kid, you'll be sore, and you might stop coming around.

Mr. Brown turns to look me up and down, as if he must have missed something the first time. He walks back toward me and starts firing questions.

How much do you play?

Every day.

No—how long do you play at one time? An hour? Couple of hours?

I see what he's doing. He wants to know how fast I get tired. He's trying to size me up, game-planning for me.

My father's back. He's got a fistful of hundreds. He waves it in the air. Suddenly Mr. Brown has had a change of heart.

Here's what we'll do, Mr. Brown tells my father. We'll play two sets, *then* decide how much to bet on the third.

Whatever you say.

We play on Court 7, just inside the door. A crowd has gathered, and they cheer themselves hoarse as I win the first set, 6–3. Mr. Brown shakes his head. He talks to himself. He bangs his racket on the ground. He's not happy, which makes two of us. Not only am I thinking, in direct violation of my father's cardinal rule, but my mind is spinning. I feel as if I might have to stop playing at any moment, because I need to throw up.

Still, I win the second set, 6–3.

Now Mr. Brown is furious. He drops to one knee, laces his sneakers.

My father approaches him.

So? Ten grand?

Naw, Mr. Brown says. Why don't we just bet $500.

Whatever you say.

My body relaxes. My mind grows quiet. I want to dance along the baseline, knowing I won't have to play for $10,000. I can swing freely now, without thinking about consequences. Without thinking at all.

Mr. Brown, meanwhile, is thinking more, playing a less relaxed game. He's suddenly junking, drop-shotting, lofting lobs, angling the ball at the corners, trying backspin and sidespin and all sorts of trickery. He's also trying to run me, back and forth, wear me out. But I'm so relieved not to be playing for the entire contents of my father's safe that I can't be worn out, and I can't miss. I beat Mr. Brown 6–2.

Sweat running down his face, he pulls a wad from his pocket and counts out five crisp hundreds. He hands them to my father, then turns to me.

Great game, son.

He shakes my hand. His calluses feel rougher—thanks to me.

He asks what my goals are, my dreams. I start to answer, but my father jumps in.

He's going to be number one in the world.

I wouldn't bet against him, Mr. Brown says.

NOT LONG AFTER BEATING MR. BROWN, I play a practice match against my father at Caesars. I'm up 5–2, serving for the match. I've never beaten my father, and he looks as if he's about to lose much more than $10,000.

Suddenly he walks off the court. Get your stuff, he says. Let's go.

He won't finish. He'd rather sneak away than lose to his son. Deep down, I know it's the last time we'll ever play.

Packing my bag, zipping the cover on my racket, I feel a thrill greater than anything I felt after beating Mr. Brown. This is the sweetest win of my life, and it will be hard to top. I'll take this win over a wheelbarrow full of silver dollars—and Uncle Isar's jewels thrown on top—because this is the win that made my father finally sneak away from me.

3

I'M TEN, playing in the nationals. Second round. I lose badly to some kid who's older, who's supposed to be the best in the country. Not that this makes it easier. How can losing hurt so much? How can anything hurt so much? I walk off the court wishing I were dead. I stagger out to the parking lot. As my father gathers our stuff and says goodbye to the other parents, I sit in the car, crying.

A man's face appears in the car window. Black guy. Smiling.

Hey there, he says. My name's Rudy.

Same name as the man who helped my father build his backyard tennis court. Strange.

What's your name?

Andre.

He shakes my hand.

Nice to meet you, Andre.

He says he works with the great champion Pancho Segura, who coaches kids my age. He comes to these big tournaments to scout kids for Pancho. He puts his arms through the window, leans heavily on the car door, sighs. He tells me that days like this are tough, he knows, very tough indeed, but in the end these days will make me stronger. His voice is warm, thick, like hot cocoa.

That kid who beat you, why, that kid's two years older than you! You've got two years to reach that kid's level. Two years is an eternity—especially when you're working hard. Do you work hard?

Yes, sir.

You've got so much ahead of you, son.

But I don't want to play anymore. I hate tennis.

Ha, ha! Sure you do. Right now. But deep down, you don't really hate tennis.

Yes, I do.

You just think you hate it.

No, I hate it.

You're saying that because you're hurting right now, hurting like heck, but that just means you care. Means you want to win. You can *use* that. Remember this day. Try to use this day as motivation. If you don't want to feel this hurt again, good, do everything you can to avoid it. Are you ready to do everything?

I nod.

Fine, fine. So go ahead and cry. Hurt a while longer. But then tell yourself, that's it, time to get back to work.

OK.

I wipe my tears on my sleeve and thank Rudy and when he walks away I'm ready to practice. Bring on the dragon. I'm ready to hit balls for hours. If Rudy were standing behind me, whispering encouragement in my ear, I think I could *beat* that dragon. Suddenly my father climbs behind the wheel of the car and we drive slowly away, like the head car in a funeral procession. The tension in the car is so thick that I curl up on the backseat and close my eyes. I think about jumping out, running away, finding Rudy and asking him to coach me. Or adopt me.

I HATE ALL THE junior tournaments, but I hate nationals most of all, because the stakes are higher, and they're held in other states, which means airfare, motels, rental cars, restaurant meals. My father is shelling out money, investing in me, and when I lose, there goes another piece of his investment. When I lose I set back the whole Agassi clan.

I'm eleven, playing nationals in Texas on clay. I'm among the best in the nation on clay, so there's no way I'm going to lose, and then I lose. In the semis. I don't even reach the final. Now I have to play a consolation match. When you lose in the semis they make you play a match to determine third and fourth place. Worse, in this particular consolation match I'm facing my archnemesis, David Kass. He's ranked just below me, but somehow becomes a different player when he sees me across that net. No matter what I do, Kass beats me, and today is no different. I lose in three sets. Again I'm shattered. I've disappointed my father. I've cost my family. I don't cry, however. I want to make Rudy proud, so I manage to choke back the tears.

At the awards ceremony a man hands out the first-place trophy, then second, then third. Then he announces that this year a sportsmanship trophy will be awarded to the youngster who exhibits the most grace on the court. Incredibly, he says my name—maybe because I've been biting my lip for an hour. He's holding the trophy toward me, waving me to come and get it. It's the last thing in the world I want, a sportsmanship trophy, but I take it from the man and thank him and something shifts inside me. It *is* an awfully cool trophy. And I *have* been a good sport. I walk out to the car, clutching the trophy to my chest, my father a step behind me. He says nothing, I say nothing. I concentrate on the click-clack of our footsteps on the cement. Finally I break the silence. I say, I don't want this stupid thing. I say it because I think it's what my father wants to hear. My father comes alongside me. He rips the trophy from my hands. He lifts it over his head and throws it on the cement. The trophy shatters. My father picks up the biggest piece and throws it on the cement, smashing it into smaller pieces. Now he collects the pieces and throws them into a nearby dumpster. I don't say a word. I know not to say a word.

IF ONLY I COULD play soccer instead of tennis. I don't like sports, but if I must play a sport to please my father, I'd much rather play soccer. I get to play three times a week at school, and I love running the soccer field with the wind in my hair, calling for the ball, knowing the world won't end if I don't score. The fate of my father, of my family, of planet earth, doesn't rest on my shoulders. If my team doesn't win, it will be the whole team's fault, and no one will yell in my ear. Team sports, I decide, are the way to go.

My father doesn't mind my playing soccer, because he thinks it helps my footwork on the court. But I recently hurt myself in a soccer scrimmage, pulled a muscle in my leg, and the injury forces me to skip tennis practice one afternoon. My father isn't happy. He looks at my leg, then me, as if I injured myself on purpose. But an injury is an injury. Even he can't argue with my body. He stomps out of the house.

Moments later my mother looks at my schedule and realizes I have a soccer game this afternoon. What do we do? she says.

The team is counting on me, I tell her.

She sighs. How do you feel?

I think I can play.

OK. Put on your soccer uniform.

Do you think Pops will be upset?

You know Pa. He doesn't need a reason to be upset.

She drives me to the soccer game and leaves me there. After a few jogs up and down the field, my leg feels good. Surprisingly good. I dart in between defenders, fluid, graceful, calling for the ball, laughing with my teammates. We're working toward a common objective. We're in this together. This feels right. This feels like me.

Suddenly I look up and see my father. He's at the edge of the parking lot, stalking toward the field. Now he's talking to the coach. Now he's yelling at the coach. The coach is waving to me. Agassi! Out of the game!

I sprint off the field.

Get in the car, my father says. And get out of that uniform.

I run to the car and find my tennis clothes on the backseat. I put them on and walk back to my father. I hand him my soccer uniform. He walks onto the field and throws the uniform at the coach's chest.

As we drive home my father says without looking at me: You're never playing soccer again.

I beg him for a second chance. I tell my father that I don't like being by myself on that huge tennis court. Tennis is lonely, I tell him. There's nowhere to hide when things go wrong. No dugout, no sideline, no neutral corner. It's just you out there, naked.

He shouts at the top of his lungs: You're a tennis player! You're going to be number one in the world! You're going to make lots of money. *That's the plan, and that's the end of it.*

He's adamant, and desperate, because that was the plan for Rita, Philly, and Tami, but things never worked out. Rita rebelled. Tami stopped getting better. Philly didn't have the killer instinct. My father says this about Philly all the time. He says it to me, to Mom, even to Philly—right to his face. Philly just shrugs, which seems to prove that Philly doesn't have the killer instinct.

But my father says far worse things to Philly.

You're a born loser, he says.

You're right, Philly says in a sorrowful tone. I am a born loser. I was born to be a loser.

You are! You feel sorry for your opponent! You don't care about being the best!

Philly doesn't bother to deny it. He plays well, he has talent, but he just isn't a perfectionist, and perfection isn't the goal in our house, it's the law. If you're not perfect, you're a loser. A born loser.

My father decided that Philly was a born loser when Philly was about my age, playing nationals. Philly didn't just lose; he didn't argue when his opponents cheated him, which made my father turn bright red and scream curses in Assyrian from the bleachers.

Like my mother, Philly takes it and takes it, and then every once in a great while he blows. The last time it happened, my father was stringing a tennis racket, my mother was ironing, and Philly was on the couch, watching TV. My father kept after Philly, mercilessly nagging him about his performance at a recent tournament. All at once, in a tone I'd never heard him use, Philly screeched, You know why I don't win? Because of you! Because you call me a born loser!

Philly started panting with anger. My mother started crying.

From now on, Philly continued, I'll just be a robot, how's that? Would you like that? I'll be a robot and feel nothing and just go out there and do everything you say!

My father stopped stringing the racket and looked happy. Almost peaceful. Jesus Christ, he said, you're finally *getting* it.

Unlike Philly, I argue with opponents all the time. I sometimes wish I had Philly's knack for shrugging off injustice. If an opponent cheats me, if he pulls a Tarango, my face gets hot. Often I get my revenge on the next point. When my cheating opponent hits a shot in the center of the court, I call it out and stare at him with a look that says: Now we're even.

I don't do this to please my father, but it surely does. He says, You have a different mentality than Philly. You got all the talent, all the fire—and the luck. *You were born with a horseshoe up your ass.*

He says this once a day. Sometimes he says it with conviction, sometimes admiration—sometimes envy. I blanch when he says it. I worry that I got Philly's good luck, that I stole it from him somehow, because if I was born with a horseshoe up my ass, Philly was born with a black cloud over his head. When Philly was twelve he broke his wrist while riding his bike, broke it in three places, and that was the beginning of a long stretch of unbroken gloom. My father was so furious with Philly that he made Philly keep playing tournaments, broken wrist and all, which worsened Philly's wrist, made the problem chronic, and ruined his game forever. Favoring his broken wrist, Philly was forced to use a one-handed backhand, which Philly believes is a terrible habit, one he couldn't break after the wrist healed. I watch Philly lose and think: Bad habits plus bad luck—deadly combination. I also watch him when he comes home after a hard loss. He feels so rotten about himself, you can see it all over his face, and my father drives that rottenness down deeper. Philly sits in a corner, beating himself up over the loss, but at least it's a fair fight, one on one. Then along comes my father. He jumps in and helps Philly gang up on Philly. There is name-calling, slapping. By rights this should make Philly a basket case. At the very least it should make him resent me, bully me. Instead, after every verbal or physical assault at the hands of himself and my father, Philly's slightly more careful with me, more protective. Gentler. He wants me spared his fate. For this reason, though he may be a born loser, I see Philly as the ultimate winner. I feel lucky to have him as my older brother. Feeling lucky to have an unlucky older brother? Is that possible? Does that make sense? Another defining contradiction.

PHILLY AND I spend all our free time together. He picks me up at school on his scooter and we go riding home across the desert, talking and laughing above the engine's insect whine. We share a bedroom at the back of the house, our sanctuary from tennis and Pops. Philly is as fussy about his stuff as I am about mine, so he paints a white line down the center of the room, dividing it into his side and mine, ad court and deuce court. I sleep in the deuce court, my bed closest to the door. At night, before we turn out the lights, we have a ritual I've come to depend on. We sit on the edges of our beds and whisper across the line. Philly, seven years older, does most of the talking. He pours out his heart, his self-doubts and disappointments. He talks about never winning. He talks about being called a born loser. He talks about needing to borrow money from Pops so that he can continue to play tennis, to keep trying to turn pro. Pops, we both agree, is not a man you want holding your marker.

Of all the things that trouble Philly, however, the great trauma of his life is his hairline. Andre, he says, I'm going bald. He says this in the same way he would tell me the doctor has given him four weeks to live.

But he won't lose his hair without a battle. Baldness is one opponent Philly will fight with all he's got. He thinks the reason he's going bald is that he's not getting enough blood to his scalp, so every night, at some point during our bedtime talks, Philly stands upside down. He puts his head on the mattress and lifts his feet, balancing himself against the wall. I pray it will work. I plead with God that my brother, the born loser, won't lose this one thing, his hair. I lie to Philly and tell him that I can see his miracle cure working. I love my brother so much, I'd say anything if I thought it would make him feel better. For my brother's sake, I'd stand on my own head all night.

After Philly tells me his troubles, I sometimes tell him mine. I'm touched by how quickly he refocuses. He listens to the latest mean thing

Pops said, gauges my level of concern, then gives me the proportionate nod. For basic fears, a half nod. For big fears, a full nod with a patented Philly frown. Even when upside down, Philly says as much with one nod as most people say in a five-page letter.

One night Philly asks me to promise him something.

Sure, Philly. Anything.

Don't ever let Pops give you any pills.

Pills?

Andre, you have to hear what I am telling you. This is really important.

OK, Philly, I hear you. I'm listening.

Next time you go away to nationals, if Pops gives you pills, don't take them.

He already gives me Excedrin, Philly. He makes me take Excedrin before a match, because it's loaded with caffeine.

Yeah, I know. But these pills I'm talking about are different. These pills are tiny, white, round. Don't take them. Whatever you do.

What if Pops makes me? I can't say no to Pops.

Yeah. Right. OK, let me think.

Philly closes his eyes. I watch the blood rushing to his forehead, turning it purple.

OK, he says. I got it. If you have to take the pills, if he *makes* you take them, play a bad match. Tank. Then, as you come off the court, tell him you were shaking so bad that you couldn't concentrate.

OK. But Philly—what are these pills?

Speed.

What's that?

A drug. Gives you lots of energy. I just know he's going to try to slip you some speed.

How do you know, Philly?

He gave it to me.

Sure enough, at the nationals in Chicago my father gives me a pill. Hold out your hand, he says. This will help you. Take it.

He puts a pill on my palm. Tiny. White. Round.

I swallow the pill and feel OK. Not much different. Slightly more alert. But I pretend to feel very different. My opponent, an older kid, poses no challenge, and still I carry him, drag out points, hand him several games. I make the match look tougher than it is. Walking off the court I tell my father I don't feel right, I want to pass out, and he looks guilty.

OK, he says, rubbing his hand across his face, that's not good. We won't try that again.

I phone Philly after the tournament and tell him about the pill.

He says, I fucking knew it!

I did just what you told me to do, Philly, and it worked.

My brother sounds the way I imagine a father is supposed to sound. Proud of me and scared for me at the same time. When I return from nationals I grab him and hug him and we spend my first night home locked in our room, whispering across the white line, cherishing our rare victory over Pops.

A short time later I play an older opponent and beat him. It's a practice match, no big deal, and I'm much better than the opponent, but once again I carry him, drag out points, make the match look tougher than it is, just as I did in Chicago. Walking off Court 7 at Cambridge—the same court on which I beat Mr. Brown—I feel devastated, because my opponent looks devastated. I should have tanked all the way. I hate losing, but I hate winning this time because the defeated opponent is Philly. Does this devastated feeling prove I don't have the killer instinct? Confused, sad, I wish I could find that old guy, Rudy, or the other Rudy before him, and ask them what it all means.

4

I'M PLAYING A TOURNAMENT at the Las Vegas Country Club, vying for a chance to go to the state championship. My opponent is a kid named Roddy Parks. The first thing I notice about him is that he too has a unique father. Mr. Parks wears a ring with an ant frozen inside a large gumdrop of yellow amber. Before the match starts, I ask him about it.

You see, Andre, when the world ends in a nuclear holocaust, ants will be the only things that survive. So *I'm* planning for my spirit to go *into* an ant.

Roddy is thirteen, two years older than I, and big for his age, with a military crew cut. But he looks beatable. Right away I see holes in his game, weaknesses. Then, somehow, he fills in the holes, papers over the weaknesses. He wins the first set.

I talk to myself, tell myself to suck it up, dig in. I take the second set.

Bearing down now, I play smarter, quicker. I feel the finish line. Roddy is mine, he's toast. What kind of name is Roddy anyway? But a few points slip away, and now Roddy is raising his arms above his head, he's won the third set, 7–5, and the match. I look into the stands for my father, and he's staring down, concerned. Not angry—concerned. I'm concerned too, but damned angry also, sick with self-loathing. I wish I were the frozen ant in Mr. Parks's ring.

I'm saying hateful things to myself as I pack my tennis bag. Out of nowhere a boy appears and interrupts my rant.

Hey, he says, don't sweat it. You didn't play your best today.

I look up. The boy is slightly older than I, a head taller, wearing an expression that I don't like. There's something different about his face. His nose and mouth are out of alignment. And, the capper, he's wearing a fruity shirt with a little man *playing polo*? I want no part of him.

Who the fuck are you? I say.

Perry Rogers.

I turn back to my tennis bag.

He won't take a hint. He drones on about how I didn't have my best game, how much better I am than Roddy, how I'll beat Roddy the next time, blah, blah. He's trying to be nice, I guess, but he's coming off like a know-it-all, like some kind of Björn Borg Jr., so I stand and pointedly do an about-face. The last thing I need is a consolation speech, which is more pointless than a consolation trophy, especially from a kid with a man playing polo on his chest. Slinging my tennis bag over my shoulder I tell him: What the fuck do you know about tennis?

Later I feel bad. I shouldn't have been so harsh. Then I find out the kid is a tennis player, that he was competing in the same tournament. I also hear he's got a crush on my sister Tami, which is undoubtedly why he talked to me in the first place. Trying to get close to Tami.

But if I feel guilty, Perry is pissed. Word spreads along the Vegas teenager grapevine: Watch your back. Perry is gunning for you. He's telling everyone that you disrespected him, and the next time he sees you, he's going to kick your ass.

WEEKS LATER TAMI SAYS the whole gang is going to see a horror flick, all the older kids, and she asks if I want to go along.

That Perry kid going?

Maybe.

Yeah, I'll go.

I love horror movies. And I have a plan.

Our mother drives us to the theater early so we can buy popcorn and licorice and find the perfect seats, dead center, middle row. I always sit dead center, middle row. Best seats in the house. I put Tami to my left and save the seat to my right. Sure enough, here comes Preppy Perry. I jump to my feet and wave. Hey Perry! Over here!

He turns, squints. I can see he's caught off guard by my friendliness. He's trying to analyze the situation, weigh his response. Then he smiles, visibly releases whatever anger he's been holding. He saunters down the aisle and slides down our row, throwing himself into the seat next to me.

Hey Tami, he says across me.

Hey Perry.

Hey Andre.

Hey Perry.

Just as the lights go down and the first coming attraction starts we give each other a look.

Peace?

Peace.

The movie is *Visiting Hours*. It's about a psycho who stalks a lady journalist, sneaks into her house, kills her maid, then for some reason puts on lipstick and pops out when the lady journalist comes home. She fights free, and somehow gets to a hospital, where she thinks she's safe, but of course the psycho is hiding in the hospital, trying to find the lady journalist's room, killing everyone who gets in his way. Cheesy, but satisfyingly creepy.

When scared, I react like a cat thrown into a room full of dogs. I freeze, don't move a muscle. But Perry apparently is the high-strung type. As the suspense builds, he twitches and fidgets and spills soda on himself. Every time the killer jumps out of a closet, Perry jumps out of his seat. Several times I turn to Tami and roll my eyes. I don't tease Perry about his reaction, however. I don't even mention it when the lights come on. I don't want to break our fragile peace accord.

We roll out of the theater and decide the popcorn and Cokes and Twizzlers weren't enough. We head across the street to Winchell's and buy a box of French crullers. Perry gets his covered with chocolate. I get mine with rainbow sprinkles. We eat the donuts at the counter, talking. Perry sure can talk. He's like a lawyer before the Supreme Court. Then, in the middle of a fifteen-minute sentence, he stops and asks the guy behind the counter, Is this place open twenty-four hours?

Yup, the counter guy says.

Seven days a week?

Uh-huh.

Three hundred sixty-five days a year?

Yeah.

Then why are there *locks* on the front door?

We all turn and look. What a brilliant question! I start laughing so hard that I have to spit out my cruller. Rainbow sprinkles are falling from my mouth like confetti. This might be the funniest, smartest thing anyone's ever said. Certainly the funniest, smartest thing said by anyone in this particular Winchell's. Even the donut guy has to smile and admit: Kid, that's a head-scratcher.

Isn't life just like that? Perry says. Full of Winchell's locks and other stuff you can't explain?

You said it.

I always thought I was the only one who noticed. But here's a kid who not only notices, he points that stuff out. When my mother comes to pick up me and Tami, I'm sad to say goodbye to my new friend Perry. I even find myself less annoyed by his polo shirt.

I ASK MY FATHER if I can sleep over at Perry's house.

No fucking way, he says.

He doesn't know Perry's family from a hole in the ground. And he doesn't trust anyone he doesn't know. My father is suspicious of everyone in the world, especially the parents of our friends. I don't bother asking why, and I don't waste my breath arguing. I just invite Perry to our house for a sleepover.

Perry is extremely polite with my parents. He's agreeable with my siblings, especially Tami, though she's gently discouraged his crush. I ask if he wants a quick tour. Sure thing, he says, so I show him the room I share with Philly. He laughs at the white stripe down the middle. I show him the court out back. He takes a turn hitting with the dragon. I tell him how much I hate the dragon, how I used to think it was a living, breathing monster. He looks sympathetic. He's seen enough horror flicks to know that monsters come in all shapes and sizes.

Since Perry is a fellow connoisseur of horror, I've got a surprise for him. I've scored a beta copy of *The Exorcist*. After seeing him jump out of his skin at *Visiting Hours,* I can't wait to see how he reacts to a genuine horror classic. After everyone's asleep we slide the movie into the machine. I suffer a minor aneurysm with every rotation of Linda Blair's head, but Perry doesn't flinch once. *Visiting Hours* gives him the shakes, but *The Exorcist* leaves him cold? I think: This dude marches to his own drummer.

Afterward, we sit up drinking sodas and talking. Perry agrees that my father's scarier than anything Hollywood can offer, but he says his father is twice as scary. His father, he says, is an ogre, a tyrant, and a narcissist—the first time I've heard this word.

Perry says, Narcissist means he thinks only about himself. It also means his son is his personal property. He has a vision of how his son's life is going to be, and he couldn't care less about his son's vision of that future.

Sounds familiar.

Perry and I agree that life would be a million times better if our fathers were like other kids' fathers. But I hear an added note of pain in Perry's voice, because he says his father doesn't love him. I've never questioned my father's love. I just wish it were softer, with more listening and less rage. In fact, I sometimes wish my father loved me less. Maybe then he'd back off, let me make my own choices. I tell Perry that having no choice, having no say about what I do or who I am, makes me crazy. That's why I put more thought, obsessive thought, into the few choices I do have—what I wear, what I eat, who I call my friends.

He nods. He gets it.

At last, in Perry, I have a friend with whom I can share these deep thoughts, a friend I can tell about the Winchell's locks in my life. I talk to Perry about playing tennis, despite hating tennis. Hating school, despite enjoying books. Feeling lucky to have Philly, despite his streak of bad luck. Perry listens, patient as Philly, but more involved. Perry doesn't just talk, then listen, then nod. He converses. He analyzes, strategizes, spitballs, helps me come up with a plan to make things better. When I tell Perry my problems, they sound jumbled and asinine at first, but Perry has a way of rearranging them, making them sound logical, which feels like the first step to making them solvable. I feel as if I've been on a desert island, with no one to talk to but the palm trees, and now a thoughtful, sensitive, like-minded castaway—albeit with a stupid polo player on his shirt—has come stumbling ashore.

Perry confides in me about his nose and mouth. He says he was born with a cleft palate. He says it's made him deeply self-conscious and painfully shy with girls. He's had surgeries to fix it, and faces one more surgery at least. I tell him it's not that noticeable. He gets tears in his eyes. He mumbles something about his father blaming him.

Most conversations with Perry eventually lead to fathers, and from fathers it's a quick segue to the future. We talk about the men we're going to be once we're rid of our fathers. We promise each other that we'll be different, not just from our fathers but from all the men we know, even the ones we see in movies. We make a pact that we'll never do drugs or drink alcohol. And when we're rich, we vow, we'll do what we can to help the world. We shake on it. A secret handshake.

Perry has a long way to go to get rich. He never has a dime. Everything we do is my treat. I don't have much—a modest allowance, plus what I hustle from guests at the casinos and hotels. But I don't care; what's mine is Perry's, because I've decided that Perry is my new *best* friend. My father gives me five dollars every day for food, and I freely spend half on Perry.

We meet every afternoon at Cambridge. After goofing off, hitting a few balls around, we go for a snack. We slip out the back door, hop the wall, and race across the vacant lot to 7-Eleven, where we play video games and eat Chipwiches, paid for by me, until it's time to go home.

A Chipwich is a new ice cream sandwich Perry recently discovered. Vanilla ice cream pressed between two doughy chocolate chip cookies— it's the greatest food in the world, according to Perry, who's a raging addict. He loves Chipwiches more than talking. He can talk for an hour about the beauty of the Chipwich—and yet a Chipwich is one of the few things that can get him to stop talking. I buy him Chipwiches by the dozens, and I feel sorry for him that he doesn't have enough money to feed his habit.

We're at 7-Eleven one day when Perry stops chewing his Chipwich and looks up at the wall clock.

Shit, Andre, we better get back to Cambridge, my mother's coming early to get me.

Your mother?

Yeah. She said to be ready and waiting out front.

We haul ass across the vacant lot.

Uh-oh, Perry shouts, there she is!

I look up the street and see two cars cruising toward Cambridge—a Volkswagen bug and a convertible Rolls-Royce. I see the bug keep going past Cambridge, and I tell Perry to relax, we have time. She missed the turn.

No, Perry says, come on, come on.

He turns on the jets, sprinting after the Rolls.

Hey! What the—? Perry, are you kidding? Your mom drives a Rolls? Are you—*rich*?

I guess so.

Why didn't you tell me?

You never asked.

For me, that's the definition of being rich: it doesn't cross your mind to mention it to your best friend. And money is such a given you don't care how you come by it.

Perry, however, is more than rich. Perry is super-rich. Perry is Richie Rich. His father, a senior partner at a major law firm, owns a local TV station. He sells *air,* Perry says. Imagine. *Selling air.* When you can sell air, man, you've got it made. (Presumably his father gives him air for an allowance.)

My father finally lets me visit Perry's house, and I discover that he doesn't live in a house, in fact, but a mega-mansion. His mother drives us there in the Rolls, and my eyes get big as we pass slowly up a massive front drive, around green rolling hills, then under enormous shade trees. We stop outside a place that looks like Bruce Wayne's stately manor. One entire wing is set aside for Perry, including a teenager's dream room, featuring a ping-pong table, pool table, poker table, big-screen TV, mini fridge, and drum set. Down a long hallway lies Perry's bedroom, the walls of which are covered with dozens and dozens of *Sports Illustrated* covers.

My head rotating on a swivel, I look at all the portraits of great athletes and I can only say one word: Whoa.

Did this all myself, Perry says.

The next time I'm at the dentist I tear off the covers of all the *Sports Illustrated*s in the waiting room and stash them under my jacket. When I hand them to Perry, he shakes his head.

No, I have this one. And this one. I have them all, Andre. I have a subscription.

Oh. OK. Sorry.

It's not just that I've never met a rich kid. I've also never met a kid with a subscription.

IF WE'RE NOT HANGING OUT AT CAMBRIDGE, or at his mansion, Perry and I are talking on the phone. We're inseparable. He's crushed, therefore, when I tell him that I'm going away for a month, to play a series of tournaments in Australia. McDonald's is putting together a team of America's elite juniors, sending us to play Australia's best.

A whole month?

I know. But I have no choice. My father.

I'm not being entirely truthful. I'm one of only two twelve-year-olds selected, so I'm honored, excited, if slightly on edge about traveling so far from home—the plane ride is fourteen hours. For Perry's sake I downplay the trip. I tell him not to worry, I'll be back in no time, and we'll have a Chipwich feast.

I fly alone to Los Angeles, and upon landing I want to go straight back to Vegas. I'm scared. I'm not sure where I'm supposed to go or how to find my way through the airport. I feel as if I stick out in my warm-up suit with the McDonald's Golden Arches on the back and my name on the chest. Now, off in the distance I see a group of kids wearing the same warm-up suit. My team. I approach the one adult in the group and introduce myself.

He flashes a big smile. He's the coach. My first real coach.

Agassi, he says. The hotshot from Vegas? Hey, glad to have you aboard!

During the flight to Australia, Coach stands in the aisle, telling us how the trip is going to work. We're going to play five tournaments in five different cities. The most important tournament, however, will be the third, in Sydney. That's where we'll pit our best against the best Australians.

There should be five thousand fans in the arena, he says, plus it's going to be televised throughout Australia.

Talk about pressure.

But here's the good news, Coach says. Every time you win a tournament, I'll let you have one cold beer.

I win my first tournament, in Adelaide, no problem, and on the bus Coach hands me an ice-cold Foster's Lager. I think of Perry and our pact. I think of how strange it is that I'm twelve and being served booze. But the beer can looks so frosty cold, and my teammates are watching. Also, I'm thousands of miles from home—fuck it. I take a sip. Delicious. I drain it in four gulps, then wrestle with my guilty conscience the rest of the afternoon. I stare out the window as the outback crawls by and I wonder how Perry will take the news, if he'll stop being my friend.

I win three of the next four tournaments. Three more beers. Each more delicious than the last. But with every sip, I taste the bitter dregs of guilt.

PERRY AND I FALL right back into our old routine. Horror movies. Long talks. Cambridge. 7-Eleven. Chipwiches. Every now and then, however, I look at him and feel the weight of my betrayal.

We're walking from Cambridge to 7-Eleven and I can't hold it in any longer. The guilt is eating away at me. We're each wearing headphones plugged into Perry's Walkman, listening to Prince. *Purple Rain.* I tap Perry on the shoulder and tell him to take off his headphones.

What's up?

I don't know how to say this.

He stares.

What is it?

Perry. I broke our pact.

No.

I had a beer in Australia.

Just one?

Four.

Four!

I look down.

He thinks. He stares off at the mountains. Well, he says, we make choices in life, Andre, and you've made yours. I guess that leaves me on my own.

But a few minutes later, he's curious. He asks how the beers tasted, and again I can't lie. I tell him they were great. I apologize again, but there's no point in pretending to be remorseful. Perry's right—I had a choice, for once, and I made it. Sure, I wish I hadn't broken our pact, but I can't feel bad about finally exercising free will.

Perry frowns like a father. Not like my father, or his father, but like a TV father. He looks as if he should be wearing a cardigan sweater and smoking a pipe. I realize that the pact Perry and I made, at its root, was a promise to become each other's fathers. To raise each other. I apologize once more, and I realize how much I missed Perry while I was gone. I make another pact, with myself, that I won't leave home again.

MY FATHER ACCOSTS ME IN THE KITCHEN. He says we need to talk. I wonder if he heard about the beer.

He tells me to sit at the table. He sits across from me. An unfinished Norman Rockwell separates us. He describes a story he caught recently on *60 Minutes*. It was all about a tennis boarding school on the west coast of Florida, near Tampa Bay. The first school of its kind, my father says. A boot camp for young tennis players, it's run by a former paratrooper named Nick Bollettieri.

So?

So—you're going there.

What!

You're not getting any better here in Las Vegas. You've beaten all the local boys. You've beaten all the boys in the West. *Andre, you've beaten all the players at the local college!* I have nothing left to teach you.

My father doesn't say the words, but it's obvious: he's determined to do things differently with me. He doesn't want to repeat the mistakes he made with my siblings. He ruined their games by holding on too long, too tight, and in the process he ruined his relationship with them. Things got so bad with Rita that she's recently run off with Pancho Gonzalez, the tennis legend, who's at least thirty years her senior. My father doesn't want to limit me, or break me, or ruin me. So he's banishing me. He's sending me away, partly to protect me from himself.

Andre, he says, you've got to eat, sleep, and drink tennis. It's the only way you're going to be number one.

I already eat, sleep, and drink tennis.

But he wants me to do my eating, sleeping, and drinking elsewhere.

How much does this tennis academy cost?

About $12,000 a year.

We can't afford that.

You're only going for three months. That's $3,000.

We can't afford that either.

It's an investment. In you. We'll find a way.

I don't want to go.

I can see from my father's face it's settled. End of story.

I try to look on the bright side. It's only three months. I can take anything for three months. Also, how bad could it be? Maybe it will be like Australia. Maybe it will be fun. Maybe there will be unforeseen benefits. Maybe it will feel like playing for a team.

What about school? I ask. I'm in the middle of seventh grade.

There's a school in the next town, my father says. You'll go in the morning, for half a day, then play tennis all afternoon and into the night.

Sounds grueling. A short time later my mother tells me that the *60 Minutes* report was actually an exposé on this Bollettieri character, who was in essence running a tennis sweatshop that employed child labor.

THEY GIVE A GOODBYE PARTY for me at Cambridge. Mr. Fong looks glum, Perry looks suicidal, my father looks uncertain. We stand around eating cake. We play tennis with the balloons, then pop them with pins. Everyone pats me on the back and says what a blast I'm going to have.

I know, I say. Can't wait to mix it up with those Florida kids.

The lie sounds like a deliberate miss, like a ball off the wooden rim of my racket.

As the day of my departure draws closer, I don't sleep well. I wake up thrashing, sweating, twisted up in the sheets. I can't eat. All at once the concept of homesickness makes perfect sense. I don't want to leave my home, my siblings, my mother, my best friend. Despite the tension of my home, the occasional terror, I'd give anything to stay. For all the pain my father has caused me, the one constant has been his presence. He's always been there, at my back, and now he won't be. I feel abandoned. I thought the one thing I wanted was to be free of him, and now that he's sending me away, I'm heartbroken.

I spend my last days at home hoping that my mother will come to my rescue. I look at her imploringly, but she looks back with a face that says: I've seen him break three kids. You're lucky to be getting out while you're whole.

My father drives me to the airport. My mother wants to go but can't miss a day of work. Perry takes her place. He doesn't stop talking the whole way. I can't decide if he's trying to cheer me up or himself. It's only three months, he says. We'll write letters, postcards. You'll see, it's going to be fine. You're going to learn so much. Maybe I'll even come visit.

I think about *Visiting Hours,* the cheesy horror movie we saw the night our friendship was born. Perry is acting now the way he acted then, the way he always reacts to fear—twitching, jumping out of his seat. And I'm reacting in my typical way. A cat thrown into a room full of dogs.

5

THE AIRPORT SHUTTLE pulls into the compound just after sunset. The Nick Bollettieri Tennis Academy, built on an old tomato farm, is nothing fancy, just a few outbuildings that look like cell blocks. They're named like cell blocks too: B Building, C Building. I look around, half expecting to find a guard tower and razor wire. More ominously, stretching off into the distance I see row after row of tennis courts.

As the sun sinks beyond the inky black marshes, the temperature plummets. I huddle into my T-shirt. I thought Florida was supposed to be hot. A staff member greets me as I step out of the van and marches me straight to my barracks, which are empty and eerily quiet.

Where is everyone?

Study hall, he says. In a few minutes it'll be free hour. That's the hour between study hall and bedtime. Why don't you go down to the rec center and introduce yourself to the others?

In the rec center I find two hundred wild boys, plus a few tough-looking girls, separated into tight cliques. One of the largest cliques is pressed around a Nerf ping-pong table, screaming insults at two boys playing. I press my back against a wall and scan the room. I recognize a few faces, including one or two from the Australia trip. That kid over there—I played him in California. That evil-looking homey right there— I played a tough three-setter against him in Arizona. Everyone looks talented, supremely confident. The kids are all colors, all sizes, all ages, and from all around the world. The youngest is seven, the oldest nineteen. After ruling Las Vegas my whole life, I'm now a tiny fish in a vast pond. Or marsh. And the biggest of the big fish are the best players in the country—teenage Supermen who form the tightest clique in a far corner.

I try to watch the ping-pong game. Even there I'm outclassed. Back home, nobody could beat me at Nerf ping-pong. Here? Half these guys would cream me.

I can't imagine how I'll ever fit in at this joint, how I'll make friends. I want to go home, right now, or at least phone home, but I'd have to call collect and I know my father wouldn't accept the charges. Just knowing I can't hear my mother's voice, or Philly's, no matter how much I need to, makes me feel panicky. When free hour ends I hurry back to the barracks and lie on my bunk, waiting to disappear into the black marsh of sleep.

Three months, I tell myself. Just three months.

PEOPLE LIKE TO CALL the Bollettieri Academy a boot camp, but it's really a glorified prison camp. And not all that glorified. We eat gruel—beige meats and gelatinous stews and gray slop poured over rice—and sleep in rickety bunks that line the plywood walls of our military-style barracks. We rise at dawn and go to bed soon after dinner. We rarely leave, and we have scant contact with the outside world. Like most prisoners we do nothing but sleep and work, and our main rock pile is drills. Serve drills, net drills, backhand drills, forehand drills, with occasional match play to establish the pecking order, strong to weak. Sometimes it feels as though we're gladiators, preparing underneath the Colosseum. Certainly the thirty-five instructors who bark at us during drills think of themselves as slave drivers.

When we're not drilling, we're studying the psychology of tennis. We take classes on mental toughness, positive thinking, and visualization. We're taught to close our eyes and picture ourselves winning Wimbledon, hoisting that gold trophy above our heads. Then we go to aerobics, or weight training, or out to the crushed-shell track, where we run until we drop.

The constant pressure, the cutthroat competition, the total lack of adult supervision—it slowly turns us into animals. A kind of jungle law prevails. It's *Karate Kid* with rackets, *Lord of the Flies* with forehands. One night two boys get into an argument in the barracks. A white boy and an Asian boy. The white boy uses a racial slur, then walks out. For a full hour the Asian boy stands in the middle of the barracks, stretching, shaking out his legs and arms, rolling his neck. He runs through a progression of judo moves, then carefully, methodically tapes his ankles. When the white boy returns, the Asian boy spins, whipsaws his leg through the air, and unleashes a kick that shatters the white boy's jaw.

The shocking part is that neither boy gets expelled, which greatly adds to the overall sense of anarchy.

Another two boys have a low-grade, long-running feud. It's mostly taunts, teases, minor stuff—until one boy ups the ante. For days he urinates and defecates into a bucket. Then, late one night, he bursts into the other boy's barracks and dumps the bucket on his head.

The jungle feeling, the constant threat of violence and ambush, is reinforced, just before lights out, by the sound of drums in the distance.

I ask one of the boys: What the hell is that?

Oh. That's just Courier. He likes to pound a drum set his parents sent him.

Who?

Jim Courier. From Florida.

Within days I get my first glimpse of the warden, founder, and owner of the Nick Bollettieri Tennis Academy. He's fiftysomething, but looks 250, because tanning is one of his obsessions, along with tennis and getting married. (He's got five or six ex-wives, no one is quite sure.) He's soaked up so much sun, baked himself so deeply beneath so many ultraviolet sunlamps, he's permanently altered his pigmentation. The one portion of his face that isn't the color of beef jerky is his mustache, a black, meticulously trimmed quasi-goatee, only without the chin hair, so it looks like a permanent frown. I see Nick striding across the compound, an angry red man in wraparound shades, berating someone who jogs alongside, trying to keep pace, and I pray that I never have to deal with Nick directly. I watch as he slides into a red Ferrari and zooms away, leaving a dorsal fin of dust in his wake.

A boy tells me it's our job to keep Nick's four sports cars washed and polished.

Our job? That's bullshit.

Tell it to the judge.

I ask some of the older boys, some of the veterans, about Nick. Who is he? What makes him tick? They say he's a hustler, a guy who makes a very nice living off tennis, but he doesn't love the game or even know it all that well. He's not like my father, captivated by the angles and numbers and beauty of tennis. Then again, he's just like my father. He's captivated by cash. He's a guy who flunked the exam for Navy pilots, dropped out of law school, then landed one day on the idea of teaching tennis. Stepped in shit. Through a bit of hard work, and a ton of luck, he's turned himself into this image of a tennis titan, mentor to prodigies. You can learn a few things from him, the other kids say, but he's no miracle worker.

He doesn't sound like a guy who can make me stop hating the game.

. . .

I'm PLAYING A PRACTICE MATCH, putting a fairly good whooping on a kid from the East Coast, when I become aware that Gabriel, one of Nick's henchmen, is behind me, staring.

After a few more points Gabriel stops the match. He asks, Has Nick seen you play yet?

No, sir.

He frowns, walks off.

Later, over the loudspeaker that carries across all the courts of the Bollettieri Academy, I hear:

Andre Agassi to the indoor supreme court! Andre Agassi, report to the indoor supreme court—immediately!

I've never been to the indoor supreme court, and I can't imagine there's a good reason for my being summoned now. I run there and find Gabriel and Nick, standing shoulder to shoulder, waiting.

Gabriel says to Nick: You've got to see this kid hit.

Nick strolls off into the shadows. Gabriel gets on the other side of the net. He puts me through drills for half an hour. I sneak occasional glances over my shoulder: I can vaguely make out the silhouette of Nick, concentrating, stroking his mustache.

Hit some backhands, Nick says. His voice is like sandpaper on Velcro.

I do as I'm told. I hit backhands.

Now hit some serves.

I serve.

Come to the net.

I come to the net.

That's enough.

He steps forward. Where are you from?

Las Vegas.

What's your national ranking?

Number three.

How do I reach your father?

He's at work. He works nights at the MGM.

How about your mother?

At this hour? She's probably at home.

Come with me.

We walk slowly to his office, where he asks for my home number. He's sitting in a tall black leather chair, turned almost away from me. My face feels redder than his face looks. He dials and speaks to my mother. She gives him my father's number. He dials again.

He's yelling. Mr. Agassi! Nick Bollettieri here! Right, right. Yes, well, listen to me. I'm going to tell you something *very* important. Your boy has more talent than anybody I've ever seen come through this academy. That's right. Ever. And I'm going to take him to the top.

What the hell is he talking about? I'm only here for three months. I'm leaving here in sixty-four days. Is Nick saying he wants me to *stay* here? Live here—forever? Surely my father won't go for that.

Nick says: That's right. No, that's no issue. I'm going to make it so you won't pay a penny. Andre can stay, free of charge. I'm tearing up your check.

My heart sinks. I know my father can't resist anything free. My fate is sealed.

Nick hangs up and spins toward me in his chair. He doesn't explain. He doesn't console. He doesn't ask if this is what I want. He doesn't say a thing besides: Go back out to the courts.

The warden has tacked several years to my sentence, and there's nothing to be done but pick up my hammer and return to the rock pile.

EVERY DAY AT THE BOLLETTIERI ACADEMY starts with the stench. The surrounding hills are home to several orange-processing plants, which give off a toxic smell of burned orange peels. It's the first thing that hits me when I open my eyes, a reminder that this is real, I'm not back in Vegas, I'm not in my deuce-court bed, dreaming. I've never cared much for orange juice, but after the Bollettieri Academy I'll never be able to look at a gallon of Minute Maid again.

As the sun clears the marshes, burning off the morning mist, I hurry to beat the other boys into the shower, because only the first boys get hot water. Actually, it's not a shower, just a tiny nozzle that shoots a narrow jet of painful needles, which hardly gets you wet, let alone clean. Then we all rush to breakfast, served in a cafeteria so chaotic, it's like a mental hospital where the nurses forgot to hand out the meds. But you'd better get there early or it might be worse. The butter will be filled with everyone else's crumbs, the bread will be gone, the plastic eggs will be ice.

Straight from breakfast we board a bus for school, Bradenton Academy, twenty-six minutes away. I divide my time between two academies, both prisons, but Bradenton Academy makes me more claustrophobic, because it makes less sense. At the Bollettieri Academy, at least I'm learning something about tennis. At Bradenton Academy, the only thing I learn is that I'm stupid.

Bradenton Academy has warped floors, dirty carpets, and a color scheme that's fourteen shades of gray. There isn't one window in the building, so the light is fluorescent and the air is stale, filled with a medley of foul odors, chiefly vomit, toilet, and fear. It's almost worse than the scorched-orange smell back at the Bollettieri Academy.

Other kids, non-tennis kids from town, don't seem to mind. Some actually thrive at Bradenton Academy, maybe because their life schedules are manageable. They don't balance school with careers as semipro athletes. They don't contend with waves of homesickness that rise and fall like nausea. They spend seven hours a day in class, then go home to eat dinner and watch TV with their families. Those of us who commute from the Bollettieri Academy, however, spend four and a half hours in class, then board the bus for the long slog back to our full-time jobs, hitting balls until after dusk, at which time we collapse in heaps on our wooden bunks, to grab a half hour of rest before returning to the original state of nature that is the rec center. Then we nod over our textbooks for a few futile hours before free hour and lights out. We're always behind on schoolwork and falling ever further behind. The system is rigged, guaranteed to produce bad students as quickly and efficiently as it produces good tennis players.

I don't like anything that's rigged, so I don't give much effort. I don't study. I don't do homework. I don't pay attention. And I don't give a damn. In every class I sit quietly at my desk, staring at my feet, wishing I were somewhere else, while the teacher drones on about Shakespeare or Bunker Hill or the Pythagorean theorem.

The teachers don't care that I've tuned them out, because I'm one of Nick's Boys, and they don't want to cross Nick. Bradenton Academy exists because the Bollettieri Academy keeps sending it a bus full of paying customers every semester. The teachers know that their jobs depend on Nick, so they can't flunk us, and we cherish our special status. We feel a lordly sense of entitlement, never realizing that the thing to which we're most entitled is the thing we're not getting—an education.

Inside the metal front doors of Bradenton Academy stands the office, the nerve center of the school and the source of much pain. Report cards and threatening letters emanate from the office. Bad boys are sent there. The office is also the lair of Mrs. G and Doc G, married coprincipals of Bradenton Academy, and, I suspect, frustrated sideshow performers.

Mrs. G is a gangly woman with no midsection. She looks as if her shoulders have been set directly on her hips. She tries to disguise this odd shape by wearing skirts, but this only accentuates the problem. On her face she wears two gobs of blush and one smear of lipstick, a symmetrical triad of three circles that she color-coordinates the way other people do their shoes and belt. Her cheeks and mouth always match, and always *almost* distract you from the hump in her back. Nothing Mrs. G wears, however, can distract you from her gargantuan hands. She has mitts the size of rackets, and the first time she shakes my hand I think I might faint.

Old Doc G is half her size but has just as many body issues. It's not hard to see what they first found in common. Frail, gamy, Doc G has a right arm that's been shriveled since birth. He ought to hide this arm, keep it behind his back or shoved in a pocket. Instead he waves it around, brandishes it like a weapon. He likes to take students aside for one-on-one chats, and whenever he does so, he swings his bad arm up onto the student's shoulder, setting it there until he's said his piece. If this doesn't give you the heebie-jeebies, nothing will. Doc G's arm feels like a pork tenderloin lying on your shoulder, and hours later you can still feel it there and you can't help but shiver.

Mrs. G and Doc G have instituted dozens of rules at Bradenton Academy, and one of the most strictly enforced is their ban on jewelry. Thus, I go out of my way to pierce my ears. It's an easy show of rebellion, which, as I see it, is my last resort. Rebellion is the one thing I get to choose every day, and this rebellion comes with the added bonus that it represents a neat little fuck-you to my father, who's always hated earrings on men. Many times I've heard my father say that earrings equal homosexuality. I can't wait for him to see mine. (I buy both studs and dangly hoops.) He'll finally regret sending me thousands of miles from home and leaving me here to be corrupted.

I make a feeble and insincere effort to hide my new accessory, wrapping a Band-Aid around it. Mrs. G notices, of course, just as I hoped she would. She pulls me out of class and confronts me.

Mr. Agassi, what is the meaning of that bandage?

I hurt my ear.

Hurt your—? Don't be ridiculous. Remove that Band-Aid.

I pull off the Band-Aid. She sees the stud and gasps.

We do not allow earrings at Bradenton Academy, Mr. Agassi. The next time I see you, I will expect the Band-Aid gone and the earring out.

By the end of the first semester I'm close to failing all my classes. Except English. I show a strange aptitude for literature, especially poetry.

Memorizing famous poems, writing original poems, it comes easily to me. We're assigned to write a short verse about our daily lives and I set mine proudly on the teacher's desk. She likes it. She reads it aloud in class. Some of the other kids later ask me to ghostwrite their homework. I dash off their assignments on the bus, no problem. The English teacher detains me after class and says I have real talent. I smile. It's different from being told by Nick that I have talent. This feels like something I'd like to pursue. For a moment I imagine what it would be like to do something besides playing tennis—something I choose. Then I go to my next class, math, and the dream dies in a cloud of algebra formulae. I'm not cut out to be a scholar. The math teacher's voice sounds as if it's coming from miles away. The next class, French, is worse. I'm *très stupide*. I transfer to Spanish, where I'm *muy estúpido*. Spanish, I think, might actually shorten my life. The boredom, the confusion, might cause me to expire in my chair. They will find me one day in my seat, *muerto*.

Gradually school goes from being hard to being physically harmful. The anxiety of boarding the bus, the twenty-six-minute ride, the inevitable confrontation with Mrs. G or Doc G, actually make me ill. What I dread most is the moment, the daily moment, when I'm exposed as a loser. An academic loser. So great is this dread that over time Bradenton Academy modifies my view of the Bollettieri Academy. I *look forward* to all those drills, and even the high-pressure tournaments, because at least I'm not at school.

Thanks to one particularly big tournament, I miss a major history test at Bradenton Academy, a test I was sure to fail. I celebrate this dodging of a bullet by eviscerating my opponents. But when I return to school my teacher says I have to take a makeup.

The injustice. I skulk down to the office for the makeup test. Along the way I duck into a dark corner and prepare a cheat sheet, which I stash in my pocket.

There is only one other student in the office, a red-haired girl with a fat, sweaty face. She doesn't blink, doesn't register my presence in any way. She seems to be in a coma. I fill out the test, fast, copying from my cheat sheet. Suddenly I feel a pair of eyes on me. I look up, and the red-haired girl is out of her coma, staring. She closes her book and strolls out. Quickly I shove the cheat sheet into the crotch of my underwear. I tear another sheet of paper from my notebook and, imitating a girlish handwriting, I write: *I think you're cute! Give me a call!* I shove the paper in my front pocket just as Mrs. G storms in.

Pencil down, she says.

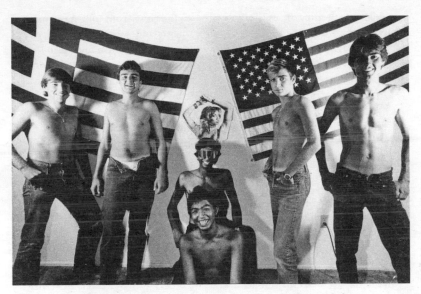

Soon after arriving at the Bollettieri Academy, I start to rebel.

What's up, Mrs. G?

Are you cheating?

On what? *This?* If I were going to cheat on something it wouldn't be this. I've got this history stuff down cold. Valley Forge. Paul Revere. Piece of cake.

Empty your pockets.

I lay out a few coins, a pack of gum, the note from my imaginary admirer. Mrs. G picks up the note and reads under her breath.

I say, I'm thinking about what I should write back. Any ideas?

She scowls, walks out. I pass the test and chalk it up as a moral victory.

MY ENGLISH TEACHER is my only advocate. She's also the daughter of Mrs. G and Doc G, so she pleads with her parents that I'm smarter than my grades and my behavior indicate. She even arranges an IQ test and the results confirm her opinion.

Andre, she says, you need to apply yourself. Prove to Mrs. G that you're not who she thinks you are.

I tell her that I *am* applying myself, that I'm doing as well as I can under the circumstances. But I'm tired all the time from playing tennis, and distracted by the pressure of tournaments and so-called challenges. Especially the challenges: once a month we play someone above us in the pecking order. I'd like any teacher to explain how you're supposed to concentrate on conjugating verbs or solving for x when you're steeling yourself for a five-set brawl with some punk from Orlando that afternoon.

I don't tell her everything, because I can't. I'd feel like a sissy talking about my fear of school, the countless times I sit in class drenched in sweat. I can't tell her about my trouble concentrating, my horror of being called on, how this horror sometimes morphs into an air bubble in my lower intestine, which grows and grows until I need to run to the bathroom. Between classes I'm often locked in a toilet stall.

Then there's the social anxiety, the doomed effort to fit in. At Bradenton Academy, fitting in takes money. Most of the kids are fashion plates, whereas I have three pairs of jeans, five T-shirts, two pairs of tennis shoes—and one cotton crewneck with gray and black squares. In class, rather than thinking about *The Scarlet Letter,* I'm thinking about how many days per week I can get away with wearing my sweater, worrying about what I'll do when the weather gets warm.

The worse I do in school, the more I rebel. I drink, I smoke pot, I act like an ass. I'm dimly aware of the inverse ratio between my grades and my rebellion, but I don't dwell on it. I prefer Nick's theory. He says I don't do well in school because I have a hard-on for the world. It might be the only thing he's ever said about me that's halfway accurate. (He typically describes me as a cocky showboater who seeks the limelight. Even my father knows me better than that.) My general demeanor does feel like a hard-on—violent, involuntary, unstoppable—and so I accept it as I accept the many changes in my body.

Finally, when my grades hit bottom, my rebellion reaches the breaking point. I walk into a hair salon in the Bradenton Mall and tell the stylist to give me a mohawk. Razor the sides, shave them to the scalp, and leave just one thick strip of spiked hair down the middle.

Are you sure, kid?

I want it high, and I want it spiky. Then dye it pink.

He works his shearer back and forth for eight minutes. Then he says, All done, and spins me around in the chair. I look in the mirror. The earring was good, this is better. I can't wait to see the look on Mrs. G's face.

Outside the mall, while I wait for the bus back to the Bollettieri Academy, no one recognizes me. Kids I play with, kids I bunk with, they look right past me. To the casual observer I've done something that seems like a desperate effort to stand out. But in fact I've rendered myself, my inner self, my true self, invisible. At least, that was the idea.

I FLY HOME FOR CHRISTMAS, and as the plane approaches the Strip, as the casinos below the canting right wing twinkle like a row of Christmas trees, the flight attendant says we're stuck in a holding pattern.

Groans.

Since we know you're all itching to hit the casinos, she says, we thought it might be fun to do a little gambling till we're clear to land.

Cheers.

Let's everybody take out a dollar and put it in this airsick bag. Then write your seat number on your ticket stub and throw it in this other airsick bag. We'll pull out one ticket stub, and that person will win the jackpot!

She collects everyone's dollar while another flight attendant collects the ticket stubs. Now she stands at the head of the plane and reaches in the bag.

And the grand prize goes to, drumroll please, 9F!

I'm 9F. I won! I won! I stand and wave. The passengers turn and see me. More groans. Great, the kid with the pink mohawk won.

The flight attendant reluctantly hands me the airsick bag full of ninety-six ones. I spend the rest of the flight counting and recounting them, thanking my lucky stars for this horseshoe up my ass.

My father, as expected, is horrified by my hair and earring. But he refuses to blame himself or the Bollettieri Academy. He won't admit that sending me away was a mistake, and he won't stand for any talk of my coming home. He simply asks if I'm a faggot.

No, I say, then go to my room.

Philly follows. He compliments my new look. Even a mohawk beats bald. I tell him about my windfall on the airplane.

Whoa! What are you going to do with all that cash?

I'm thinking about spending it on an ankle bracelet for Jamie. She's a girl who goes to school with Perry. She let me kiss her the last time I was home. But I don't know—I desperately need new clothes for school. I can't make it much farther with one gray-black sweater. I want to fit in.

Philly nods. Tough call, bro.

He doesn't ask why, if I want to fit in, I got a mohawk and an earring.

He treats my dilemma as serious, my contradictions as coherent, and helps me work through the options. We decide that I should spend the money on the girlfriend, forget about the new clothes.

The moment I have the anklet in my hands, however, I'm filled with regret. I picture myself back in Florida, rotating my few articles of clothing. I tell Philly, and he gives a half nod.

In the morning I open one eye and find Philly hovering over me, grinning. He's staring at my chest. I look down and find a stack of bills.

What's this?

Went out and played cards last night, bro. Hit a lucky streak. Won $600.

So—what's this?

Three hundred bucks. Go buy yourself some sweaters.

DURING SPRING BREAK my father wants me to play semipro tournaments, called satellites, which are open qualification, meaning anyone can show up and play at least one match. They're held in out-of-the-way towns, *way* out of the way, burgs like Monroe, Louisiana, and St. Joe, Missouri. I can't travel by myself; I'm just fourteen. So my father sends Philly along to chaperone me. Also, to play. Philly and my father still cling to the belief that he can do something with his tennis.

Philly rents a beige Omni, which quickly becomes a mobile version of our bedroom back home. One side his, one side mine. We log thousands of miles, stopping only for fast-food joints, tournament sites, and sleep. Our lodging is free, because in every town we stay with strangers, local families who volunteer to host players. Most of the hosts are pleasant enough, but they're overly enthusiastic about the game. It's awkward enough to stay with strangers, but it's a chore to make tennis talk over pancakes and coffee. For me, that is. Philly will talk to anyone, and I often have to nudge and pull him when it's time to go.

Philly and I both feel like outlaws, living on the road, doing whatever we please. We throw fast-food wrappers over our shoulders into the backseat. We listen to loud music, curse all we want, say whatever is on our minds, without fear of being corrected or ridiculed. Still, we never mention our very different goals for this trip. Philly wants only to earn one ATP point, just one, so he can know what it feels like to be ranked. I want only to avoid playing Philly, in which case I'll have to beat my beloved brother again.

At the first satellite I rout my opponent and Philly gets routed by his.

Afterward, in the rental car, in the parking garage beside the stadium, Philly stares at the steering wheel, looking stunned. For some reason this loss hurt more than the others. He balls his fist and punches the steering wheel. Hard. Then punches it again. He begins talking to himself, so low that I can't hear. Now he's talking louder. Now he's shouting, calling himself a born loser, hitting the steering wheel again and again. He's hammering the wheel so hard that I'm sure he's going to break a bone in his hand. I think of our father, shadowboxing the steering wheel after knocking out the trucker.

Philly says, It would be better if I broke my fucking fist! At least then it would all be over! Dad was right. I *am* a born loser.

All at once he stops. He looks at me and becomes resigned. Calm. Like our mother. He smiles; the storm has passed, the poison is gone.

I feel better, he says with a laugh and a snuffle.

Driving out of the parking garage, he gives me pointers on my next opponent.

DAYS AFTER I RETURN to the Bollettieri Academy, I'm at the Bradenton Mall. I take a chance and place a collect call home. Pfew: Philly answers. He sounds the way he did in the parking garage.

So, he says. We got a letter from the ATP.

Yeah?

You want to know your ranking?

I don't know—do I?

You're number 610.

Really?

Six-ten in the world, bro.

Which means there are only 609 people better than me in the entire world. On planet earth, in the solar system, I'm number 610. I slap the wall of the phone booth and shout for joy.

The line is silent. Then, in a kind of whisper, Philly asks, How does it feel?

I can't believe how thoughtless I've been, shouting in Philly's ear when he must feel bitterly disappointed. I wish I could throw half of my ATP points on his chest. In a tone of supreme boredom, stifling a pretend yawn, I tell him: You know what? It's no big deal. It's overrated.

6

WHAT MORE CAN I DO? Nick, Gabriel, Mrs. G, Doc G—no one seems to notice my antics anymore. I've mutilated my hair, grown my nails, including one pinky nail that's two inches long and painted fire-engine red. I've pierced my body, broken rules, busted curfew, picked fistfights, thrown tantrums, cut classes, even slipped into the girls' barracks after hours. I've consumed gallons of whiskey, often while sitting brazenly atop my bunk, and as an extra dash of audacity I've built a pyramid from my dead soldiers. A three-foot tower of empty Jack Daniel's bottles. I chew tobacco, hardcore weed like Skoal and Kodiak, soaked in whiskey. After losses I stick a plum-sized wad of chew inside my cheek. The bigger the loss, the bigger the wad. What rebellion is left? What new sin can I commit to show the world I'm unhappy and want to go home?

Each week, the only time I'm not plotting rebellion is free hour, when I can goof off in the rec center, or Saturday night, when I can go to the Bradenton Mall and flirt with girls. That adds up to ten hours per week that I'm happy, or at least not wracking my brain to think up some new form of civil disobedience.

When I'm still fourteen the Bollettieri Academy hires a bus and ships us upstate to a major tournament in Pensacola. The Bollettieri Academy travels several times each year to tournaments like this one, throughout Florida, because Nick thinks they're good tests. Measuring sticks, he calls them. Florida is tennis heaven, Nick says, and if we're better than Florida's best, then we must be tops in the world.

I have no trouble reaching the final in my bracket, but the other kids don't fare as well. They all get knocked out early. Thus they're all forced to gather and watch my match. They have no choice, nowhere else to go. When I'm done, we'll get back on the bus, en masse, and drive the twelve hours home to the Bollettieri Academy.

Take your time, the kids joke.

No one is eager to spend twelve more hours on that slow stinky bus.

For laughs, I decide to play the match in jeans. Not tennis shorts, not warm-up pants, but torn, faded, dirty dungarees. I know it won't affect the outcome. The kid I'm playing is a chump. I can beat him with one hand tied behind my back, wearing a gorilla costume. For good measure I pencil on some eyeliner and put in my gaudiest earrings.

I win the match in straight sets. The other kids cheer wildly. They award me bonus points for style. On the ride back to the Bollettieri Academy I get extra attention, slaps on the back and attaboys. I feel at last as though I'm fitting in, becoming one of the cool kids, one of the alphas. Plus I got the W.

The next day, right after lunch, Nick calls a surprise meeting.

Everyone gather around, he bellows.

He directs us to a back court with bleachers. When all two hundred full-time kids are settled in and quiet he starts pacing before us, talking about what the Bollettieri Academy means, how we should feel privileged to be here. He built this place from nothing, he says, and he's proud to have it bear his name. The Bollettieri Academy stands for excellence. The Bollettieri Academy stands for class. The Bollettieri Academy is known and respected the world over.

He pauses.

Andre, would you stand up for a minute?

I stand.

All that I've just said about this place, Andre, you have vi-o-lated. You have *defiled* this place, shamed it with your little stunt yesterday. Wearing jeans and makeup and earrings during your final? Boy, I'm going to tell you something very important: If you're going to act like that, if you're going to dress like a girl, then here's what I'm going to do. In your next tournament I'm going to have you wear a skirt. I've contacted Ellesse, and I've asked them to send a bunch of skirts for you, and you will wear one, yes sirree, because if that's who you are, then that is how we're going to treat you.

All two hundred kids are looking at me. Four hundred eyes, fixed tight on me. Many of the kids are laughing.

Nick keeps going. Your free time, he says, is hereby revoked. Your free time is now my time. You're on detail, Mr. Agassi. Between nine and ten you'll clean every bathroom on the property. When the toilets are scrubbed, you'll police the grounds. If you don't like it, well, it's simple.

Leave. If you're going to act like you did yesterday, we don't want you here. If you're incapable of showing that you care about this place as much as we do, *buh-bye.*

This last word, *buh-bye,* rings out, echoes across the empty courts.

That's it, he says. Everyone get back to work.

All the kids scurry away. I stand stock still, trying to decide what to do. I could curse out Nick. I could threaten to fight him. I could start bawling. I think of Philly, then Perry. What would they have me do? I think of my father, sent to school in girl clothes when his mother wanted to humiliate him. The day he became a fighter.

There is no more time to decide. Gabriel says my punishment begins right now. For the rest of the afternoon, he says—on your knees. Weed.

AT DUSK, relieved of my weed sack, I walk to my room. No more indecision. I know exactly what I'm going to do. I throw my clothes in a suitcase and start for the highway. The thought crosses my mind that this is Florida, any maniac halfwit could pick me up and I'd never be heard from again. But I'd be better off with a maniac halfwit than with Nick.

In my wallet I have one credit card, which my father gave me for emergencies, and I'm thinking this is a bona fide Code Red. I'm headed for the airport. By this time tomorrow I'll be sitting in Perry's bedroom, telling him the story.

I keep my eyes peeled for searchlights. I listen for the yelps of distant bloodhounds. I stick out my thumb.

A car pulls up. I open the door, wind up to toss my suitcase in the backseat. It's Julio, the disciplinarian on Nick's staff. He says my father is on the phone back at the Bollettieri Academy and wants to speak to me—now.

I'd prefer the bloodhounds.

I TELL MY FATHER that I want to come home. I tell him what Nick has done.

You dress like a fag, my father says. Sounds like you deserved it.

I move to Plan B.

Pops, I say, Nick's ruining my game. It's all about hitting from the baseline—we never work on my net game. We never work on serve and volley.

My father says he'll talk to Nick about my game. He also says Nick has given his assurance that I'll only be punished for a few weeks, to prove that Nick is in charge of the place. They can't have one kid flouting the rules. They need to maintain some show of discipline.

In conclusion my father says again that I'm staying. I have no choice. Click. Dial tone.

Julio shuts the door. Nick takes the receiver from my hand and says my father told him to take away my credit card.

No way I'm giving up my credit card. My only means of ever getting out of here? Over my dead body.

Nick tries to negotiate with me and I suddenly realize: He needs me. He sent Julio after me, he phoned my father, now he's trying to get my credit card? He told me to leave, and when I left, he fetched me back. I called his bluff. Despite the trouble I cause, I'm apparently worth something to this guy.

BY DAY, I'M THE MODEL PRISONER. I pick weeds, clean toilets, wear the proper tennis clothes. By night I'm the masked avenger. I steal a master key to the Bollettieri Academy, and after everyone's asleep I go marauding with a group of other disgruntled inmates. While I confine my vandalism to minor stuff, like throwing shaving cream bombs, my cohorts spray walls with graffiti, and on the door to Nick's office they paint *Nick the Dick*. When Nick has the door repainted, they do it again.

My primary cohort on these late-night sprees is Roddy Parks, the boy who beat me that long-ago day when Perry introduced himself. Then Roddy gets caught. His bunkmate drops a dime. I hear that Roddy's been expelled. So now we know what it takes to get expelled. *Nick the Dick.* To his credit, Roddy takes the fall. He doesn't rat out anyone.

Aside from petty vandalism, my main act of insurrection is silence. I vow that, as long as I live, I'll never speak to Nick. This is my code, my religion, my new identity. This is who I am, the boy who won't speak. Nick, of course, doesn't notice. He strolls by the courts and says something to me and I don't answer. He shrugs. But other kids see me not answer. My status rises.

One reason for Nick's oblivion is that he's busy organizing a tournament, which he hopes will attract top juniors from throughout the nation. This gives me a great idea, another way to stick it to Nick. I pull aside one of his staff and mention a kid back in Vegas who'd be perfect for the tournament. He's unbelievably talented, I say. He gives me problems whenever we play.

What's his name?

Perry Rogers.

It's like laying fresh bait in a Nick trap. Nick lives to discover new stars and showcase them in his tournaments. New stars generate buzz. New stars add to the aura of the Bollettieri Academy, and bolster Nick's image as the great tennis mentor. Sure enough, days later, Perry receives a plane ticket and a personal invite to the tournament. He flies down to Florida and takes a cab to the Bollettieri Academy. I meet him in the compound and we throw our arms around each other, cackling at the fast one we're pulling on Nick.

Who do I have to play?

Murphy Jensen.

Oh no. He's great!

Don't worry about it. That's not for a few days. For now, let's party.

One of the many perks for kids playing in the tournament is a field trip to Busch Gardens in Tampa. On the bus to the amusement park I bring Perry up to speed, tell him about my public humiliation, describe how miserable I am at the Bollettieri Academy. And at Bradenton Academy. I tell him I'm close to failing. That's where I lose him. For once he's not able to make my problem sound coherent. He loves school. He dreams of attending a fine Eastern college, then law school.

I change the subject. I grill him about Jamie. Did she ask about me? How does she look? Does she wear my ankle bracelet? I tell Perry I want to send him back to Vegas with a special present for Jamie. Maybe something nice from Busch Gardens.

That would be cool, he agrees.

We're not at Busch Gardens ten minutes before Perry sees a booth filled with stuffed animals. On a high shelf sits an enormous black-and-white panda, its legs sticking left and right, its tiny red tongue hanging out.

Andre—you need to get Jamie *that*!

Well, sure, but it's not for sale. You have to win the grand prize to get that panda, and no one wins this game. It's rigged. I don't like things that are rigged.

Nah. You just have to toss two rubber rings around the neck of a Coke bottle. We're *athletes*. We've got this.

We try for half an hour, scattering rubber rings all over the booth. Not one ring comes close to lassoing a Coke bottle.

OK, Perry says. Here's what we do. You distract the lady running the booth, I'll sneak back there and put two of these rings on the bottles.

I don't know. What if we get caught?

But then I remember: It's for Jamie. Anything for Jamie.

I call out to the booth lady: Excuse me, ma'am, I have a question.

She turns. Yes?

I ask something inane about the rules of ringtoss. In my peripheral vision I see Perry tiptoe into the booth. Four seconds later he leaps back.

I won! I won!

The booth lady spins around. She sees two Coke bottles with rubber rings around their necks. She looks shocked. Then skeptical.

Now wait just a minute, kid—

I won! Give me my panda!

I didn't see—

That's your problem if you didn't see. That's not the rule, you have to see. Where does it say you have to see? I want to talk to your supervisor! Get Mr. Busch Gardens himself down here! I'm taking this whole amusement park to court. What kind of a gyp is this? I paid a dollar to play this game, and that's an implied contract. You owe me a panda. I'm suing. My father is suing. You have exactly three seconds to get me my panda, which I won fair and fucking square!

Perry is doing what he loves, talking. He's doing what his father does, selling air. And the booth lady is doing what she hates, manning a booth at an amusement park. It's no contest. She doesn't want any trouble and she doesn't need this headache. With a long stick she snatches down the big panda and forks it over. It's nearly as tall as Perry. He grabs it like a giant Chipwich and we run off before she changes her mind.

For the rest of the night we're a threesome: Perry, me, and the panda. We bring the panda to the snack bar, into the boys' room, on the roller coaster. It's like we're babysitting a comatose fourteen-year-old. A real panda couldn't be more trouble. When the time comes to board the bus, we're both weary and glad to dump the panda in its own seat, which it fills. Its girth is as shocking as its height.

I say, I hope Jamie appreciates this.

Perry says, She's going to love it.

A little girl sits behind us. She's eight or nine. She can't take her eyes off the panda. She coos and pets its fur.

What a pretty panda! Where did you get it?

We won it.

What are you going to do with it?

I'm giving it to a friend.

She asks to sit with the panda. She asks if she can cuddle it. I tell her to help herself.

I hope Jamie likes the panda half as much as this girl does.

PERRY AND I are hanging out in the barracks the next morning when Gabriel pokes his head in.

The Man wants to see you.

What about?

Gabriel shrugs.

I walk slowly, taking my time. I stop at the door to Nick's office and with a thin smile I remember. *Nick the Dick.* You'll be missed, Roddy.

Nick is sitting behind his desk, leaning back in his tall black leather chair.

Andre, come in, come in.

I sit in a wooden chair across from him.

He clears his throat. I understand, he says, that you were at Busch Gardens yesterday. Did you have fun?

I say nothing. He waits. Then clears his throat again.

Well, I understand you came home with a very large panda.

I continue to stare straight ahead.

Anyway, he says, my daughter apparently has fallen in love with that panda. Ha ha.

I think of the little girl on the bus. Nick's daughter—of course. How could I have missed that?

She can't stop talking about it, Nick says. So here's the thing. I'd like to buy that panda from you.

Silence.

You hear me, Andre?

Silence.

Can you understand?

Silence.

Gabriel, why isn't Andre saying anything?

He's not speaking to you.

Since when?

Gabriel frowns.

Look, Nick says, just tell me how much you want for it, Andre.

I don't move my eyes.

I know. Why don't you *write down* how much you want for it?

He slides a piece of paper toward me. I don't move.

How about if I give you $200.

Deep silence.

Gabriel tells Nick that he'll talk to me later about the panda.

Yeah, Nick says. OK. Have a think about it, Andre.

YOU'LL NEVER BELIEVE THIS, I tell Perry at the barracks. He wanted the Panda. For his daughter. That little girl on the bus was Nick's daughter.

You're kidding. And what did you say?

I said nothing.

What do you mean, nothing?

Vow of silence, remember? Forever.

Andre, you misplayed that. No, no, that's a miss. You've got to revisit this, quickly. Here's the play. You take the panda, you give it to Nick and tell him you don't want his money, you just want an opportunity to succeed and get out of this place. You want wild cards, bids to tournaments, different rules to live by. Better food, better everything. Above all—you don't want to go to school. This is your chance to break free. You've got real leverage now.

I can't give that fucking guy my panda. I just can't. Besides, what about Jamie?

We'll worry about Jamie later. This is your future we're talking about. You have to give that panda to Nick!

We talk until long after lights out, arguing in heated whispers. Finally Perry convinces me.

So, he says, yawning, you're going to give it to him tomorrow.

No. Bullshit. I'm going to his office right now. I'm going to let myself in with the master key, then put the panda on Nick's tall leather chair, ass up.

THE NEXT MORNING, before breakfast, Gabriel comes for me again.

Office. On the double.

Nick is in his chair. The panda is now in the corner, leaning, staring into space. Nick looks at the panda, then me. He says, You don't talk. You wear makeup. You wear jeans in a tournament. You get me to invite your friend Perry to the tourney, even though he can't play, he can barely chew gum and walk at the same time. And that hair. Don't get me started on that hair. And now you give me something I ask for, but you break into my office in the middle of the night and put it ass-up in my fucking chair? How the fuck did you get in my office? Jesus, boy, what is your problem?

You want to know what my problem is?

Even Nick is shocked by the sound of my voice.

I shout, *You* are my fucking problem. You. And if you haven't figured that out, then you're stupider than you look. Do you have any idea what it's like here? What it's like to be three thousand miles from home, living in this prison, waking up at six thirty, having thirty minutes to eat that shitty breakfast, getting on that broken-down bus, going to that lousy school for four hours, hurrying back and having thirty minutes to eat more crap before going on the tennis court, day after day after *day*? Do you? The only thing you have to look forward to, the only real fun you have every week, is Saturday night at the Bradenton Mall—and then that gets taken away! *You took that from me!* This place is hell, and I want to burn it down!

Nick's eyes are wider than the panda's. But he's not angry. Or sad. He's mildly pleased, because this is the only language he understands. He reminds me of Pacino in *Scarface,* when a woman tells him, Who, why, when, and how I fuck is none of your business, and Pacino says, Now you're *talking* to me, baby.

Nick, I realize, likes it rough.

OK, he says, you made your point. What do you want?

I hear Perry's voice.

I want to quit school, I say. I want to start doing correspondence school, so I can work on my game full-time. I want your help, instead of the bullshit you've been giving me. I want wild cards, bids to tournaments. I want to take real steps toward turning pro.

Of course none of this is really what I want. It's what Perry tells me I want, and it's better than what I've got. Even as I demand it, I feel ambivalent. But Nick looks at Gabriel, and Gabriel looks at me, and the panda looks at all of us.

I'll think about it, Nick says.

HOURS AFTER PERRY LEAVES FOR VEGAS, Nick sends word via Gabriel that my first wild card will be the big tournament at La Quinta. Also, he's going to get me into the next Florida satellite. Furthermore, I'm to consider myself hereby dismissed and excused from Bradenton Academy. He'll set up a correspondence program of some sort, when he gets around to it.

Gabriel walks off, smirking. You won, kid.

I watch everyone else board the bus for Bradenton Academy, and as it rumbles away, spewing black smoke, I sit on a bench, basking in the sunshine. I tell myself: You're fourteen years old, and you never have to go to school again. From now on, every morning will feel like Christmas and the first day of summer vacation, combined. A smile spreads across my face, my first in months. No more pencils, no more books, no more teacher's dirty looks. You're free, Andre. You'll never have to learn anything again.

7

I PUT IN MY EARRING and run down to the hard courts. The morning is mine, mine, and I spend it hitting balls. Hit *harder*. I hit for two hours, channeling my newfound freedom into every swing. I can feel the difference. The ball explodes off my racket. Nick appears, shaking his head. I pity your next opponent, he says.

Meanwhile, back in Vegas, my mother begins correspondence school on my behalf. Her first actual correspondence is a letter to me, in which she says that her son might not go to college, but he's damn sure going to graduate high school. I write back and thank her for doing my homework and taking my tests. But when she earns the degree, I add, she can keep it.

In March 1985, I fly to Los Angeles and stay with Philly, who's living in someone's guest cottage, giving tennis lessons, searching for what he wants to do with his life. He helps me train for La Quinta, one of the year's biggest tournaments. The guest cottage is tiny, smaller than our room back in Vegas, smaller than our rented Omni, but we don't mind, we're thrilled to be reunited, hopeful about my new direction. There's just one problem: We have no money. We subsist on baked potatoes and lentil soup. Three times a day we bake two potatoes and heat a can of generic lentil soup. We then pour the soup over the potatoes and voilà— breakfast, lunch, or dinner is served. The whole meal costs eighty-nine cents and keeps hunger at bay for about three hours.

THE DAY BEFORE THE TOURNAMENT, we drive Philly's beat-up jalopy over to La Quinta. The car produces enormous clouds of black smoke. It feels like driving in a portable summer storm.

Maybe we should stick a potato in the tailpipe, I tell Philly.

Our first stop is the grocery store. I stand before the bin of potatoes and my stomach rolls. I can't face another spud. I walk off, wander up and down the aisles, and find myself in the frozen-food section. My eye lands on one particularly enticing treat. Oreo ice cream sandwiches. I reach for them like a sleepwalker. I take a box of ice cream sandwiches from the case and meet my brother in the express lane. Slipping behind him I gently set the ice cream sandwiches on the conveyor belt.

He looks down, then looks at me.

We can't afford that.

I'll have this instead of my potato.

He picks up the box, looks at the price, lets out a low whistle. Andre, this costs as much as ten potatoes. We can't.

I know. Fuck.

Walking back to the frozen-food case, I think: I hate Philly. I love Philly. I hate potatoes.

Woozy with hunger, I go out and beat Broderick Dyke in the first round at La Quinta, 6–4, 6–4. In the second round I beat Rill Baxter, 6–2, 6–1. In the third round I beat Russell Simpson, 6–3, 6–3. Then I win my first round in the main draw against John Austin, 6–4, 6–1. Down a break in the first set, I come storming back. I'm fifteen years old, beating grown men, beating them senseless, churning my way through the ranks. Everywhere I walk people are pointing at me, whispering. *There he is. That's the kid I was telling you about—the prodigy.* It's the prettiest word I've ever heard applied to me.

Prize money for reaching the second round at La Quinta, is $2,600. But I'm an amateur, so I get nothing. Still, Philly learns that the tournament will reimburse players for expenses. We sit in his jalopy and make up an itemized list of imaginary expenses, including our imaginary first-class flight from Vegas, our imaginary five-star-hotel room, our imaginarily lavish restaurant meals. We think we're shrewd, because our expenses equal exactly $2,600.

Philly and I have the balls to ask for so much because we're from Vegas. We've spent our childhoods in casinos. We think we're born bluffers. We think we're high rollers. After all, we did learn to double down before we were potty-trained. Recently, while walking through Caesars, Philly and I passed a slot machine just as it began to play that old Depression-era song We're in the Money. We knew the song from Pops, so we felt it was a sign. It didn't occur to us that the slot machine played that song all day long. We sat down at the nearest blackjack table—and won. Now, with the same swagger born of naïveté, I walk our list of expenses into the office of the tournament director, Charlie Pasarell, while Philly waits in the car.

Charlie is a former player. In fact, back in 1969 he played Pancho Gonzalez in the longest men's singles match ever at Wimbledon. Pancho is now my brother-in-law—he recently married Rita. Another sign that Philly and I are in the money. But the biggest sign of all: one of Charlie's oldest friends is Alan King, who hosted the very same Vegas tournament where I saw Caesar and Cleopatra and the wheelbarrow full of silver dollars, where I worked as a ball boy with Wendi, where I first stepped onto a professional tennis court in an official capacity. Signs, signs, everywhere signs. I place the list on Charlie's desk and stand back.

Huh, Charlie says, looking over the list. Very interesting.

Sorry?

Expenses don't usually work out so neat.

I feel a hot flash.

Your expenses, Andre, are exactly the same amount as the prize money you'd be able to collect if you were a pro.

Charlie looks at me over the top of his glasses. I feel my heart shrivel to the size of a lentil. I consider making a run for it. I imagine Philly and me living in that guest cottage for the rest of our lives. But Charlie suppresses a smile, reaches into a strongbox, and removes a wad of bills.

Here's two grand, kid. Don't grind me for the other six hun.

Thank you, sir. Thank you very much.

I run outside and dive into Philly's car. He peels out as if we've just held up the First Bank of La Quinta. I count out $1,000 and throw it at my brother.

Your cut of the loot.

What? No! Andre, you worked hard for this, bro.

Are you kidding? *We* worked. Philly, I couldn't have done this without you! Impossible! We're in this together, man.

In the back of our minds we're both thinking of the morning I woke up with $300 on my chest. We're also thinking of all those nights, sitting in the ad court–deuce court of our bedroom, sharing everything. He leans over, while driving, and gives me a hug. Then we talk about where we're going to eat dinner. We're drooling as we bandy names of restaurants about. In the end we agree that this is a special occasion, a once-in-a-lifetime occasion, which calls for something truly fancy.

Sizzler.

I can already taste that rib eye, Philly says.

I'm not going to bother with a plate. I'm just going to shove my head into the salad bar.

They have an all-you-can-eat shrimp special.

They're going to be sorry they ever came up with that idea!

You said it, bro!

We gnaw through the La Quinta Sizzler, not leaving a single seed or crouton in our wake, then sit around and stare at the money we have left over. We line up the bills, stack them, stroke them. We talk about our new buddy, Benjamin Franklin. We're so drunk on calories, we break out the steam iron and run it lightly over each bill, gently smoothing out the wrinkles in Ben's face.

8

I CONTINUE TO LIVE AND TRAIN at the Bollettieri Academy, with Nick as my coach and sometime travel companion, though he feels more like a sounding board. And, honestly, a friend. Our makeshift truce has turned into a surprisingly harmonious working relationship. Nick respects the way I stood up to him, and I respect him for being true to his word. We're working hard to achieve a common goal, to conquer the tennis world. I don't expect much from Nick in the way of Xs and Os; I look to him for cooperation, not information. Meanwhile, he looks to me for headline-generating wins which help his academy. I don't pay him a salary, because I can't, but it's understood that when I turn pro I'll give him bonuses based on what I earn. He considers this more than generous.

Early spring, 1986. I tramp all over Florida, playing a series of satellite tournaments. Kissimmee. Miami. Sarasota. Tampa. After a year of working hard, focusing exclusively on tennis, I play well, making it to the fifth tournament of the series, the Masters. I reach the final and, though I lose, I'm entitled to a finalist check of $1,100.

I want to take it. I yearn to take it. Philly and I sure could use the money. Still, if I take that check I'm a professional tennis player, forever, no turning back.

I phone my father back in Vegas and ask him what I should do.

My father says, What the hell do you mean? Take the money.

If I take the money, there's no turning back. I'm pro.

So?

If I cash this check, Pops, that's it.

He acts as if we have a bad connection.

You've dropped out of school! You have an eighth-grade education. What are your choices? What the hell else are you going to do? Be a doctor?

None of this comes as news, but I hate the way he puts it.

I tell the tournament director I'll take the money. As the words leave my mouth I feel a shelf of possibilities fall away. I don't know what those possibilities might be, but that's the point—I never will know. The man hands me a check, and as I walk out of his office I feel as if I'm starting down a long, long road, one that seems to lead into a dark, ominous forest.

It's April 29, 1986. My sixteenth birthday.

In disbelief, all day long, I tell myself: You're a professional tennis player now. That's what you are. That's *who* you are. No matter how many times I say it, it just doesn't sound right.

The one unequivocally good thing about my decision to turn pro is that my father sends Philly on the road with me full-time, to help with the minutiae, the endless details and arrangements of being a pro, from renting cars to reserving hotel rooms to stringing rackets.

You need him, my father says. But all three of us know that Philly and I need each other.

The day after I turn pro, Philly gets a call from Nike. They want to meet with me about an endorsement deal. Philly and I meet the Nike man in Newport Beach, at a restaurant called the Rusty Pelican. His name is Ian Hamilton.

I call him Mr. Hamilton, but he says I should call him Ian. He smiles in a way that makes me trust him instantly. Philly, however, remains wary.

Boys, Ian says, I think Andre has a very bright future.

Thank you.

I'd like Nike to be a part of that future, to be a *partner* in that future.

Thank you.

I'd like to offer you a two-year contract.

Thank you.

During which time Nike will provide all your gear, and pay you $20,000.

For both years?

For *each* year.

Ah.

Philly jumps in. What would Andre have to do in exchange for this money?

Ian looks confused. Well, he says. Andre would have to do what Andre has been doing, son. Keep being Andre. And wear Nike stuff.

Philly and I look at each other, two Vegas kids who still think they know how to bluff. But our poker faces are long gone. We left them back at Sizzler. We can't believe this is happening, and we can't pretend to feel otherwise. At least Philly still has the presence of mind to ask Ian if we may be excused. We need a few moments in private to discuss his offer.

We speed-walk to the back of the Rusty Pelican and dial my father from the pay phone.

Pops, I whisper, Philly and I are here with the guy from Nike and he's offering me $20,000. What do you think?

Ask for more money.

Really?

More money! More money!

He hangs up. Philly and I rehearse what we're going to say. I play me, he plays Ian. Men passing us on their way in and out of the men's room think we're doing a skit. At last we walk casually back to the table. Philly spells out our counteroffer. More money. He looks grave. He looks, I can't help but notice, like my father.

OK, Ian says. I think we can manage that. I have the budget for $25,000 for the second year. Deal?

We shake his hand. Then we all walk out of the Rusty Pelican. Philly and I wait for Ian to drive off before jumping up and down, singing We're in the Money.

Can you believe this is happening?

No, Philly says. Honestly? No, I can't.

Can I drive back to L.A.?

No. Your hands are shaking. You'll plow us straight into a median, and we can't have that. You're worth twenty grand, bro!

And twenty-five next year.

All the way back to Philly's place, item one on our agenda is what model of cool but cheap car we're going to buy. The main thing is to buy a car with a tailpipe that doesn't blow black clouds. Pulling up to Sizzler in a car that doesn't smoke—now *that* would be the height of luxury.

MY FIRST TOURNAMENT as a pro is in Schenectady, New York. I reach the final of the $100,000 tournament, then lose to Ramesh Krishnan, 6–2, 6–3. I don't feel bad, however. Krishnan is great, better than his ranking of forty-something, and I'm an unknown teenager, playing in the final of a fairly important tournament. It's that ultimate rarity—a painless loss. I feel nothing but pride. In fact, I feel a trace of hope, because I know I could have played better, and I know Krishnan knows.

Next I travel to Stratton Mountain, Vermont, where I beat Tim Mayotte, who's ranked number twelve. In the quarterfinal I play John McEnroe, which feels like playing John Lennon. The man is a legend. I've grown up watching him, admiring him, though I've often rooted against him, because his archrival, Borg, was my idol. I'd love to beat Mac, but this is his first tournament after a brief hiatus. He's well rested, raring to go, and he was recently ranked number one in the world. Moments before we take the court I wonder why a player as polished and accomplished as Mac needs a hiatus. Then he shows me. He demonstrates the virtue of rest. He beats me soundly, 6–3, 6–3. During the loss, however, I manage to hit one atomic winner, a forehand return of Mac's serve that explodes past him. At the post-match news conference, Mac announces to reporters: I've played Becker, Connors, and Lendl, and no one ever hit a return that hard at me. I never even saw the ball.

This one quote, this ringing endorsement of my game from a player of Mac's status, puts me on the national map. Newspapers write about me. Fans write to me. Philly suddenly finds himself deluged with requests for interviews. He giggles every time he fields another.

Nice to be popular, he says.

My ranking, meanwhile, keeps pace with my popularity.

I GO TO MY FIRST U.S. OPEN in the late summer of 1986, feeling eager for the step up in competition. Then I see the New York skyline from the airplane window and my eagerness evaporates. It's a beautiful sight, but intimidating for someone who grew up in the desert. So many people. So many dreams.

So many opinions.

Up close, at street level, New York is less intimidating than irritating. The nasty smells, the ear-splitting sounds—and the tipping. Raised in a house that depended on tips, I believe in tips, but in New York the tip takes on a brand new dimension. It costs me a hundred dollars just to get from the airport to my hotel room. By the time I've greased the palm of the cabbie, the doorman, the bellhop, and the concierge, I'm tapped out.

Also, I'm late for everything. I continually underestimate the time it takes to travel in New York from Point A to Point B. One day, right before the start of the tournament, I'm due to practice at two o'clock. I leave my hotel in what I think is plenty of time to reach the arena in Flushing Meadows. I board a charter bus outside the hotel, and by the time we navigate the midtown gridlock and cross the Triborough I'm horribly late. A woman tells me they've given away my court.

I stand before her, pleading for another practice time.

Who are you?

I show her my credentials, flash a weak smile.

Behind her is a chalkboard, covered with a sea of players' names, which she consults skeptically. I think of Mrs. G. She runs her fingers up and down the left column.

OK, she says. Four o'clock, Court 8.

I peer at the name of the player I'll be practicing with.

I'm sorry. I can't practice with that guy. I'm possibly going to play that guy in the second round.

She consults the chalkboard again, sighing, annoyed, and now I wonder if Mrs. G has a long-lost sister. At least I'm no longer rocking a mohawk, which would make me even more offensive to this woman. On the other hand, my current hairstyle is only slightly less outrageous. A fluffy, spiky, two-toned mullet, with black roots and frosted tips.

OK, she says. Court 17, five o'clock. But you'll have to share with three other guys.

I tell Nick: It feels as if I'm in over my head in this town.

Nah, he says. You'll be fine.

The whole place looks a lot better from a distance.

What doesn't?

In the first round I face Jeremy Bates, from Great Britain. We're on a back court, far from the crowds and the main action. I'm excited. I'm proud. Then I'm terrified. I feel as if it's the final Sunday of the tournament. My butterflies are flying in tight formation.

Because it's a Grand Slam, the energy of the match is different from anything I've experienced. More frenetic. The play is moving at warp speed, a rhythm with which I'm unfamiliar. Plus, the day is windy, so points seem to be flying past like the gum wrappers and dust. I don't understand what's happening. This doesn't even feel like tennis. Bates isn't a better player than I, but he's playing better, because he came in knowing what to expect. He beats me in four sets, then looks up at my box, where Philly is sitting with Nick, and shoves his fist into the crook of his arm, the international sign for *Up yours.* Apparently Bates and Nick have a history.

I feel disappointed, slightly embarrassed. But I know that I wasn't prepared for my first U.S. Open or New York. I see a gap between where I am and where I need to be, and I feel reasonably confident that I can close that gap.

You're going to get better, Philly says, putting an arm around me. It's just a matter of time.

Thanks. I know.

And I do know. I really do. But then I begin to lose. Not just lose, but lose badly. Weakly. Miserably. In Memphis I get knocked out in the first round. In Key Biscayne, first round again.

Philly, I say, what's going on? I have no clue out there. I feel like a hacker, a weekend player. I'm lost.

The low point is at the Spectrum in Philadelphia. It's not a tennis facility but a converted basketball arena, and barely that. Cavernous, poorly lit, it's got two tennis courts, side by side, and two matches taking place simultaneously. At the same moment I'm returning serve, somebody is returning serve in the next court, and if his serve goes wide at the same moment mine kicks, we both need to worry about colliding head-on. My concentration is fragile enough without factoring in collisions with other players. I don't know yet how to tune out distractions. After one set I can't think and can't hear anything but my own heartbeat.

Also, my opponent is bad, which puts me at a disadvantage. I'm at my worst against lesser opponents. I play down to their level. I don't know how to maintain my game while adjusting for an opponent's, which feels like inhaling and exhaling at the same time. Against great players I rise to the challenge. Against bad players I press, which is the tennis term for not letting things flow. Pressing is one of the deadliest things you can do in tennis.

Philly and I stagger back to Vegas. We're discouraged, but a more immediate problem is that we're broke. I've made no money in months, and with all the traveling and hotels, all the rental cars and restaurant meals, I've burned through nearly all my Nike money. From the airport I drive straight to Perry's house. We hole up in his bedroom with a couple of sodas. As soon as his door is closed I feel safer, saner. I notice that the walls are plastered with a few dozen more covers of *Sports Illustrated*. I study the faces of all the great athletes, and I tell Perry that I always believed I'd be a great athlete, whether I wanted to be one or not. I took it for granted. It was my life, and though I hadn't chosen it, my sole consolation was its certainty. At least fate has a structure. Now I don't know what the future holds. I'm good at one thing, but it looks as though I'm not as good at that one thing as I thought. Maybe I'm finished before I've started. In which case, what the hell are Philly and I going to do?

I tell Perry that I want to be a normal sixteen-year-old, but my life keeps getting more abnormal. It's abnormal to be humiliated at the U.S. Open. It's abnormal to run around the Spectrum worrying about a head-on collision with some giant Russian. It's abnormal to be shunned in locker rooms.

Why are you shunned?

Because I'm sixteen and in the top hundred. Also, Nick isn't well liked, and I'm associated with Nick. I have no friends, no allies. I have no girl-friend.

Jamie and I are done. My latest crush, Jillian, another schoolmate of Perry's, doesn't return my calls. She wants a boyfriend who isn't on the road all the time. I can't blame her.

Perry says, I had no idea you were dealing with all this.

But here's the topper, I tell him. I'm broke.

What happened to the twenty grand from Nike?

Travel. Expenses. It's not just me on the road, it's Philly, Nick—it adds up. When you're not winning it adds up faster. You can burn through twenty grand fast.

Can you ask your father for a loan?

No. Absolutely not. Help from him comes with a cost. I'm trying to break free of him.

Andre, everything will be fine.

Yeah, sure.

Really, it's about to get so much better. Before you know it, you're going to be winning again. Blink your eyes and your face will be on one of these *Sports Illustrated* covers.

Pff.

It will! I know it. And Jillian? Please. She's small time. You'll always have girl problems. That's the nature of the beast. But soon the girl giving you problems will be—Brooke Shields.

Brooke Shields? Where do you get Brooke Shields?

He laughs.

I don't know, I just read about her in *Time*. She's graduating from Princeton. She's the most beautiful woman in the world, she's brilliant, she's famous, and someday you're going to date her. Don't get me wrong, your life might never be normal—but soon the abnormal will be cool.

Buoyed by Perry, I go to Asia. I have just enough cash to get Philly and me there and back. I play the Japan Open, win a few matches before falling to Andrés Gómez in the quarters. I then go to Seoul, where I reach the final. I lose, but my share of the prize money is $7,000, enough to fund another three months of searching for my game.

As Philly and I land in Vegas, I feel relieved. I feel buoyant. Our father is meeting us at the airport, and I tell Philly as we walk through McCar-ran International Airport that I've made a momentous decision. I'm going to hug Pops.

Hug him? What for?

I feel *good*. I'm happy, damn it. Why not? I'm going to do it. You only live once.

Our father is at the gate, wearing a baseball cap and sunglasses. I rush toward him, wrap my arms around him, and squeeze. He doesn't move. He stiffens. It feels like hugging the pilot.

I release him and tell myself I'll never try that again.

PHILLY AND I GO TO ROME in May 1987. I'm in the main draw, so our rooms will be comped. We can upgrade from the dump Philly booked, which doesn't have TVs or shower curtains, to the swank Cavalieri, which sits atop a main hill overlooking the city.

In our free days before the tournament we get out and see the sights. We go to the Sistine Chapel and gaze at the frescoes of Christ handing St. Peter the keys to the kingdom of Heaven. We stare at Michelangelo's ceiling and learn from the tour guide that he was a tormented perfectionist, eaten up with rage whenever he discovered that his work—or even materials on which he planned to work—had the tiniest flaws.

We spend a day in Milan, stopping in churches and museums. We stand for half an hour before Leonardo da Vinci's *The Last Supper*. We learn about da Vinci's notebooks, with their minute observations of the human form, and their futuristic plans for helicopters and toilets. Both of us are floored that one man could have been so *inspired*. To be inspired, I tell Philly—that's the secret.

The Italian Open is on red clay, a surface that feels unnatural to me. I've only played on green clay, which is sort of fast. Red clay, I tell Nick, is hot glue and wet tar laid across a bed of quicksand. You can't put a guy away on this red-clay shit, I complain at our first practice.

He smirks. You're going to be fine, he says. You just have to get used to it. Don't be impatient, don't try to finish every point.

I don't have the slightest idea what he means. I lose in the second round.

We fly to Paris for the French Open. More red clay. I manage to win my first-rounder, but get spanked in the second. Again, Philly and I try to see something of the city, to improve ourselves. We go to the Louvre. The sheer number of paintings and sculptures daunts us. We don't know where to turn, how to stand. We can't comprehend all that we're seeing. We pass from room to room, dumbstruck. Then we come to a piece that we understand all too well. It's a painting from the Italian Renaissance and it depicts a young man, naked, standing on a cliff. With one hand he clutches a bare, breaking tree limb. With the other he holds a woman and two infants. Wrapped around his neck is an old man, perhaps his father, who also grasps a sack of what looks like money. Below them lies an abyss strewn with the bodies of those who couldn't hold on. Everything depends on this one naked man's strength—his grip.

The longer you look, I tell Philly, the tighter that old guy's arm around the hero's neck feels.

Philly nods. He looks up at the man on the cliff and says softly: Hang in there, bro.

IN JUNE 1987 we go to Wimbledon. I'm scheduled to play a Frenchman, Henri Leconte, on Court 2, known as the Graveyard Court because so many players have suffered fatal losses there. It's my first time at the most hallowed venue in tennis, and from the moment we arrive I dislike it. I'm a sheltered teenager from Las Vegas with no education. I reject all that's alien, and London feels as alien as a place can be. The food, the buses, the venerable traditions. Even the grass of Wimbledon smells different from the grass back home, what little there is of it.

More off-putting, Wimbledon officials appear to take a haughty, high-handed pleasure in telling players what to do and what not to do. I resent rules, but especially arbitrary rules. Why must I wear white? I don't want to wear white. Why should it matter to these people what I wear?

Above all, I take offense at being barred and blocked and made to feel unwanted. I need to show a badge to get into the locker room—and not the main locker room at that. I'm playing in this tournament, but I'm treated as an intruder, not even allowed to practice on the courts where I'll be competing. I'm restricted to indoor courts up the street. Consequently the first time I ever hit a ball on grass is the first time I play Wimbledon. And what a shock. The ball doesn't bounce right, doesn't bounce at all, because this grass isn't grass, but ice slathered with Vaseline. And I'm so afraid of slipping that I tiptoe. When I look around, to see if the British fans have noticed my discomfort, I get a scare: they're right on top of me. The building is like a dollhouse. Add my name to the list of those who've expired on Graveyard Court. Leconte euthanizes me. I tell Nick that I'm never coming back. I'll hug my father again before I embrace Wimbledon.

· · ·

STILL IN A FOUL MOOD, I travel several weeks later to Washington, D.C. In the first round, playing Patrick Kuhnen, I come up empty. Bone dry. After the long slog across Europe I have nothing left. The travel, the losses, the stress, it's all sapped me. Plus, the day is oppressively hot and I'm not physically fit. I'm wholly unprepared, so I become *unpresent*. When we're tied at one set apiece, I leave the court, mentally. My mind departs my body and goes floating out of the arena. I'm long gone when the third set starts. I lose 6–0.

I walk to the net and shake Kuhnen's hand. He says something, but I can't see or hear him. He's a blob of energy at the end of a tube. I grab my tennis bag and stumble out of the arena. I walk across the street, into Rock Creek Park, into some woods, and when I feel sure no one is around, I berate the trees.

I can't take this shit anymore! I'm fucking done! I quit!

I keep walking, walking, until I come to a clearing, where I find myself surrounded by a group of homeless men. Some are sitting on the ground, some are stretched out on logs, sleeping. Two are playing cards. They all look like trolls in a fairy tale. I walk up to one who seems fairly alert. I unzip my bag and remove several Prince rackets.

Here, man, you want these? Do you? Because I don't have any use for them anymore.

The man isn't sure what's happening, but he's pretty confident that he's finally met someone crazier than himself. His buddies shuffle over and I tell them, Gather round, fellas, gather round. It might be a hundred degrees in the shade, but it's Christmas Eve.

I dump out my tennis bag, pull out the rest of the rackets, each one worth hundreds of dollars, and pass them around.

Here, help yourselves! I sure as hell won't be needing them!

Then, reveling in how much *lighter* my tennis bag feels, I walk to the hotel where Philly and I are staying. I sit on one bed and Philly sits on the other, just like old times, in more ways than one. I tell him I've had it. I can't do this anymore.

He doesn't argue. He understands. Who better to understand? We knuckle down to details, making a plan. How to tell Nick, how to tell my father, how I can earn a living.

What do you want to do instead of playing tennis?

I don't know.

We go out for dinner, talk it over, analyze where I stand financially—a few hundred dollars above zero. We joke that we're getting close to potato-and-lentil-soup territory.

Back at the hotel the phone in our room is flashing. I have one message. The organizers of a tennis exhibition in North Carolina phoned to say a player canceled on them. They want to know if I can play. If I do, they'll guarantee me $2,000.

Philly agrees it would be nice to walk away from tennis with a little coin in my pocket.

OK, I say. One last tournament. I better get some more rackets.

IN THE FIRST ROUND I draw a kid named Michael Chang. I grew up playing him. I played him all through juniors, and I've never lost to him. I've never even had problems with him. Also, he's only fifteen, two years younger than I. He comes up to my navel. So this is just what the doctor ordered for my bruised psyche. A preordained beat-down. I walk onto the court, smiling.

Chang, however, has undergone some kind of metamorphosis since our last meeting. He's made a quantum leap in his game, and now he plays like a flea on speed. It takes everything I've got to beat him. Still, I do beat him. My first win in months. I decide to postpone my retirement. Just a few more weeks. I tell Philly I want to go to Stratton Mountain, where I did well last year. Stratton will be a fitting place for my last hurrah.

We fly up to Vermont with two fellow players, Peter Doohan and Kelly Evernden. Kelly says he grabbed the Stratton draw right before we left.

Anyone want to hear who he'll be playing?

I do.

No, Andre. You don't.

Uh-oh. Who did I draw?

Luke Jensen.

Fuck.

Luke's the best junior in the world, by far the most promising kid on the tour. I sink in my seat and watch the clouds. Should have quit while I was ahead. Should have retired after Chang.

LUKE SERVES BOTH lefty and righty, which is why they call him Dual Hand Luke, and he can bring it 130 miles an hour from either side. But today, against me, his first serve is off, and I cane his second. I'm more surprised than he is when I scrape by him in three sets and advance.

Next up is Pat Cash—who just won Wimbledon, twelve days after I met my demise on Graveyard Court. Cash is a machine, a finely tuned athlete who moves well and covers the net like a hydra. I don't even think about beating him, only about holding my own. But in the early going I find that he doesn't have a lot of top on his ball, so I'm getting nice, clean, eye-level looks, hitting one winner after another. Since I have no chance to win, since I want only to be credible, I'm free, loose, and this makes Cash tight. He appears shocked by what's unfolding. He's missing first serves, which lets me cheat in a half step, put everything I've got behind my return. Every time I hit a ball past him, Cash glares across the net with an expression that says, This wasn't in the plan. You're not supposed to be doing this.

Foolishly, somewhat arrogantly, he spends more and more time at the net looking surprised, rather than going back to the baseline and thinking up a new strategy. After one of my better returns, he hits a so-so volley, and I pass him again. He stands with his hands on his hips, staring at me, radiating a sense of injustice.

Keep staring, I think. Keep it up.

Toward the end he's giving me painfully easy targets, making his ball so beautifully hittable, so marvelously strikable, that it all seems unfair. I have a legit chance of hitting a winner on every point. I just wanted to leave a mark, but I'm leaving a gash. I score a shocking upset, 7–6, 7–6.

Stratton Mountain, I conclude, is my magic mountain. My anti-Wimbledon. Last year I played above my level here, now I'm playing twice as well. The setting is breathtaking, laid back—and quintessentially American. Unlike those snooty Brits, these Strattonites know me, or at least the idealized me I want them to know. They don't know about my struggles of the last twelve months, about my giving rackets to homeless men, about my pending retirement. And if they knew they wouldn't hold it against me. They cheered me during my match with Jensen, but after I outclass Cash, they adopt me. This guy is *our* guy. This guy does well here. Inspired by their raucous encouragement, I reach the semis against Ivan Lendl, who's ranked number one. My biggest match ever. My father flies in from Vegas.

An hour before the match, Lendl is walking around the locker room wearing only his tennis shoes. Seeing him so relaxed, so remarkably nude, right before facing me, I know what's coming. The beat-down to end all beat-downs. I lose in three sets. Still, I walk away feeling encouraged, because I won the second set. For half an hour, I gave the best in the world all he wanted. I can build on that. I feel good.

That is, until I see what Lendl has to say about me in the newspapers. Asked about my game, he sniffs: *A haircut and a forehand.*

9

I FINISH 1987 WITH A BANG. I win my first tournament as a pro, in Itaparica, Brazil, all the more impressive because I do it before a crowd of initially hostile Brazilians. After I beat their top player, Luiz Mattar, the fans don't seem to hold a grudge. In fact they make me an honorary Brazilian. They rush the court, hoist me on their shoulders, throw me in the air. Many have come to the arena straight from the beach. They're slathered with cocoa butter, and consequently so am I. Women in bikinis and thongs cover me with kisses. Music plays, people dance, someone hands me a bottle of champagne and tells me to spray it into the crowd. The carnival atmosphere is the perfect complement to my inner Mardi Gras. I finally broke through. I won five matches in a row. (To win a slam, I realize with some alarm, I'll need to win seven.)

A man hands me the winner's check. I have to look twice at the number. In the amount of: $90,000.

With the check still folded in my jeans pocket, I stand two days later in my father's living room and employ a bit of remedial psychology. Pops, I say, how much do you think I'm going to make next year?

Ho ho, he says, beaming. Millions.

Good—then you won't mind if I buy a car.

He frowns. Checkmate.

I know just the kind I want. A white Corvette with all the extras. My father insists that he and my mother go with me to the dealership, to make sure the salesman doesn't screw me. I can't say no. My father is my landlord and keeper. I no longer live full-time at the Bolletieri Academy, so once again I live under my father's roof, and thus under his control. I'm traveling the world, making good money, winning a measure of fame, and yet my old man essentially keeps me on an allowance. It's inappropriate, but hell, my whole life is inappropriate. I'm only seventeen, not ready to live on my own, barely ready to stand alone on a tennis court, and yet I was just in Rio, holding a girl in a thong with one hand and a $90,000 check with the other. I'm an adolescent who's seen too much, a man-child without a checking account.

At the car dealership my father goes back and forth with the salesman, and the negotiation quickly turns contentious. Why am I not surprised? Every time my father makes a new offer the salesman walks off to consult his manager. My father clenches and unclenches his fists.

The salesman and my father eventually agree on a price. I'm seconds from owning my dream car. My father puts on his glasses, gives the paperwork a last look. He runs his finger down the itemized list of charges. Wait, what's this? A charge for $49.99?

Small fee for the paperwork, the salesman says.

Ain't my fucking paper. That's your fucking paper. Pay for your own fucking paper.

The salesman doesn't care for my father's tone. Hard words are exchanged. My father gets that look in his eye, the same look he had before dropping the trucker. Just the sight of all these cars is giving him the old road rage.

Pops, the car costs $37,000, and you're flipping out about a $50 fee?

They're screwing you, Andre! They're screwing me. The world is trying to screw me!

He storms out of the salesman's office and into the main showroom, where the managers sit along a high counter. He screams at them: You think you're safe back there? You think you're safe behind that counter? Why don't you come out from behind there?

His dukes are up. He's ready to fight five men at once.

My mother puts an arm around me and says the best thing we can do now is go outside and wait.

We stand on the sidewalk and watch my father's tirade through the plate-glass window of the dealership. He's pounding the desk. He's waving his hands. It's like watching a terrible silent movie. I'm mortified, but also slightly envious. I wish I possessed some of my father's rage. I wish I could tap into it during tough matches. I wonder what I could do in tennis if I could access that rage and aim it across the net. Instead, whatever rage I have, I turn on myself.

Mom, I ask, how do you take it? All these years?

Oh, she says, I don't know. He hasn't gone to jail yet. And nobody's killed him yet. I think we're pretty lucky, all things considered. Hopefully we'll get through this incident without either of those two things happening, and move on.

Along with my father's rage, I wish I had a fraction of my mother's calm.

Philly and I go back to the dealership the next day. The salesman hands me the keys to my new Corvette, but treats me with pity. He says I'm nothing like my father, and though he means it as a compliment, I feel vaguely offended. Driving home, the thrill of my new Corvette is dampened. I tell Philly that things are going to be different from now on. Weaving in and out of traffic, gunning the engine, I tell him: The time has come. I need to take control of my money. I need to take control of my fucking life.

I'M RUNNING OUT of steam in long matches. And for me every match is long, because my serve is average. I can't serve my way out of trouble, I get no easy points off my serve, so every opponent takes me the full twelve rounds. My knowledge of the game is improving, but my body is breaking down. I'm skinny, brittle, and my legs give out quickly, followed in short order by my nerve. I tell Nick that I'm not fit enough to compete with the best in the world. He agrees. Legs are everything, he says.

I find a trainer in Vegas, a retired military colonel named Lenny. Tough as burlap, Lenny curses like a sailor and walks like a pirate, the result of being shot in a long-ago war he doesn't like to talk about. After one hour with Lenny I wish someone would shoot me. Few things give Lenny more pleasure than abusing me and hurling obscenities at me in the process.

In December 1987 the desert turns unseasonably cold. The blackjack dealers wear Santa hats. The palm trees are strung with lights. The hookers on the Strip wear Christmas ornaments for earrings. I tell Perry I can't wait for this new year. I feel strong. I feel as if I'm starting to *get* tennis.

I win the first tournament of 1988, in Memphis, and the ball sounds alive as it leaves my racket. I'm growing into my forehand. I'm hitting the ball *through* opponents. Each one turns to me with a look that says, Where the hell did that come from?

I notice something on the faces of fans too. The way they watch me and ask for my autograph, the way they scream as I enter an arena, makes me uncomfortable, but also satisfies something deep inside me, some hidden craving I didn't know was there. I'm shy—but I like attention. I cringe when fans start dressing like me—but I also dig it.

Dressing like me in 1988 means wearing denim shorts. They're my signature. They're synonymous with me, mentioned in every article and profile. Oddly, I didn't choose to wear them; they chose me. It was 1987, in Portland, Oregon. I was playing the Nike International Challenge and Nike reps invited me up to a hotel suite to show me the latest demos and clothing samples. McEnroe was there, and of course he was given first choice. He held up a pair of denim shorts and said, What the fuck are these?

My eyes got big. I licked my lips and thought, *Whoa*. Those are cool. If you don't want those, Mac, I've got dibs.

The moment Mac set them aside, I scooped them up. Now I wear them at all my matches, as do countless fans. Sportswriters murder me for it. They say I'm trying to stand out. In fact—as with my mohawk— I'm trying to hide. They say I'm trying to change the game. In fact I'm trying to prevent the game from changing me. They call me a rebel, but I have no interest in being a rebel, I'm only conducting an everyday, run-of-the-mill teenage rebellion. Subtle distinctions, but important. At heart, I'm doing nothing more than being myself, and since I don't know who that is, my attempts to figure it out are scattershot and awkward— and, of course, contradictory. I'm doing nothing more than I did at the Bollettieri Academy. Bucking authority, experimenting with identity, sending a message to my father, thrashing against the lack of choice in my life. But I'm doing it on a grander stage.

Whatever I'm doing, for whatever reasons, it strikes a chord. I'm routinely called the savior of American tennis, whatever that means. I think it has to do with the atmosphere at my matches. Besides wearing my outfits, fans come sporting my hairdo. I see my mullet on men *and* women. (It looks better on the women.) I'm flattered by the imitators, embarrassed, thoroughly confused. I can't imagine all these people trying to be like Andre Agassi, since I don't want to be Andre Agassi.

Now and then I start to explain this in an interview, but it never comes out right. I try to be funny, and it falls flat or offends someone. I try to be profound, and I hear myself making no sense. So I stop, fall back on pat answers and platitudes, tell journalists what they seem to want to hear. It's the best I can do. If I can't understand my motivations and demons, how can I hope to explain them to journalists on deadline?

To make matters worse, journalists write down exactly what I say, while I'm saying it, word for word, as if this represented the literal truth. I want to tell them, Hold it, don't write that down, I'm only thinking out loud here. You're asking about the subject I understand least—me. Let me edit myself, contradict myself. But there isn't time. They need black-

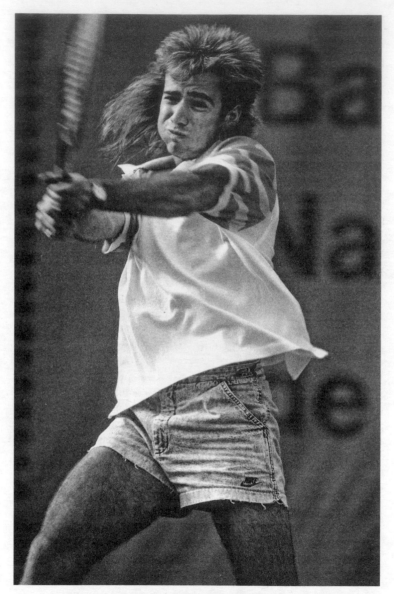

Eighteen years old, wearing a frosted mullet and denim shorts,
my first signature look

and-white answers, good and evil, simple plot lines in seven hundred words, and then they're on to the next thing.

If I had time, if I were more self-aware, I would tell journalists that I'm trying to figure out who I am, but in the meantime I have a pretty good idea of who I'm not. I'm not my clothes. I'm certainly not my game. I'm not anything the public thinks I am. I'm not a showman simply because I come from Vegas and wear loud clothes. I'm not an *enfant terrible,* a phrase that appears in every article about me. (I think you can't be something you can't pronounce.) And, for heaven's sake, I'm not a *punk rocker.* I listen to soft, cheesy pop, like Barry Manilow and Richard Marx.

Of course the key to my identity, the thing I know about myself but can't bring myself to tell journalists, is that I'm losing my hair. I wear it long and fluffy to conceal its rapid departure. Only Philly and Perry know, because they're fellow sufferers. In fact Philly recently flew to New York to meet with an owner of Hair Club for Men, to buy himself a few toupees. He's finally given up on the headstands. He phones to tell me about the astonishing variety of toupees the Hair Club offers. It's a hair smorgasbord, he says. It's like the salad bar at Sizzler, only all hair.

I ask him to pick one up for me. Every morning I find a little more of my identity on my pillow, in my sink, in my drain.

I ask myself: You're going to wear a hairpiece? During *tournaments*?

I answer: What choice do I have?

AT INDIAN WELLS, in February 1988, I blaze my way to the semis, where I meet Boris Becker, from West Germany, the most famous tennis player in the world. He cuts an imposing figure, with a shock of hair the color of a new penny and legs as wide as my waist. I catch him at the peak of his powers, but win the first set. Then I lose the next two, including a hard, tough third. We walk off the court glowering at each other like rutting bulls. I promise myself I won't lose to him the next time we meet.

In March, at Key Biscayne, I face an old schoolmate from the Bollettieri Academy, Aaron Krickstein. We're often compared to each other, because of our connection with Nick and our precocious skills. I'm up two sets to none and then wear out. Krickstein wins the next two sets. As the fifth set starts I'm cramping. I'm still not where I need to be, physically, to reach the next level. I lose.

I go to Isle of Palms, near Charleston, and win my third tournament. In the middle of the tournament I turn eighteen. The tournament director rolls a cake out to center court, and everyone sings. I've never liked birthdays. No one ever took note of my birthday when I was growing up. But this feels different. I'm legal, everyone keeps saying. In the eyes of the law, you're a grown-up.

Then the law is an ass.

I go to New York City, the Tournament of Champions, a significant milestone because it's a clash of the top players in the world. Once more I square off against Chang, who's developed a bad habit since we last met. Every time he beats someone, he points to the sky. He thanks God— credits God—for the win, which offends me. That God should take sides in a tennis match, that God should side against me, that God should be in Chang's box, feels ludicrous and insulting. I beat Chang and savor every blasphemous stroke. Then I take revenge on Krickstein. In the final I face Slobodan Zivojinovic, a Serb better known for his doubles play. I beat him in straight sets.

I'm winning more often. I should be happy. Instead I'm uptight, because it's over. I've enjoyed a triumphant hard-court season, my body wants to keep playing on hard courts, but clay season is starting. The sudden switch from one surface to another changes everything. Clay is a different game, thus your game must become different, and so must your body. Instead of sprinting from side to side, stopping short and starting, you must slide and lean and dance. Familiar muscles now play supporting roles, dormant muscles dominate. It's painful enough, under the best of circumstances, that I don't know who I am. To suddenly become a different person, a clay person, adds another degree of frustration and anxiety.

A friend tells me that the four surfaces in tennis are like the four seasons. Each asks something different of you. Each bestows different gifts and exacts different costs. Each radically alters your outlook, remakes you on a molecular level. After three rounds of the Italian Open, in May 1988, I'm no longer Andre Agassi. And I'm no longer in the tournament.

I go to the 1988 French Open expecting more of the same. Walking into the locker room at Roland Garros, I see all the clay experts leaning against the walls, leering. Dirt rats, Nick calls them. They've been here for months, practicing, waiting for the rest of us to finish hard courts and fly into their clay lair.

Disorienting as the new surface is, Paris itself is more of a shock to the system. The city has all the same logistical problems of New York and London, the large crowds and cultural anomalies, but with an added language barrier. Also, the presence of dogs in restaurants unsettles me. The first time I walk into a café, on the Champs-Élysées, a dog raises its leg and unleashes a stream of pee against the table next to mine.

Roland Garros provides no escape from the strangeness. It's the only place I've ever played that reeks of cigars and pipes. While I'm serving, at a critical point in a match, a finger of pipe smoke curls under my nose. I want to find the person smoking that pipe and admonish him, and yet I don't want to find that person, because I can't imagine what sort of gnarled hobbit is sitting at an outdoor tennis match puffing on a pipe.

Despite my unease, I manage to beat my first three opponents. I even beat the great clay master Guillermo Pérez-Roldán in the quarterfinal. In the semis I run into Mats Wilander. He's ranked number three in the world, but to my mind he's the player of the moment. When one of his matches is on TV, I stop whatever I'm doing and watch. He's on his way to an astounding year. He's already won the Australian Open and is the favorite to win this tournament. I manage to take him to a fifth set, then lose 6–0, cramping badly.

I remind Nick that I'm skipping Wimbledon. I say, Why switch to grass and expend all that energy? Let's take a month off, rest, get ready for the hard courts of summer.

He's more than happy not to go to London. He doesn't like Wimbledon any more than I do. Besides, he wants to hurry back to the U.S. and find me a better trainer.

NICK HIRES A CHILEAN STRONGMAN named Pat who never asks me to do anything he's not willing to do himself, which I respect. But Pat also has a habit of spitting on me when he talks, and leaning over me while I'm lifting weights, drizzling sweat on my face. I feel as if I should show up for Pat's workout sessions in a plastic poncho.

The mainstay of Pat's training regimen is a brutal daily run up and down a hill outside Vegas. The hill is remote and sunbaked, and gets hotter as you near the top, as if it's an active volcano. It's also an hour from my father's house, which seems unnecessarily far. Nothing like driving to Reno for a run. Pat insists, however, that this hill is the answer to all my physical problems. When we get to the base and pile out of the car, he starts running straight up, and orders me to follow. Within minutes I'm holding my side, sweat rolling off me. By the time we reach the summit I can't breathe. According to Pat, this is good. This is healthy.

A battered truck appears one day as Pat and I crest the hill. An ancient Native American man climbs out. He comes toward us with a pole. If he wants to kill me, I won't be able to fend him off, because I can't lift my arms. And I won't be able to run away, because I can't draw breath.

The man asks, What are you doing here?

We're training. What are you doing here?

Catching me some rattlesnakes.

Rattlesnakes! There are rattlesnakes out here?

There's training out here?

When I stop laughing the Indian says, more or less, that I must have been born with a horseshoe up my ass, because this is Rattlesnake Fucking Hill. He catches twelve rattlers every day on this hill, and he expects to catch twelve more this morning. It's a flat-out miracle that I haven't stepped on one, big and plump and ready to strike.

I look at Pat, and feel an urge to spit on him.

IN JULY I GO to Argentina as one of the youngest men ever to play for the U.S. Davis Cup team. I play well against Martín Jaite, from Argentina, and the crowd gives me its grudging respect. I'm leading two sets to none, ahead 4–0 in the third, waiting for Jaite's serve. I'm hunched against the cold, because it's the dead of winter in Argentina. The temperature must be thirty degrees. Jaite hits a let serve, then hits a bending unreturnable serve that I reach up and catch with my hand. A riot breaks out. The crowd thinks I'm trying to show up their countryman, disrespecting him. They boo me for several minutes.

The next day's newspapers kill me. Rather than defend myself, I react with truculence. I say I've always wanted to do something like that. The truth is, I was just cold and not thinking. I was being stupid, not cocky. My reputation takes a major hit.

THE CROWD AT STRATTON MOUNTAIN welcomes me days later, however, like a prodigal. I play to please them. I play to thank them for banishing the memory of Argentina. Something about these people, these emerald mountains, this Vermont air—I win the tournament. I wake soon after to discover that I'm number four in the world. But I'm too spent to celebrate. Between Pat and Davis Cup and the grind of the tour, I'm sleeping twelve hours a night.

I fly to New York in the late summer to play a minor tournament in New Jersey, a tune-up for the 1988 U.S. Open. I reach the final and face Tarango. I beat him soundly, a delicious victory, because I can still close my eyes and see Tarango cheating me when I was eight. My first loss. I'll never forget. Each time I hit a winner I think, Fuck you, Jeff. Fuck. You.

At the U.S. Open I reach the quarters. I'm due to face Jimmy Connors. Before the match I approach him meekly in the locker room and remind him that we once met. In Las Vegas? I was four? You were playing at Caesars Palace? We hit some balls together?

Nope, he says.

Oh. Well. Actually, we met again, several times, when I was seven. I used to deliver rackets to you? My father strung your rackets whenever you came to town, and I'd bring them to you at your favorite restaurant on the Strip?

Nope, he says again, then lies back on a bench and pulls a long white towel over his legs and closes his eyes.

Dismissed.

This gibes with everything I've heard about Connors from other players. Asshole, they say. Rude, condescending, egomaniac prick. But I thought he'd treat me differently, I thought he'd show me some love, given our longtime connection.

Just for that, I tell Perry, I'm beating this guy in three easy sets—and he's going to win no more than nine games.

The crowd is pulling for Connors. It's the opposite of Stratton. Here, I'm cast as the bad guy. I'm the impertinent upstart who dares to oppose the elder statesman. The crowd wants Connors to defy the odds, and Father Time, and I'm standing in the way of that dream scenario. Each time they cheer I think: Do they realize what this guy is like in the locker room? Do they know what his peers say about him? Do they have any concept of how he responds to a friendly hello?

I'm cruising, winning easily, when a man in the upper bleachers calls out, *C'mon, Jimmy, he's a punk—you're a legend!* The words hang in midair for a moment, bigger and louder than the Goodyear Blimp overhead, and then twenty thousand fans guffaw. Connors cracks a sly smile, nods, and hits a ball as a souvenir to the man who yelled.

Now the crowd erupts. A standing ovation.

Running on adrenaline and anger, I punk the legend in the final set, 6–1.

After the match, I tell reporters about my pre-match prediction, and then they tell Connors.

He says: I enjoy playing guys who could be my children. Maybe he's one of them. I spent a lot of time in Vegas.

In the semis I lose again to Lendl. I take him to a fourth set, but he's too strong. Trying to wear him out, I wear myself out. Despite the best efforts of Limping Lenny and Pat the Spitting Chilean, I'm not able to stay with a man of Lendl's caliber. I tell myself that when I get back to Vegas, the search must continue for someone, anyone, who can make me battle ready.

BUT NO ONE CAN MAKE me ready for the battle with the media, because it's not really a battle, it's a massacre. Each day brings another anti-Agassi screed in another magazine or newspaper. A dig from a fellow player. A diatribe from a sportswriter. A fresh piece of libel, served up as analysis. I'm a punk, I'm a clown, I'm a fraud, I'm a fluke. I have a high ranking because of a conspiracy, a cabal of networks and teenagers. I don't rate the attention I get because I haven't won a slam.

Millions of fans like me, apparently. I get potato sacks full of fan mail, including naked pictures of women with their phone numbers scrawled along the margin. And yet each day I'm vilified because of my look, because of my behavior, because of no reason at all. I absorb the role of villain-rebel, accept it, grow into it. The role seems like part of my job, so I play it. Before long, however, I'm being typecast. I'm to be the villain-rebel forever, in every match and every tournament.

I turn to Perry. I fly back east and visit him for a weekend. He's studying business at Georgetown. We go out for big dinners, and he takes me to his favorite local bar, the Tombs, and over beers he does what Perry has always done. He reshapes my anguish, makes it more logical and articulate. If I'm a returner, he's a reworder. First, he redefines the problem as a negotiation between me and the world. Then he clarifies the terms of the negotiation. He grants that it's horrible to be a sensitive person who's publicly excoriated every day, but he insists it's only temporary. There's a time limit to this torture. Things will get better, he says, the moment I start to win Grand Slams.

Win? What's the point? Why should winning change people's minds about me? Win or lose, I'll still be the same person. That's why I need to win? To shut people up? To satisfy a bunch of sportswriters and reporters who don't know me? Those are the terms of this negotiation?

PHILLY SEES THAT I'M SUFFERING, that I'm searching. He's searching too. He's been searching all his life, and recently he's stepped up the search. He tells me he's been going to a church, or a kind of church, in an office complex on the west side of Vegas. It's nondenominational, he says, and the pastor is different.

He drags me to the church and I have to admit, he's right, the pastor, John Parenti, is different. He wears jeans, a T-shirt and he has long, sandy-brown hair. He's more surfer than pastor. He's unconventional, which I respect. He's—no other way to say it—a rebel. I also like his prominent aquiline nose, his sad canine eyes. Above all, I like the casual vibe of his service. He simplifies the Bible. No ego, no dogma. Just common sense and clear thinking.

Parenti is so casual, he doesn't want to be called Pastor Parenti. He insists we call him J.P. He says he wants his church to feel unlike a church. He wants it to feel like a home where friends gather. He doesn't have any answers, he says. He just happens to have read the Bible a few dozen times, front to back, and he has some observations to share.

I think he has more answers than he's letting on. And I need answers. I consider myself a Christian, but J.P.'s church is the first one where I've felt truly close to God.

I attend with Philly every week. We time our arrival so that we walk in just as J.P. starts talking, and we always sit in the back, slouched low, so we don't get recognized. One Sunday Philly says he wants to meet J.P. I hang back. Part of me would like to meet J.P. too, but part of me is wary of strangers. I've always been shy, but the recent avalanche of bad press has made me borderline paranoid.

Days later I'm driving around Vegas, feeling gutted after reading the latest attacks on me. I find myself parked outside J.P.'s church. It's late, all the lights are off—except one. I peer in the window. A secretary is doing some paperwork. I knock at the door and tell the woman I need to speak with J.P. She says he's at home. She doesn't say, *Where you should be.* With a shaky voice I ask if she could please phone him. I really need to talk to him. To somebody. She dials J.P. and hands me the receiver.

Hello? he says.

Hi. Yes. You don't know me. My name is Andre Agassi, I'm a tennis player, and, well, it's just—

I know you. I've seen you in church the last six months. I recognized you, of course. I just didn't want to bother you.

I thank him for his discretion, for respecting my privacy. I haven't been getting that kind of respect lately. I say, Look, I wonder if we could spend some time together. Talk.

When?

Now?

Oh. Well, I guess I could come down to the office and meet you.

With all due respect, can I come to wherever you are? I have a fast car, and I think I can get there faster than you can get here.

He pauses. OK, he says.

I'm there in thirteen minutes. He meets me on his doorstep.

Thanks for agreeing to see me. I feel like I have nowhere else to turn.

What is it you need?

I wonder if we can just, um, get to know each other?

He smiles. Listen, he says, I don't do father figure real well.

I nod, laugh at myself. I say, Right, right. But maybe you could give me some assignments? Life assignments? Reading assignments?

Like a mentor?

Yeah.

I don't do mentor real well either.

Oh.

Talking, listening, fellowship—those things I can do.

I frown.

Look, J.P. says, my life is as screwed up as the next guy's. Maybe more. I can't offer much in the way of shepherding. I'm not that kind of pastor. If you're looking for advice, I'm sorry. If you're looking for a friend, that we can do, maybe.

I nod.

He holds open the door, asks if I'd like to come in. But I ask if he'd like to go for a drive. I think better when I drive.

He cranes his neck and sees my white Corvette. It looks like a small private plane parked in his driveway. The color drains a bit from his face.

I drive J.P. all over Vegas, up and down the Strip, then into the mountains that circle the town. I show him what the Vette can do, open up the engine on a lonely stretch of highway, then open up myself. I tell him my story, in a ragged and disorderly fashion, and he has Perry's knack for saying it all back to me, artfully reworded. He understands my contradictions, and reconciles a few of them.

You're a kid who still lives with his parents, he says, but you're known around the planet. That's got to be hard. You're trying to express yourself freely and creatively and artistically, and you're slammed at every turn. That's *very* hard.

I tell him about the knock on me, that I've snuck up on my high ranking, that I've never beaten anyone good, that I've been lucky. Horseshoe up my ass. He says I'm experiencing backlash, and never even got to enjoy the lash.

I laugh.

He says it must be bizarre to have strangers think they know me, and love me beyond reason, while others think they know me and resent me beyond reason—all while I'm a relative stranger to myself.

What makes it perverse, I tell him, is that it all revolves around tennis, and I hate tennis.

Right, sure. But you don't actually hate tennis.

Yes. Yes, I do.

I talk about my father. I tell J.P. about the yelling, the pressure, the rage, the abandonment. J.P. gets a funny look on his face. You do realize, don't you, that God isn't anything like your father? You know that—don't you?

I almost drive the Corvette onto the shoulder.

God, he says, is the opposite of your father. God isn't mad at you all the time. God isn't yelling in your ear, harping on your imperfections. That voice you hear all the time, that angry voice? That's not God. That's still your father.

I turn to him: Do me a favor? Say that again.

He does. Word for word.

Say it once more.

He does.

I thank him. I ask about his own life. He tells me that he hates what he does. He can't abide being a pastor. He no longer wants to be responsible for people's souls. It's a round-the-clock job, he says, and it leaves him no time for reading and reflection. (I wonder if this is a slight jab at me.) He's also hounded by death threats. Prostitutes and drug pushers come to his church and reform, and then their pimps and junkies and families, who've depended on that stream of income, blame J.P.

What do you think you'd like to do instead?

Actually, I'm a songwriter. A composer. I'd like to make music for a living.

He says he's written a song, When God Ran, that's a huge hit on the Christian charts. He sings a few bars. He has a nice voice and the song is moving.

I tell him that if he wants it bad enough, and works hard enough, he'll succeed.

When I start talking like a motivational speaker, I know I'm tired. I look at my watch. Three in the morning. Wow, I say, stifling a yawn, if you don't mind, can you just drop me off at my parents' house? I live right up here at the corner and I'm exhausted. I can't drive another minute. Take my car, take yourself home, bring it back to me when you can.

I don't want to take your car.

Why not? Fun car. Goes like the wind.

I see that. But what if I wreck it?

If you wreck it, as long as you're okay, I would laugh. I don't give a shit about the car.

How long do you want me to—I mean, when should I bring it back? Whenever.

He brings it back the next day.

Driving to church in this thing was awkward enough, he says, tossing me the keys. But, Andre, I officiate at funerals. You cannot drive up to a funeral in a white Corvette.

I INVITE J.P. TO MUNICH for Davis Cup. I look forward to Davis Cup, because it's not about me, it's about country. I imagine it's as close as I'll ever get to playing on a team, so I expect the trip to be a pleasant diversion, the matches to be easy, and I want to share the experience with my new friend.

Early on I find myself pitted against Becker, who's attained godlike status in West Germany. The fans are bringing down the house, twelve thousand Germans cheering his every swing, booing me. And yet I'm unfazed, because I'm in a zone. Maybe not *the* zone, but *my* zone. I can't miss. Also, I promised myself months ago that I'd never again lose to Becker, and I'm making good on that promise. I jump out to a two-set lead. J.P. and Philly and Nick are the only people cheering for me, and I can hear them. A fine day in Munich.

Then I lose my concentration, followed by my confidence. I drop a game and head for my chair during the changeover, discouraged.

Suddenly several German officials are gabbling at me. They're calling me back onto the court.

The game isn't over.

Come back, Mr. Agassi, *come back*.

Becker giggles. The audience roars with laughter.

I walk back onto the court, feeling my eyes throb. Once again I'm at the Bollettieri Academy, being humiliated by Nick in front of the other kids. I have enough trouble being laughed at in the press, but I can't handle being laughed at in person. I lose the game. I lose the match.

Showered, climbing into a car outside the arena, I ignore J.P. and turn to Nick and Philly. I tell them: The first person who talks to me about tennis is fired.

I SIT ON THE BALCONY of my Munich hotel room, alone, staring out over the city. Without thinking, I begin lighting things on fire. Paper, clothes, shoes. For years this has been one of my furtive ways of coping with extreme stress. I don't do it consciously. An impulse comes over me and I reach for the matches.

Just as I've got a small bonfire going, J.P. appears. He watches, then calmly adds a piece of hotel stationery to my bonfire. Then a napkin. I add the room-service menu. We feed the bonfire for fifteen minutes, neither of us saying a word. As the last flame dies down he asks, Do you want to go for a walk?

We wind our way through the beer gardens of downtown Munich. Everywhere we look, people are being boisterous, festive. They're drinking from one-liter tankards, singing and laughing. The laughter gives me the shakes.

We come to a large stone bridge with a cobblestone walkway. We cross. Far below is a rushing river. At the apex of the bridge we stop. No one is around. The singing and laughter have subsided. We hear nothing but the rushing water. I stare into the river and ask J.P.: What if I'm no good? What if today wasn't a bad day, but my best day? I'm always making excuses when I lose. I could have beaten him if such-and-such. *If* I'd wanted it. *If* I'd had my A game. *If* I'd gotten the calls. But what if I'm playing my best, and I care, and I want it, and I'm still not the best in the world?

Well—what if?

I think I'd rather die.

I lean against the railing, sobbing. J.P. has the decency, the wisdom, to say and do nothing. He knows there is nothing to say, nothing to do, but to wait for this fire to burn out.

I FACE CARL-UWE STEEB, another German, the following afternoon. Spent, physically and emotionally, I play Steeb exactly the wrong way. Yes, I'm attacking his backhand, which is his weakest shot, but I'm doing it with pace. If I were to give him no pace, he'd have to generate his own, and his backhand would be much weaker. His greatest flaw would be on display. Using my pace, however, he can hit a low slice that stays down on this fast surface. I'm making him better than he is, all because I'm trying to hit bigger than I need to, trying to be perfect. With a cordial smile Steeb accepts my gifts, settling into his legs and his Agassi-augmented backhand, having a marvelous time. Later, the captain of the Davis Cup team accuses me of tanking, as does a prominent sportswriter.

PART OF THE PROBLEM with my game in 1989 is my racket. I've always used a Prince, but Nick has convinced me to sign with a new company, Donnay. Why? Because Nick's got money troubles, and for delivering me to Donnay he gets a lucrative contract for himself.

Nick, I tell him—I love my Prince.

You could play with a broomstick, he says. It wouldn't matter.

Now, with the Donnay, I feel as if I *am* playing with a broomstick. I feel as if I'm playing left-handed, as if I've suffered a brain injury. Everything is slightly off. The ball doesn't listen to me. The ball doesn't do what I say.

I'm in New York, hanging out with J.P. It's well after midnight. We're sitting in a seedy deli with garish fluorescent lights and loud countermen arguing in several Eastern European languages. We're each having a cup of coffee and I'm holding my head in my hands, telling J.P. over and over: When I hit the ball with this new racket, I don't know where it's going.

You'll find a solution, J.P. says.

How? What?

I don't know. But you will. This is a momentary crisis, Andre. One of many. As sure as we're sitting here, there will be others. Bigger, smaller, and everything in between. Treat this crisis as practice for the next crisis.

And then the crisis is resolved *during* a practice. Days later, I'm in Florida, hitting at the Bollettieri Academy and someone hands me a new Prince. I hit three balls, just three, and it's something like a religious experience. Every ball goes like a laser to the spot where I want it to go. The court opens before me like Xanadu.

I don't care about any deals, I tell Nick. I can't sacrifice my life to a deal.

I'll handle it, he says.

He doctors a Prince racket, stencils it to look like a Donnay, and I cruise to several easy victories at Indian Wells. I lose in the quarters, but I don't care, because I have my racket back, my game back.

The next day, three Donnay execs descend on Indian Wells.

This is unacceptable, they say. It's clear to everyone that you're playing with a doctored Prince. You're going to ruin us. You're going to be liable for the destruction of our company.

Your racket is going to be liable for the destruction of me.

Seeing that I'm unrepentant, and not budging, the Donnay execs say they'll build me a better racket. They go away and duplicate a Prince, just as Nick did, but make it look more convincing. I take my faux Donnay to Rome and play a kid I recognize from juniors, Pete Something. Sampras, I think. Greek kid from California. When I played him in juniors, I beat him handily. I was ten, he was nine. The next time I saw him was some months ago, at a tournament. I can't recall which one. I was sitting on a beautiful grassy hill beside my hotel, just after winning my match. Philly and Nick were sitting alongside me. We were stretched out, enjoying the fresh air, and watching Pete, who'd just taken a beating in his match. He was on the hotel court for a post-match practice, and nearly every ball he hit looked bad. He missed three of every four swings. His backhand was awkward, and one-handed, which was new. Someone had tinkered with his backhand, and it was clearly going to cost him a career.

This guy will never make it on the tour, Philly said.

He'll be lucky to qualify into tournaments, I said.

Whoever did that to his game should be ashamed, Nick said.

They should be indicted, Philly said. He has all the physical gifts. He's six foot one, moves great, but someone has turned him into a mess. Someone is responsible for that shit. *Someone should pay.*

At first I was taken aback by Philly's vehemence. Then I realized: Philly was projecting. He was seeing himself in Pete. He knew what it was like to try and fail to make it on tour, particularly with an involuntary one-handed backhand. In Pete's plight, in Pete's fate, Philly saw his own.

Now, in Rome, I see that Pete has improved since that day, but not much. He has a big serve, but not extraordinary, not a Becker serve. He has a fast arm, good action, an easy motion, and comes close to his spots. He wants to ace you out wide, and when he misses it's not by much—he's not one of these players who try to ace you out wide and serve it by mistake into your chest. His real problem comes after his serve. He's inconsistent. He can't keep three balls in a row between the lines. I beat him, 6–2, 6–1, and as I walk off the court I think to myself that he's got a long and painful slog ahead. I feel bad for the guy. He seems like a good soul. But I don't expect to see him again on the tour, ever.

I go on to reach the final. I face Alberto Mancini. Strong, stocky, with tree-trunk legs, he pounds the ball with tremendous weight, penetration, and a tornado spin that causes it to hit your racket like a medicine ball. I have match point against him in the fourth set, but I lose the point— then fall apart. Somehow I lose the match.

Back in my hotel I sit in my room for hours, watching Italian TV, setting things on fire. People, I think, don't understand the pain of losing in a final. You practice and travel and grind to get ready. You win for one week, four matches in a row. (Or, at a slam, two weeks, six matches.) Then you lose that final match and your name isn't on the trophy, your name isn't in the record books. You lost only once, but you're a loser.

I go to the 1989 French Open and in the third round I face Courier, my schoolmate from the Bollettieri Academy. I'm the chalk, the heavy favorite, but Courier scores the upset, then rubs my nose in it. He pumps his fist, glares at me and Nick. Moreover, in the locker room, he makes sure everyone sees him lacing up his running shoes and going for a jog. Message: Beating Andre just didn't provide enough cardio.

Later, when Chang wins the tournament, and thanks Jesus Christ for making the ball go over the net, I feel sickened. How could Chang, of all people, have won a slam before me?

Again, I skip Wimbledon. I hear another chorus of jeers from the media. Agassi doesn't win the slams he enters, and then he skips the slams that matter most. But it feels like a drop in the ocean. I'm becoming desensitized.

EVEN THOUGH I'M A PUNCHING BAG for sportswriters, big companies beg me to pose with their products. In the middle of 1989 one of my corporate sponsors, Canon, schedules a series of photo shoots, including one in the wilds of Nevada, in the Valley of Fire. I like the sound of that. I walk every day through a valley of fire.

Since the ad campaign is for a camera, the director wants a colorful setting. Vivid, he says. Cinematic. He builds an entire tennis court in the middle of the desert, and as I watch the workmen I can't help thinking of my father building his tennis court in his desert. I've come a long way. Or have I?

For a full day the director films me playing tennis by myself, the flame-red mountains and orange rock formations in the background. I'm weary, sunburned, ready for a break, but the director isn't done with me. He tells me to take off my shirt. I'm known for taking off my shirt, in moments of teenage exuberance, and throwing it into crowds.

Then he wants to film me in a cave, hitting a ball at the camera, as if to shatter the lens.

Then, at Lake Mead, we film several scenes against the watery backdrop.

It all seems silly, goofy, but harmless.

Back in Vegas we do a series of shots on the Strip, then around a swimming pool. As luck would have it, they choose the pool at good old Cambridge Racquet Club. Finally, we set up for one last shot at a Vegas country club. The director puts me in a white suit, then has me drive up to the front portico in a white Lamborghini. Step out of the car, he says, turn to the camera, lower your black sunglasses, and say, *Image Is Everything.*

Image Is Everything?

Yes. Image Is Everything.

Between takes I look around and in the crowd of spectators I see Wendi, the former ballgirl, my childhood crush, all grown up. Now *she's* definitely come a long way since the Alan King tournament.

She's carrying a suitcase. She's just dropped out of college and she's just come home. You were the first person I wanted to see, she says.

She looks beautiful. Her brown hair is long, curly, and her eyes are impossibly green. She's all I can think about while the director is ordering me around. As the sun goes down, the director yells, Cut! That's a wrap! Wendi and I jump into my new Jeep, the doors and top off, and go roaring away like Bonnie and Clyde.

Wendi says, What was that slogan they kept making you say into the camera?

Image Is Everything.

What's that supposed to mean?

Beats me. It's for a camera company.

WEEKS LATER I BEGIN TO HEAR this slogan twice a day. Then six times a day. Then ten. It reminds me of those Vegas windstorms, the kind that begin with a faint, ominous rustling of leaves, and ultimately turn into high-pitched, gale-force, three-day blows.

Overnight the slogan becomes synonymous with me. Sportswriters liken this slogan to my inner nature, my essential being. They say it's my philosophy, my religion, and they predict it's going to be my epitaph. They say I'm nothing but image, I have no substance, because I haven't won a slam. They say the slogan is proof that I'm just a pitchman, trading on my fame, caring only about money and nothing about tennis. Fans at my matches begin taunting me with the slogan. *Come on, Andre—image is everything!* They yell this if I show any emotion. They yell it if I show no emotion. They yell it when I win. They yell it when I lose.

This ubiquitous slogan, and the wave of hostility and criticism and sarcasm it sets off, is excruciating. I feel betrayed—by the advertising agency, the Canon execs, the sportswriters, the fans. I feel abandoned. I feel the way I did when I arrived at the Bollettieri Academy.

The ultimate indignity, however, is when people insist that I've *called myself* an empty image, that I've proclaimed it, simply because I spoke the line in a commercial. They treat this ridiculous throwaway slogan as if it's my Confession, which makes as much sense as arresting Marlon Brando for murder because of a line he uttered in *The Godfather*.

As the ad campaign widens, as this insidious slogan creeps its way into every article about me, I change. I develop an edge, a mean streak. I stop giving interviews. I lash out at linesmen, opponents, reporters— even fans. I feel justified, because the world is against me, the world is trying to screw me. I'm becoming my father.

When crowds boo, when they yell, *Image is everything,* I yell back. *As much as you don't want me here, that's how much I don't want to be here!* In Indianapolis, after a particularly bad loss, and a sonorous booing, a reporter asks me what went wrong. You didn't seem like yourself today, he says with a smile that isn't a smile. Something bothering you?

I tell him, in so many words, to kiss my ass.

No one counsels me that you should never snap at reporters. No one bothers to explain that snapping, baring your fangs, makes reporters more rabid. Don't show them fear, but don't show them your fangs, either. Even if someone were to give me this sensible advice, I don't know that I could take it.

Instead I hide. I act like a fugitive, and my accomplices in seclusion are Philly and J.P. We go every night to an old coffee shop on the Strip, a place called the Peppermill. We drink bottomless cups of coffee and eat slabs of pie and talk and talk—and sing. J.P. has made the leap from pastor to composer-musician. He's moved to Orange County and rededicated his life to music. Along with Philly we belt out our favorite songs until the other customers at the Peppermill turn and stare.

J.P. is also a frustrated comedian, a devotee of Jerry Lewis, and he slips in and out of slapstick routines that leave Philly and me weak from laughter. We then try to out-slapstick J.P. We dance around the waitress, crawl along the floor, and eventually the three of us are laughing so hard that we can't breathe. I laugh more than I've laughed since I was a boy, and even though it's tinged with hysteria, the laughter has healing properties. For a few hours, late at night, laughter makes me feel like the old Andre, whoever that is.

10

NOT FAR FROM MY FATHER'S HOUSE is the sprawling concrete campus of the University of Nevada–Las Vegas, which in 1989 is gaining a reputation for its sports teams. The basketball squad is a powerhouse, with NBA-ready stars, and the football team is vastly improved. The Runnin' Rebels are known for their speed and superb conditioning. Plus, they're the Rebels—that's my kind of mascot. Pat says there might be someone at UNLV who can help me get in shape when he's not in town.

We drive to the campus one day and make our way to the gym, a new building that I find as daunting as the Sistine Chapel. So many perfect bodies. So many full-grown men. I'm five foot eleven, 148 pounds, and my Nike clothes hang off me. I tell myself this was a mistake. Apart from feeling woefully undersized, I still feel edgy in a school, any kind of school.

Pat, who am I kidding? I don't belong here.

We're here, he says, spitting.

We find the office of the school's strength coach. I tell Pat to wait, I'll go in and talk to the guy. I poke my head in the doorway, and there, across the office, in the far corner, behind a desk the size of my Corvette, I see a real-life giant. He looks like the statue of Atlas fronting Rockefeller Center, which I saw during my first U.S. Open, except this Atlas has long black hair and black eyes as large and round as the weights neatly stacked in the gym. He looks as if he'll flatten the first person who disturbs him.

I jump back through the doorway.

You go, Pat.

He walks in. I hear him say something. I hear a deep baritone rumble in response. It sounds like a truck engine. Then Pat calls to me.

I hold my breath and again go through the doorway.

Hello, I say.

Hello, the giant says.

Um, yeah, well, my name is Andre Agassi. I play tennis, and uhh, I live here in Vegas, and—

I know who you are.

He stands. He's six feet tall, with a chest at least fifty-six inches around. For a moment I think he might tip the desk over in anger. Instead he comes around from behind and extends his hand. The largest hand I've ever seen. A hand that goes with his shoulders, biceps, and legs, also record-setters in my personal experience.

Gil Reyes, he says.

Nice to meet you, Mr. Reyes.

Call me Gil.

OK. Gil. I know you must be very busy. I don't want to take up your time. I was just wondering—that is, Pat and I were wondering—if we could talk to you about using your facilities now and then. I'm really struggling to improve my conditioning.

Sure, he says. His voice makes me think of the bottom of the ocean and the core of the earth. But it's also a voice as soft as it is deep.

He shows us around, introduces us to several student-athletes. We talk about tennis, basketball, the differences, the similarities. Then the football team walks in.

Excuse me, Gil says. I need to speak with the fellas. Make yourself at home. Use whatever machines or weights you want to use. But please, be careful. And be discreet. Technically speaking, you know, it's against the rules.

Thank you.

Pat and I do a few bench presses, leg lifts, sit-ups, but I'm more interested in watching Gil. The football players gather before him and gaze up at him with awe. He's like a Spanish general addressing his conquistadors. He gives them their orders. You—take this bench. You—grab that machine. You—that squat rack. While he's speaking, no one looks away. He doesn't demand their attention, he simply compels it. Lastly, he tells them to gather round, closer, reminds them that hard work is the answer, the only answer. Everyone bring it in. Hands together. One two three—
Rebels!

They break, then fan out and hit the weights. I'm reminded how much better off I'd be on a team.

. . .

PAT AND I GO BACK to the gym at UNLV every day, and while doing curls and bench presses I can feel Gil keeping tabs on us. I sense that he's noting my bad form. I sense that the other athletes are noticing too. I feel amateurish, and often want to leave, but Pat always stops me.

After a few weeks, Pat needs to fly back east. Family emergency. I knock at the door to Gil's office and tell him that Pat is gone, but he left a regimen for me to follow. I hand Gil the piece of paper with Pat's regimen and ask if he might be willing to help me go through it.

Sure, Gil says. But he sounds put upon.

With each exercise, Gil arches an eyebrow. He looks over Pat's regimen, turns the paper in his hands, frowns. I encourage him to tell me what's on his mind, but he only frowns more deeply.

He asks, What's the point of this exercise?

I'm not sure.

Tell me again, how long have you been doing this?

Long time.

I beg him to speak his mind.

I don't want to step on anybody's toes, he says. I don't want to speak out of turn. But I can't lie to you: if somebody can write down your routine on a piece of paper, it isn't worth the piece of paper it's written on. You're asking me to put you through a workout here that leaves no room for where you are, how you're feeling, what you need to focus on. It doesn't allow for *change*.

That makes sense. Could you help me? Maybe give me some tips?

Well, look, what are your goals?

I tell him about my recent loss to Alberto Mancini, from Argentina. He out-physicalled me, pushed me around like an old-time bully at the beach kicking sand in my face. I had the match won, I had my foot on the man's neck, but I couldn't finish him off. I was serving for the match, and Mancini broke me, then won the tiebreak, then broke me three times in the fifth set. I had nothing left. I need to get strong so that I never let that happen again. Losing is one thing; being outgunned is another. I can't bear that feeling anymore.

Gil listens, not moving, not interrupting, soaking it all in.

That fuzzy ball takes some fuzzy bounces, I tell him, and I can't control it all the time. But one thing I think maybe I can control is my body. At least, I could, maybe, if I had the right information.

Gil fills his fifty-six-inch chest with air and then breathes out slowly. He says, What's your schedule?

I'll be gone the next five weeks. Summer hard courts. But when I get back, I'd really consider it an honor if we could work together.

All right, Gil says. We'll figure something out. Good luck on your road trip. I'll see you when you get back.

AT THE 1989 U.S. OPEN I play Connors again in the quarters. It's the first five-set win of my career, after five straight losses. Somehow it only earns me a new wave of criticism: I should have finished Connors off in three. Someone claims to have heard me yelling to Philly in my box: I'm going to take him five sets and give him some pain!

Mike Lupica, a columnist for the New York *Daily News*, points to my nineteen unforced errors in the third set and says I carried Connors merely to prove that I was tough enough to go the distance. If they're not trashing me for losing on purpose, they're ragging me for the way I win.

WHEN I WALK BACK INTO the gym, I see from Gil's face that he's been expecting me. We shake hands. The start of something.

He walks me over to the weight racks and tells me that many of the exercises I've been doing are wrong, dead wrong, but the way I've been doing them is worse. I'm courting disaster. I'm going to hurt myself.

He gives me a fast primer on the mechanics of the body, the physics and hydraulics and architecture of human anatomy. To know what your body wants, he says, to understand what it needs and what it doesn't, you need to be part engineer, part mathematician, part artist, part mystic.

I don't fare well in lectures, but if all lectures were like Gil's, I'd still be in school. I soak up every fact, every insight, confident that I'll never forget a single word.

It's amazing, Gil says, how many fallacies there are about the human body, how little we know about our own bodies. For instance: guys do incline benches for their upper pecs. It's not an efficient use of time, he says. I haven't done an incline in thirty years. Is it possible that my chest would be bigger if I did inclines?

No, sir.

The step-ups you're doing, the exercises where you hold a heavy weight on your back as you walk upstairs? You're asking for a catastrophic injury. You're lucky you haven't already ruined your knee.

How so?

It's all about angles, Andre. At one angle, you're engaging your quad. Fine, great. At another angle, you're engaging your knee, putting loads of pressure on that knee. Engage that knee too many times—it'll break off the engagement.

The best exercises, he says, exploit gravity. He tells me how to use gravity and resistance to break down a muscle, so it will come back stronger. He shows me how to do a proper, safe bicep curl. He walks me over to a dry-erase board and diagrams my muscles, arms, joints, tendons. He talks about a bow and arrow, shows me the pressure points along a bow as it's pulled taut, then uses this model to explain my back, why it hurts after matches and workouts.

I tell him about my spine, my spondylolisthesis, the vertebra that's out of sync. He jots a note, says he'll look up the condition in the medical books and learn all about it for me.

Bottom line, he says, if you keep doing what you're doing, you're going to have a short career. Big-time back problems, knee problems. Plus, keep doing curls the way I saw you doing them, you're going to have elbow problems.

While spelling it all out, Gil sometimes literally spells it out. He likes to emphasize a point by spelling the key word. He likes to break words down for me, crack them open, reveal the knowledge inside, like the meat inside a nut. *Calorie,* for instance. He says it comes from the Latin *calor,* which is a measure of heat. People think calories are bad, Gil says, but calories are just measures of heat, and we need heat. With food, you feed your body's natural furnace. How can that be bad? It's *when* you eat, *how much* you eat, the *choices* you make—that's what makes all the difference.

People think eating is bad, he says, but we need to stoke our internal fire.

Yes, I think. My internal fire needs stoking.

Speaking of heat, Gil mentions casually that he hates the warm weather. He can't bear it. He's unusually sensitive to high temperatures, and his idea of torture is sitting under the direct sun. He turns up the air-conditioning.

I make a note.

I tell him about running with Pat on Rattlesnake Hill, how I feel I've hit a plateau. He asks, How much do you run every day?

Five miles.

Why?

I don't know.

Have you ever run five miles in a match?

No.

How often in a match do you run more than five steps in one direction before stopping?

Not very.

I don't know anything about tennis, but it seems *to me* that, by the third step, you'd better be thinking about stopping. Otherwise you're going to hit the ball and keep running, which means you'll be out of position for your next shot. The trick is to throttle down, then hit, then slam on the brakes, then hustle back. The way I see it, your sport isn't about running, it's about starting and stopping. You need to focus on building the muscles necessary for starting and stopping.

I laugh and tell him that might be the smartest thing I've ever heard anyone say about tennis.

When it's time to lock up for the night, I help Gil clean the gym, turn off the lights. We sit in my car and talk. Eventually, he notices that my teeth are chattering.

Doesn't this fancy car have a heater?

Yes.

Why don't you turn it on?

Because you said you're sensitive to heat.

He stammers. He says he can't believe I remembered. And he can't bear to think I've been suffering all this time. He turns up the car heater full blast. We continue talking, and soon I notice that beads of sweat are forming on Gil's brow and upper lip. I turn off the heat and roll down the windows. We talk for another half hour, until he notices that I'm starting to turn blue. He turns on the heater full blast. In this way, back and forth, we talk, and demonstrate our respect for each other, until the early hours of the morning.

I tell Gil a little about my story. My father, the dragon, Philly, Perry. I tell him about being banished to the Bollettieri Academy. Then he tells me his story. He talks about growing up outside Las Cruces, New Mexico. His people were farmworkers. Pecans and cotton. Hard work. Wintertime, pick the pecans. Summertime, cotton. Then they moved to East L.A., and Gil grew up fast on the hard streets.

It was war, he says. I got shot. Still have the bullet hole in my leg. Also, I didn't speak English, only Spanish, so I'd sit in school, self-conscious, not talking. I learned English by reading Jim Murray in the *Los Angeles Times* and listening to Vin Scully calling Dodger games on the radio. I had a little transistor. KABC, every night. Vin Scully was my English teacher.

After mastering English, Gil decided to master the body God gave him.

He says, Only the strong survive, right? Well, we couldn't afford weights in our neighborhood, so we made our own. Guys who'd been in the joint showed us how. For instance, we filled coffee cans with cement, stuck them on the ends of a pole, and that's how we made a bench press. We used milk crates for the actual bench.

He tells me about getting his black belt in karate. He tells me about some of his twenty-two professional fights, including one in which he got his jaw shattered. But I wasn't knocked out, he says proudly.

When it's time to say goodnight, because the sky is growing lighter, I reluctantly shake Gil's hand and tell him I'll be back tomorrow.

I know, he says.

I WORK WITH GIL throughout the fall of 1989. The gains are big, and our bond is strong. Eighteen years older than I, Gil can tell that he's a father figure. On some level I also sense that I'm the son he never had. (He has three children, all daughters.) It's one of the few things that go unspoken between us. Everything else gets hashed out, spelled out.

Gil and his wife, Gaye, have a lovely tradition. Thursday nights, everyone in the family can order whatever they want for dinner and Gaye will cook it. One daughter wants hot dogs? Fine. Another wants chocolate chip pancakes? No problem. I make a habit of stopping by Gil's house on Thursdays, eating off everyone's plates. Before long I'm eating at Gil's every other night. When it's late, when I don't feel like driving home, I crash on his floor.

Gil has another tradition. No matter how uncomfortable a person looks, if they're asleep, they can't be all that uncomfortable, you should leave them be. So he never wakes me. He just throws a light afghan over me and lets me sleep until morning.

Listen, Gil says one day, we love having you here, you know that. But I have to ask. Good-looking kid, wealthy kid, kid who can be lots of places—and yet you come to my house for Thursday-night hot dogs. You sleep curled on my floor.

I like sleeping on floors. My back feels better.

I'm not talking about the floor. I mean, here. Are you sure you want to be—here? You must have better places to be.

Can't think of anywhere else I'd rather be, Gil.

He gives me a hug. I thought I knew what a hug was, but you've really never been hugged until you've been hugged by a man with a fifty-six-inch chest.

On Christmas Eve, 1989, Gil asks if I'd like to come over to the house, celebrate the holiday with his family.

Thought you'd never ask.

While Gaye bakes cookies, while their daughters are upstairs sleeping, Gil and I sit on the living-room floor putting together toys and train sets from Santa. I tell Gil that I don't know when I've felt so peaceful.

You wouldn't be happier at a party? With friends?

I'm right where I want to be.

I stop putting together the toy in my hand and fix Gil with a look. I tell him my life has never for one day belonged to me. My life has always belonged to someone else. First, my father. Then Nick. And always, always, tennis. Even my body wasn't my own until I met Gil, who is doing the one thing fathers are supposed to do. Making me stronger.

So being here, Gil, with you and your family, I feel for the first time in my life that I'm where I belong.

Enough said. I'll never ask again. Merry Christmas, son.

11

IF I MUST PLAY TENNIS, the loneliest sport, then I'm sure as hell going to surround myself with as many people as I can off the court. And each person will have his specific role. Perry will help with my disordered thoughts. J.P. will help with my troubled soul. Nick will help with the basics of my game. Philly will help with details, arrangements, and always have my back.

Sportswriters rip me about my *entourage*. They say I travel with all these people because it feeds my ego. They say I need this many people around me because I can't be alone. They're half right. I don't like to be alone. But these people around me aren't an entourage, they're a team. I need them for company, for counsel, and for a kind of rolling education. They're my crew, but also my gurus, my blue-ribbon panel. I study them and steal from them. I take an expression from Perry, a story from J.P., an attitude or gesture from Nick. I learn about myself, create myself, through imitation. How else could I do it? I spent my childhood in an isolation chamber, my teen years in a torture chamber.

In fact, rather than make my team smaller, I want to grow it. I want to add Gil, formally. I want to hire him, full-time, to help me with my strength and conditioning. I phone Perry at Georgetown and tell him my problem.

What problem? he says. You want to work with Gil? So hire Gil.

But I've got Pat. The Spitting Chilean. I can't just *fire* the guy. I can't fire anyone. And even if I could, how do I then ask Gil to leave a high-profile, high-paying job with UNLV—to work exclusively for me? Who the fuck am I?

Perry tells me to have Nick reassign Pat to work with the other tennis players Nick coaches. Then, he says, sit down with Gil and put it to him. Let him decide.

In January 1990 I ask Gil if he would do me the great honor of working with me, traveling with me, training me.

Leave my job here at UNLV?

Yes.

But I don't know anything about tennis.

Don't worry, I don't either.

He laughs.

Gil, I think I can accomplish a lot. I think I can do—*things.* But after our short time together, I'm reasonably certain that I can only do them with your help.

He doesn't need a hard sell. Yes, he says. I would like to work with you.

He doesn't ask how much I'll pay him. He doesn't mention the word *money.* He says we're two kindred spirits, embarking on a great adventure. He says he's known it almost from the day we met. He says I have a destiny. He says I'm like Lancelot.

Who's that?

Sir Lancelot. You know, King Arthur. Knights of the Round Table. Lancelot was Arthur's greatest knight.

Did he kill dragons?

Every knight kills dragons.

There is only one obstacle in our path. Gil doesn't have a gym at his house. He'll need to convert his garage into a full-scale gym—which will take lots of time, because he wants to build the weight machines himself.

Build them?

I want to weld the metal, make the ropes and pulleys, with my own hands. I don't want to leave anything to chance. I won't have you injured. Not on my watch.

I think of my father, building his ball machines and blowers, and wonder if this is the one and only thing he and Gil have in common.

Until Gil's gym is complete, we continue to work out at UNLV. He keeps his job, works with the Rebels basketball team through a brilliant season, culminating in a blowout win over Duke for the national title. When his duties are done, when his home gym is *almost* done, Gil says he's ready.

Andre, now, are *you* ready? One last time, are you sure you want to do this?

Gil, I am more sure about this than I've ever been about anything I've ever done.

Me too.

He says he's going to drive to the college this morning and turn in his keys.

Hours later, as he walks outside the college, there I am, waiting. He laughs when he sees me, and we go for cheeseburgers, to celebrate new beginnings.

SOMETIMES A WORKOUT WITH GIL is actually a conversation. We don't touch a single weight. We sit on the free benches and free-associate. There are many ways, Gil says, of getting strong, and sometimes talking is the best way. When he's not teaching me about my body, I'm teaching him about tennis, the life on tour. I tell him how the game is organized, the circuit of minor tournaments and the four majors, or Grand Slams, that all players use as yardsticks. I tell him about the tennis calendar, how we start the year on the other side of the world, at the Australian Open, and then just chase the sun. Next comes clay season, in Europe, which culminates in Paris with the French Open. Then comes June, grass season, and Wimbledon. I stick out my tongue and make a face. Then come the dog days, the hard-court season, which concludes with the U.S. Open. Then the indoor season—Stuttgart, Paris, the World Championships. It's all very *Groundhog Day*. Same venues, same opponents, only the years and scores are different, and over time the scores all run together like phone numbers.

I try to tell Gil about my psyche. I start at the beginning, the central truth.

He laughs. You don't actually *hate* tennis, he says.

I do, Gil, I really do.

He gets a look on his face, and I wonder if he's thinking he might have quit his job at UNLV too soon.

If that's true, he says, why play?

I'm not suited for anything else. I don't know how to do anything else. Tennis is the only thing I'm qualified for. Also, my father would have a fit if I did anything different.

Gil scratches his ear. This is a new one on him. He's known hundreds of athletes, but he's never known one who hated athletics. He doesn't know what to say. I reassure him that there's nothing to be said. I don't understand it myself. I can only tell him how it is.

I also tell Gil about the *Image Is Everything* debacle. I feel, somehow, that he needs to know, so he'll understand what he's got himself into. The whole thing still makes me angry, but now the anger has seeped down deep. Hard to talk about, hard to reach. It feels like a spoonful of acid in the pit of my stomach. Hearing about it, Gil feels angry too, but he has less trouble accessing his anger. He wants to act on it, right now. He wants to punch out an advertising exec or two. He says: Some slap-dick on Madison Avenue puts together a silly ad campaign, and gets you to say a line into a camera, and it means something about you?

Millions of people think so. And say so. And write so.

They took advantage of you, he says. Plain and simple. Not your fault. You didn't know what you were saying, you didn't know how it would be taken and twisted and misinterpreted.

Our talks carry beyond the weight room. We go out for dinner. We go out for breakfast. We're on the phone six times a day. I call Gil late one night and we talk for hours. As the conversation winds down he says, Do you want to come over tomorrow and get in a workout?

I'd love to, but I'm in Tokyo.

We've been talking for three hours and you're in Tokyo? I thought you were across town. I feel guilty, man. I've been keeping you all this—.

He stops himself. He says, You know what? I don't feel guilty. Nah. I feel honored. You needed to talk to me, and it doesn't matter if you're in Tokyo or Timbuktu. I get it. All right, man, I get it.

From the start, Gil keeps a careful record of my workouts. He buys a brown ledger and marks down every rep, every set, every exercise—every day. He records my weight, my diet, my pulse, my travel. In the margins he draws diagrams and even pictures. He says he wants to chart my progress, compile a database he can refer to in the coming years. He's making a study of me, so he can rebuild me from the ground up. He's like Michelangelo appraising a block of marble, but he's not put off by my flaws. He's like da Vinci getting it all down in his notebooks. I see in Gil's notebooks, in the care he takes with them, in the way he never skips a day, that I inspire him, and this inspires me.

It goes without saying that Gil will travel with me to many tournaments. He needs to watch my conditioning in matches, monitor my food, make sure I'm always hydrated. (But not just hydrated. Gil has a special concoction of water, carbs, salt, and electrolytes that I need to drink the night before every match.) His training doesn't end on the road. If anything, it becomes more important on the road.

Our first trip together, we agree, will be February 1990, to Scottsdale. I tell Gil we'll need to be there a couple of nights before the tournament starts, for the hit-and-giggle.

Hit-and-what?

It's an exhibition with some celebrities to raise money for charity, to make corporate sponsors feel good, to entertain the fans.

Sounds fun.

What's more, I tell him, we're going to drive over in my new Corvette. I can't wait to show him how fast it goes.

But when I pull up to Gil's house I realize that I might not have thought this all the way through. The car is very small, and Gil is very big. The car is so small that it makes Gil look twice as big. He contorts himself to fit into the passenger side, and even then he needs to tilt sideways, and even then his head touches the roof. The Corvette looks as if, at any moment, it might burst apart.

Seeing Gil squished and uncomfortable, I'm motivated to go very fast. Of course I don't need extra motivation in the Corvette. The car is supersonic. We crank the music and fly out of Vegas, across Hoover Dam, down toward the craggy Joshua tree forests of northwest Arizona. We decide to stop for lunch outside Kingman. The prospect of food, combined with the speed of the Corvette, and the loud music, and the presence of Gil, makes me mash the gas. We hit Mach 1. I see Gil make a face and twirl a finger. I look in the rearview mirror—a highway patrol car inches from my back fender.

The patrolman quickly gives me a speeding ticket.

Not my first, I tell Gil, who shakes his head.

In Kingman we stop at Carl's Jr. and eat an enormous lunch. We both love to eat, and we both have a secret weakness for fast food, so we fall off the nutrition wagon, ordering French fries, then ordering seconds, refilling our sodas. When I squeeze Gil back into the Corvette I realize we're well behind schedule. We need to make up time. I floor it and zoom back onto U.S. 95. Two hundred miles to Scottsdale. Two hours of driving.

Twenty minutes later, Gil makes the same twirling gesture.

A different patrolman this time. He takes my license and registration and asks, Have you received a speeding ticket recently?

I look at Gil. He frowns.

Well, if you consider an hour ago recent, then yes, Officer, I have.

Wait right here.

He walks back to his car. One minute later, he returns.

The judge wants you back in Kingman.

Kingman? What?

Come with me, sir.

Come with—what about the car?

Your friend can drive it.

But, but, can't I just follow you?

Sir, you are going to listen to everything I say and do everything I say and that's why you're not going back to Kingman in handcuffs. You will sit in the back of my car and your friend will follow us. Now. Step out.

I'm in the back of a police car, Gil following in a Corvette that fits him like a whalebone corset. We're in the middle of nowhere and I'm hearing the crazy-ass plinking banjos from *Deliverance*. It takes forty-five minutes to reach Kingman Municipal Court. I follow the patrolman into a side door and find myself before the small, elderly judge, who wears a cowboy hat and a belt buckle the size of a pie tin.

The banjos are getting louder.

I look around for a certificate on the wall, something to prove that this is in fact a courthouse and he's a real judge. All I see are heads of dead animals.

The judge begins by rattling off a series of random questions.

You're playing in Scottsdale?

Yes, sir.

You've played that tournament before?

Uh—yes, sir.

What kind of draw do you have?

Pardon?

Who do you play in the first round?

The judge, it turns out, is a tennis fan. Also, he's followed my career closely. He thinks I should've beaten Courier at the French Open. He has a slew of opinions about Connors, Lendl, Chang, the state of the game, the scarcity of great American players. After sharing his opinions with me, liberally, for twenty-five minutes, he asks, Would you mind signing something for my kids?

No problem, sir. Your honor.

I sign everything he puts before me, then await sentencing.

All right, the judge says. I sentence you to go give 'em hell down in Scottsdale.

Sorry? I don't under— . I mean, your honor, I drove back here, thirty-some miles, sure I was going to be sent to jail, or at least fined.

No! No, no, no, I just wanted to meet you. But you'd better have your friend out there drive you to Scottsdale, because one more ticket today and I will have to keep you in Kingman until the cows come home.

I walk out of the courthouse but sprint to the Corvette, where Gil is waiting. I tell him the judge is a tennis buff who wanted to meet me. Gil thinks I'm lying. I beg him to please just drive us away from this court-house. He pulls away—slowly. Under normal circumstances, Gil is a cautious driver. But so unnerved is he by our run-in with Arizona law enforcement that he keeps the car in sixth gear and goes fifty-four miles per hour all the way to Scottsdale.

Naturally I'm late to the hit-and-giggle. As we roll into the parking lot of the stadium, I pull on my tennis gear. We stop at the security hut and tell the guard I'm expected, I'm one of the players. He doesn't believe me. I show him my driver's license, which I feel fortunate to still have in my possession. He waves our car through.

Gil says, Don't worry about the car, I'll take care of it. Just go.

I grab my tennis bag and sprint through the parking lot. Gil tells me later that when I entered the arena, he heard the applause. The windows of the Corvette were rolled up, but he still heard the crowd. In that moment he had a sense of what I'd been trying to tell him. After the command performance for the Old West judge, after hearing the stadium greet my arrival with a frenzied roar, he understood. He confesses that until this trip, he didn't realize the life was so—*insane*. He really didn't know what he was signing on for. I tell him that makes two of us.

WE HAVE A WONDERFUL TIME in Scottsdale. We learn about each other, fast, the way you learn about people on the road. During one mid-day match I halt play and wait for a tournament official to hurry an umbrella over to where Gil is sitting. He's in direct sunlight, perspiring fiercely. When the official hands Gil the umbrella, Gil looks confused. Then he looks down, sees me waving, understands. He flashes a fifty-six-inch smile, and we both laugh.

We go to dinner one night at the Village Inn. It's late, we're eating a combo platter of dinner and breakfast. Four guys burst into the restaurant and sit one booth away. They talk and laugh about my hair, my clothes.

Probably gay, one says.

Definitely homo, says his buddy.

Gil clears his throat, wipes his mouth with a paper napkin, tells me to enjoy the rest of my meal. He's done.

Aren't you going to eat, Gilly?

No, man. Last thing I want during a fight is a full stomach.

When I'm finished, Gil says he has some business to take care of at the next table. If anything happens, he says, I shouldn't worry—he knows the way home. He stands very slowly. He sidles over to the four guys. He leans on their table. The table groans. He fans his chest in their faces and says, You enjoy ruining people's meals? That's how you like to spend your time, huh? Gee, I'm going to have to try that myself. What are you having there? Hamburger?

He picks up the man's burger and eats half in one bite.

Needs ketchup, Gil says, his mouth full. You know what? Now I'm thirsty. I think I'll take a sip of your soda. Yeah. And then I think I'll spill it all over the table as I set it down. I want—*I want*—one of you to try to stop me.

Gil takes a long sip, then slowly, almost as slowly as he drives, pours the rest of the soda over the table.

Not one of the four guys moves.

Gil sets down the empty glass and looks at me. Andre, are you ready to go?

I DON'T WIN THE TOURNAMENT, but it doesn't matter. I'm content, happy as we start back on the road to Vegas. Before leaving town we stop for a bite at Joe's Main Event. We talk about all that's happened in the last seventy-two hours, and we agree that this trip feels like the start of a bigger trip. In his da Vinci notebook Gil draws a picture of me in handcuffs.

Outside, we stand in the parking lot and look at the stars. I feel such overwhelming love, and gratitude, for Gil. I thank him for all he's done, and he tells me I never need to thank him again.

Then he gives a speech. Gil, who learned English from newspapers and baseball games, delivers a flowing, lilting, poetic monologue, right outside Joe's, and one of the great regrets of my life is that I don't have a tape recorder with me. Still, I remember it nearly word for word.

Andre, I won't ever try to change you, because I've never tried to change anybody. If I could change somebody, I'd change myself. But I know I can give you structure and a blueprint to achieve what you want. There's a difference between a plow horse and a racehorse. You don't treat them the same. You hear all this talk about treating people equally, and I'm not sure equal means the same. As far as I'm concerned, you're a racehorse, and I'll always treat you accordingly. I'll be firm, but fair. I'll lead, never push. I'm not one of those people who expresses or articulates feelings very well, but from now on, just know this: It's on, man. It is *on*. You know what I'm saying? We're in a fight, and you can count on me until the last man is standing. Somewhere up there is a star with your name on it. I might not be able to help you find it, but I've got pretty strong shoulders, and you can stand on my shoulders while you're looking for that star. You hear? For as long as you want. Stand on my shoulders and reach, man. Reach.

12

AT THE 1990 FRENCH OPEN I make headlines by wearing pink. It's on the front page of the sports pages, and in some cases the news pages. *Agassi in the Pink.* Specifically, pink compression pants under acid-washed shorts. I tell reporters: It's not pink, it's technically Hot Lava. I'm astonished by how much they care. I'm astonished by how much I care that they get it right. But my feeling is, let them write about the color of my shorts rather than the flaws in my character.

Gil and Philly and I don't want to deal with the press, the crowds, Paris. We don't enjoy feeling alien, getting lost, having people stare at us because we speak English. So we lock ourselves in my hotel room, turn up the air-conditioning and send out for McDonald's and Burger King.

Nick, however, gets a nasty case of cabin fever. He wants to go out, see the sights. Guys, he says, we're in Paris! Eiffel Tower? The frickin' Louvre?

Been there, done that, Philly says.

I don't want to go near the Louvre. And I don't have to. I can close my eyes and see the scary painting of the man hanging from the cliff while his father clutches at his neck and his other loved ones hang from his limbs.

I tell Nick, I don't want to see anything or anyone. I just want to win this fucking thing and go home.

I MARCH THROUGH THE EARLY ROUNDS, playing well, and then run into Courier again. He wins the first set in a tiebreak but falters and gives me the second. I take the third and then, in the fourth, he curls up and dies, 6–0. His face turns red. His face turns Hot Lava. I want to tell him: I hope that was enough cardio for you. But I don't. Maybe I'm maturing. Without question I'm getting stronger.

Next up is Chang. The defending champ. I play with a chip on my shoulder, because I still can't believe he's won a slam before me. I envy his work ethic, admire his court discipline—but I just don't like the guy. He continues to say without compunction that Christ is on his side of the court, a blend of egotism and religion that chafes me. I beat him in four.

In the semis I play Jonas Svensson. He has a massive serve that kicks like a mule, and he's never afraid to come to the net. He plays better on fast surfaces, however, so I feel good about catching him on the clay. Since he has a big, looping forehand, I decide early that I'm going to bum-rush his backhand. Again and again I go to that vulnerable backhand, seizing a quick lead, 5–1. Svensson doesn't recover. Set, Agassi. In the second set I grab a 4–0 lead. He breaks back to 3–4. That's as close as I let him get. To his credit, he finds a ray of confidence and wins the third set. Normally I'd be rattled. But this year I look to my box and see Gil. I replay his parking lot speech, and win the fourth set, 6–3.

I'm in the final—at last. My first final at a slam. I'm facing Gómez, from Ecuador, whom I just beat weeks ago. He's thirty, on the verge of retiring—in fact, I thought he *was* retired. At last, the newspapers say, Agassi is going to realize his potential.

THEN, CATASTROPHE STRIKES. The night before the final, I'm taking a shower and I feel the hairpiece Philly bought me suddenly disintegrate in my hands. I must have used the wrong kind of conditioner. The weave is coming undone—the damned thing is falling apart.

In a state of abject panic I summon Philly to my hotel room.

Fucking disaster, I tell him. My hairpiece—look!

He examines it.

We'll let it dry, then clip it in place, he says.

With what?

Bobby pins.

He runs all over Paris looking for bobby pins. He can't find any. He phones me and says, What the hell kind of city is this? No bobby pins?

In the hotel lobby he bumps into Chris Evert and asks her for bobby pins. She doesn't have any. She asks why he needs them. He doesn't answer. At last he finds a friend of our sister Rita, who has a bag full of bobby pins. He helps me reconfigure the hairpiece and set it in place, and keeps it there with no fewer than twenty bobby pins.

Will it hold? I ask.

Yeah, yeah. Just don't move around a lot.

We both laugh darkly.

Of course I could play without my hairpiece. But after months and months of derision, criticism, mockery, I'm too self-conscious. *Image Is Everything?* What would they say if they knew I've been wearing a hairpiece all this time? Win or lose, they wouldn't talk about my game. They would talk only about my hair. Instead of a few kids at the Bollettieri Academy laughing at me, or twelve thousand Germans at Davis Cup, the whole world would be laughing. I can close my eyes and almost hear it. And I know I can't take it.

WARMING UP BEFORE THE MATCH, I pray. Not for a win, but for my hairpiece to stay on. Under normal circumstances, playing in my first final of a slam, I'd be tense. But my tenuous hairpiece has me catatonic. Whether or not it's slipping, I imagine that it's slipping. With every lunge, every leap, I picture it landing on the clay, like a hawk my father shot from the sky. I can hear a gasp going up from the crowd. I can picture millions of people suddenly leaning closer to their TVs, turning to each other and in dozens of languages and dialects saying some version of: Did Andre Agassi's *hair* just fall off?

My game plan for Gómez reflects my jangled nerves, my timidity. Knowing he doesn't have young legs, knowing he'll fold in a fifth set, I plan to stretch out the match, orchestrate long rallies, grind him down. As the match begins, however, it's clear that Gómez also knows his age, and thus he's trying to speed everything up. He's playing quick, risky tennis. He wins the first set in a hurry. He loses the second set, but also in a hurry. Now I know that the longest we'll be out here is three hours, rather than four, which means conditioning won't play a role. This is now a shot-making match, the kind Gómez can win. With two sets completed, and not much time off the clock, I'm facing a guy who's going to be fresh throughout, even if we go five.

Of course my game plan was fatally flawed from the start. Pathetic, really. It couldn't work, no matter how long the match, because you can't win the final of a slam by playing not to lose, or waiting for your opponent to lose. My attempt to orchestrate long rallies merely emboldens Gómez. He's a veteran who knows this might be his last shot at a slam. The only way to beat him is to take away his belief and his desire, by being aggressive. When he sees me playing conservative, orchestrating instead of dominating, it gives him heart.

He wins the third set. As the fourth set begins I realize I've made yet another miscalculation. Most players, when they tire late in a match, lose some zip on their serve. They have trouble getting up high on tired legs. But Gómez has a slingshot serve. He never gets up high on his legs. He leans into the ball. When he tires, therefore, he leans that much more, and his natural slingshot action becomes more pronounced. I've been waiting for his serve to weaken, and instead it's getting sharper.

Upon winning the match, Gómez is exceedingly gracious and charming. He weeps. He waves to the cameras. He knows he'll be a national hero in his native Ecuador. I wonder what it's like in Ecuador. Maybe I'll move there. Maybe that's the only place I'll be able to hide from the shame I feel at this moment. I sit in the locker room, head bowed, imagining what the hundreds of columnists and headline writers will say, not to mention my peers. I can hear them now. Image Is Everything, Agassi Is Nothing. Mr. Hot Lava Is a Hot Mess.

Philly walks in. I see in his eyes that he doesn't just sympathize—he lives it. This was his defeat too. He aches. Then he says the right thing, striking the right tone, and I know I'll always love him for it.

Let's get the fuck outta this town.

GIL PUSHES THE BIG TROLLEY with our bags through Charles de Gaulle Airport. I'm walking a step ahead. I stop to look at the Arrivals and Departures. Gil keeps going. The trolley has a sharp metal edge, and it pushes into my soft, exposed Achilles—I'm wearing loafers with no socks. A jet of my blood spurts onto the glassy floor. Then another. The Achilles is gushing. Gil hurries to get a bandage out of his bag, but I tell him to relax, take his time. It's good, I say. It's fitting. There should be a pint of my blood from my Achilles' heel on the floor before we leave Paris.

I SKIP WIMBLEDON AGAIN, train hard with Gil all summer. His home garage is finished, filled with a dozen handmade machines and many other unique touches. In the window he's mounted a massive air-conditioner. On the floor he's nailed a spongy Astroturf. And in the corner he's put an old pool table. We shoot nine-ball between reps and sets. Many nights we're in the gym until four in the morning, Gil searching for new ways to build up my mind, my confidence, along with my body. He's shaken by the French Open, as am I. One morning, before the sun comes up, he passes along some words his mother always tells him.

Qué lindo es soñar despierto, he says. How lovely it is to dream while you are awake. Dream while you're awake, Andre. Anybody can dream while they're asleep, but you need to dream all the time, and say your dreams out loud, and believe in them.

In other words, when in the final of a slam, I must dream. I must play to win.

I thank him. I give him a gift. It's a necklace with a gold pyramid, and inside the pyramid are three hoops. It represents the Father, the Son, and the Holy Ghost. I designed it, had a jeweler in Florida make it for me, and I have an earring that matches.

He puts it around his neck, and I can tell it will be a cold day in hell before he takes it off.

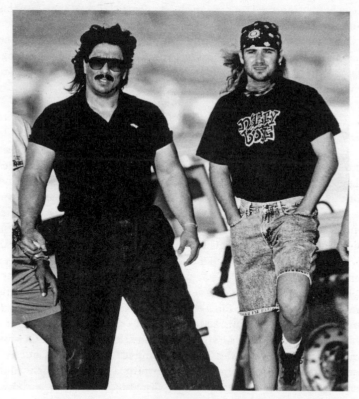

With Gil in the desert outside Las Vegas, not long after we started working together full-time in 1990

Gil likes to yell at me when I'm working out, but it's nothing like my father's yelling. Gil yells love. If I'm trying to set a new personal best, if I'm preparing to lift more than I've ever lifted, he stands in the background and yells, *Come on, Andre! Let's go! Big Thunder!* His yelling makes my heart club against my ribs. Then, for an added dash of inspiration, he'll sometimes tell me to step aside, and he'll lift his personal best—550 pounds. It's an awesome sight to see a man put that much iron above his chest, and it always makes me think that anything is possible. How beautiful to dream. But dreams, I tell Gil, in one of our quiet moments, are so damned tiring.

He laughs.

I can't promise you that you won't be tired, he says. But please know this. There's a lot of good waiting for you on the other side of tired. Get yourself tired, Andre. That's where you're going to know yourself. On the other side of tired.

Under Gil's care and close supervision I pack on ten pounds of muscle by August 1990. We go to New York for the U.S. Open and I feel lean and rangy and dangerous. I take out Andrei Cherkasov, from the Soviet Union, in an easy three-setter. I punch and scratch my way to the semis, beat Becker in four furious sets, and still have plenty of rocket fuel in my tank. Gil and I drive back to the hotel and watch the other men's semi to see who I'll get tomorrow. McEnroe or Sampras.

It doesn't seem possible, but the kid I thought I'd never see again has reconstituted his game. And he's giving McEnroe the fight of his life. Then I realize he's not giving McEnroe a fight—McEnroe is giving him a fight, and losing. My opponent tomorrow, incredibly, will be Pete.

The camera moves close on Pete's face, and I see that he has nothing left. Also, the commentators say his heavily taped feet are covered with blisters. Gil makes me drink Gil Water until I'm ready to throw up, and then I go to bed with a smile, thinking about all the fun I'm going to have, running Pete's ass off. I'll have him sprinting from side to side, left to right, from San Francisco to Bradenton, until those blisters bleed. I think of my father's old maxim: *Put a blister on his brain.* Calm, fit, cocksure, I sleep like a pile of Gil's dumbbells.

In the morning I feel ready to play a ten-setter. I have no hairpiece issues—because I'm not wearing my hairpiece. I'm using a new, low-maintenance camouflaging system that involves a thicker headband and brightly colored highlights. There's simply no way I can lose to Pete, that hapless kid I watched with sympathy last year, that poor klutz who couldn't keep the ball in the court.

Then a different Pete shows up. A Pete who doesn't ever miss. We're playing long points, demanding points, and he's flawless. He's reaching everything, hitting everything, bounding back and forth like a gazelle. He's serving bombs, flying to the net, bringing his game right to me. He's laying wood to my serve. I'm helpless. I'm angry. I'm telling myself: This is not happening.

Yes, this is happening.

No, this cannot be happening.

Then, instead of thinking how I can win, I begin to think of how I can avoid losing. It's the same mistake I made against Gómez, with the same result. When it's all over I tell reporters that Pete gave me a good old-fashioned New York street mugging. An imperfect metaphor. Yes, I was robbed. Yes, something that belonged to me was taken away. But I can't fill out a police report, and there is no hope of justice, and everyone will blame the victim.

HOURS LATER MY EYES FLY OPEN. I'm in bed at the hotel. It was all a dream. For a splendid half second I believe that I must have fallen asleep on that breezy hill while Philly and Nick were laughing about Pete's ruined game. I dreamed that Pete, of all people, was beating me in the final of a slam.

But no. It's real. It happened. I watch the room slowly grow lighter, and my mind and spirit grow palpably darker.

13

EVER SINCE WENDI CAME to watch me film the *Image Is Everything* commercial, she and I have been a couple. She travels with me, takes care of me. We're a perfect match, because we grew up together, and we figure we can keep growing up together. We come from the same place, want the same things. We love each other madly, though we agree that ours should be an *open* relationship—her word. She says we're too young to make a commitment, too confused. She doesn't know who she is. She grew up Mormon, then decided she didn't believe the tenets of that religion. She went to college, then discovered that it was the completely wrong college for her. Until she knows who she is, she says, she can't give herself to me completely.

In 1991 we're in Atlanta with Gil, celebrating my twenty-first birthday. We're in a bar, a seedy old place in Buckhead, with cigarette-scorched pool tables and plastic beer mugs. The three of us are laughing, drinking, and even Gil, who never touches the stuff, is letting himself get tipsy. To record this night for posterity, Wendi has brought her camcorder. She hands it to me and tells me to film her shooting baskets at one of those tented arcade games. She's going to school me, she says. I film her shooting for three seconds and then let the camera pan slowly down her body.

Andre, she says, please get the camera off my ass.

In comes a mob of loudmouths. Roughly my age, they look like a local football or rugby team. They make several rude remarks about me, then focus their attention on Wendi. They're drunk, crude, trying to embarrass me in front of her. I think of Nastase, doing the same thing fourteen years ago.

The rugby team slaps a stack of quarters on the edge of our pool table. One of them says, We got next. They walk off, smirking.

Gil puts down his plastic mug, picks up the quarters, and walks slowly to a vending machine. He buys a bag of peanuts and comes back to the table. Slowly he works his way through the peanuts, never taking his eyes off the rugby players, until they wisely decide to try another bar.

Wendi giggles and suggests that, in addition to his many functions and duties, Gil should be my bodyguard.

He already is, I tell her. And yet that word doesn't cut it. That word isn't adequate to what he is. Gil guards my body, my head, my game, my heart, my girlfriend. He's the one immovable object in my life. He's my life guard.

I particularly enjoy when people—reporters, fans, kooks—ask Gil if he's my bodyguard. A smile always plays across his lips as he says, Touch him and find out.

At the 1991 French Open I batter my way through six rounds and reach the final. My third slam final. I'm facing Courier, and I'm favored. Everyone says I'll beat him. I say I'll beat him. I *need* to beat him. I can't imagine what it would feel like to make three slam finals in a row and not win.

The good news is, I know how to beat Courier. I beat him just last year at this same tournament. The bad news is, it's personal, which makes me tight. We began in the same place, in the same barracks at the Bollettieri Academy, our bunk beds a few feet apart. I was so much better than Courier, so much more favored by Nick, that losing to him in the final of a slam will feel like the hare losing to the tortoise. Bad enough that Chang has won a slam before me. And Pete. But Courier too? I can't let that happen.

I come out playing to win. I've learned from my mistakes at the last two slams. I cruise through the first set, winning 6–3, and in the second set, leading 3–1, I have break point. If I win this point I'll have a choke hold on the set and match. Suddenly the rain starts to fall. Fans cover themselves and run for shelter. Courier and I retreat to the locker room, where we both pace like caged lions. Nick comes in and I look to him for advice, encouragement, but he says nothing. *Nothing.* I've known for some time that I continue with Nick out of habit and loyalty, and not for any real coaching. Still, in this moment, it's not coaching I need but a show of humanity, which is one of the duties of any coach. I need some recognition of the adrenaline-charged moment in which I find myself. Is that too much to ask?

After the rain delay, Courier stations himself farther behind the baseline, hoping to take some of the steam off my shots. He's had time to rest, and reflect, and recharge, and he storms back to keep me from breaking, then wins the second set. Now I'm angry. Furious. I win the third set, 6–2. I establish in Courier's mind, and in my own, that the second set was a fluke. Up two sets to one, I can feel the finish line pulling me. My first slam. Six little games away.

As the fourth set opens, I lose twelve of the first thirteen points. Am I unraveling or is Courier playing better? I don't know. I'll never know. But I do know that this feeling is familiar. Hauntingly familiar. This sense of inevitability. This weightlessness as momentum slips away. Courier wins the set, 6–1.

In the fifth set, tied 4–4, he breaks me. Now, all at once, I just want to lose.

I can't explain it any other way. In the fourth set I lost the will, but now I've lost the desire. As certain as I felt about victory at the start of this match, that's how certain I am now of defeat. And I want it. I long for it. I say under my breath: Let it be fast. Since losing is death, I'd rather it be fast than slow.

I no longer hear the crowd. I no longer hear my own thoughts, only a white noise between my ears. I can't hear or feel anything except my desire to lose. I drop the tenth and decisive game of the fifth set, and congratulate Courier. Friends tell me it's the most desolate look they've ever seen on my face.

Afterward, I don't scold myself. I coolly explain it to myself this way: You don't have what it takes to get over the line. You just quit on yourself—you need to quit this game.

THE LOSS LEAVES A SCAR. Wendi says she can almost see it, a mark as if I've been struck by lightning. That's about all she says on the long flight back to Vegas.

As we walk through the front door of my parents' house, my father meets us in the foyer. He starts right in on me. Why didn't you make adjustments after the rain delay? Why didn't you hit to his backhand? I don't answer. I don't move. I've been expecting his tirade for the last twenty-four hours and I'm already numb to it. But Wendi isn't. She does something no one's ever done, something I always hoped my mother would do. She throws herself between us. She says, Can we just not talk about tennis for two hours? Two hours—no tennis?

My father stops, gapes. I fear that he'll slap her. But then he wheels and storms up the hall to his bedroom.

I gaze at Wendi. I've never loved her more.

. . .

I DON'T TOUCH MY RACKETS. I don't open my tennis bag. I don't train with Gil. I lie around watching horror movies with Wendi. Only horror movies can distract me, because they capture something of the feeling in that fifth set against Courier.

Nick nags me to play Wimbledon. I laugh in his tanned face.

Back on the horse, he says. It's the only way, my boy.

Fuck that horse.

Come on, Wendi says. Honestly, how much worse can it get?

Too depressed to argue, I let Nick and Wendi push me onto a plane to London. We rent a beautiful two-story house, hidden from the main road, close to the All England Lawn Tennis and Croquet Club. It has a charming garden in the back, with pink roses and every variety of songbird, a little haven where I can sit and nearly forget why I'm in England. Wendi makes the house feel like home. She fills it with candles, groceries—and her perfume. She fixes delicious meals at night, and in the morning she packs box lunches for me to bring to the practice courts.

The tournament is delayed five days by rain. On the fifth day, though the house is cozy, we're going stir crazy. I want to get out on the court. I want to get rid of the bad taste in my mouth from the French Open, or else lose and go home. Finally the rain lets up. I play Grant Connell, a serve-and-volleyer who's made his living off fast surfaces. It's an awkward first-round opponent for my first grass match in years. He's expected to trounce me. Somehow I eke out a five-set win.

I reach the quarters, where I play David Wheaton. I'm up two sets to one, up two breaks in the fourth set, and all of a sudden I pull something in my hip flexor, the muscle that bends the joint. Hobbled, it's all I can do to finish the match. Wheaton wins easily.

I tell Wendi that I could have won the thing. I started to feel better than I'd felt at the French Open. Damned hip.

The good news, I suppose, is that I wanted to win. Maybe I've got my desire turned around and pointed in the right direction.

I'M A FAST HEALER. After a few days my hip is fine. My mind, however, continues to throb. I go to the U.S. Open and lose in the first round. *The first round.* But the scary part is the way I lose. I play Krickstein, good old Krickstein, and again I just don't want it. I know I can beat him, and yet it's not worth the trouble. I don't expend the necessary energy. I feel a strange clarity about my lack of effort. It's lack of inspiration, plain and simple. I don't question it. I don't bother wishing it away. While Krickstein is running and leaping and lunging, I'm watching him with only mild interest. Only afterward does the shame set in.

I NEED TO DO SOMETHING RADICAL, something to break the seductive grip that losing seems to have on me. I decide to move out on my own. I buy myself a three-bedroom tract home in southwest Vegas and turn it into the ultimate bachelor pad, almost a parody of a bachelor pad. I make one bedroom an arcade, with all the classic games— Asteroids, Space Invaders, Defender. I'm terrible at them, but I intend to get better. I turn the formal living room into a movie theater, with state-of-the-art sound equipment and woofers in the couches. I turn the dining room into a billiard room. Throughout the house I scatter fantastically plush leather chairs, except in the main living room, where I install a massive, modular, green chenille, double-stuffed goosedown couch. In the kitchen I place a soda machine stocked with Mountain Dew, my favorite, and beer taps. Out back I install a hot tub and a black-bottomed lagoon.

Best of all, I make the bedroom a cave, everything jet black, with blackout curtains that don't admit the tiniest slit of daylight. It's the house of an arrested adolescent, a boy-man determined to shut out the world. I walk around this new house, this deluxe playpen, daring to think how grown-up I am.

I skip the Australian Open again at the start of 1992. I've never played it, and now doesn't seem like the time to start. Still, I play Davis Cup and do fairly well, maybe because it's in Hawaii. We face Argentina. I win both my matches. Then, the night before the last day, Wendi and I go out drinking with McEnroe and his wife, Tatum O'Neal. We overdo it, and I go to bed at four in the morning, assuming someone will take my place on Sunday, in a meaningless match, often called a dead rubber.

Apparently that's not the case. Though I'm hungover and dehydrated, I need to go out and play Jaite, whose serve I once caught with my hand. Happily, Jaite's hungover too. It's fitting that this is a dead rubber; we both look dead and rubbery. To conceal my bloodshot eyes I play wearing Oakley sunglasses, and somehow I play well. I play relaxed. I walk off the court a winner, wondering if there's a lesson in this. Can I tap this sort of relaxation when the stakes are real, when it's a slam? Should I just go into every match hungover?

162

The next week I find myself on the cover of *Tennis* magazine, hitting a winner in my Oakley glasses. Hours after the magazine hits the newsstands, Wendi and I are at the bachelor pad when a delivery truck pulls up to the door. We go outside. Sign here, the deliveryman says.

What is this?

Gift. From Jim Jannard, founder of Oakley.

The back of the truck comes down, and a red Dodge Viper slowly descends.

Nice to know that, even if I've lost my game, I can still move product.

MY RANKING PLUMMETS. I fall out of the top ten. The only time I feel fairly competent on the court is when I play Davis Cup. In Fort Meyers I help the U.S. beat Czechoslovakia, winning both matches. Otherwise, the only game at which I show any improvement is Asteroids.

At the 1992 French Open I beat Pete, which feels good. Then I run into Courier again, this time in the semis. The memories of last year are still fresh, still painful, and I lose again—in straight sets. Once again Courier laces up his running shoes and goes for a jog afterward. I still can't burn enough calories for him.

I limp to Florida and crash at Nick's house. I don't pick up a racket the whole time I'm there. Then, reluctantly, I have one short practice on a hard court at the Bollettieri Academy, and we all fly to Wimbledon.

The talent assembled in London in 1992 is stunning. There's Courier, ranked number one, fresh off two slam victories. There's Pete, who keeps getting better. There's Stefan Edberg, who's playing out of his mind. I'm the twelfth seed, and the way I've been playing I should be seeded lower.

In my first-round match, against Andrei Chesnokov, from Russia, I play like a low seed. I lose the first set. Frustrated, I rip into myself, curse myself, and the umpire gives me an official warning for saying *fuck*. I almost turn to him and fire a few *fuck-fuck-fucks*. Instead I decide to shock him, shock everyone, by taking a breath and being composed. Then I do something more shocking. I win the next three sets.

I'm in the quarters. Against Becker, who's reached six of the last seven Wimbledon finals. This is his de facto home court, his honey hole. But I've been seeing his serve well lately. I win in five sets, played over two days. Memories of Munich, put to rest.

In the semis I face McEnroe, three-time Wimbledon champion. He's thirty-three, nearing the end of his career, and unseeded. Given his underdog status, and his legendary accomplishments, the fans want him to win, of course. Part of me wants him to win also. But I beat him in three sets. I'm in the final.

I'm expecting to face Pete, but he loses his semifinal match to Goran Ivanisevic, a big, strong serving machine from Croatia. I've played Ivanisevic twice before, and both times he's shellacked me in straight sets. So I feel for Pete, and I know I'll be joining him soon. I have no chance against Ivanisevic. It's a middleweight versus a heavyweight. The only suspense is whether it will be a knockout or a TKO.

AS POWERFUL AS Ivanisevic's serve is under normal circumstances, today it's a work of art. He's acing me left and right, monster serves that the speed gun clocks at 138 miles an hour. But it's not just the speed, it's the trajectory. They land at a 75-degree angle. I try not to care. I tell myself that aces happen. Each time he serves a ball past me, I say under my breath that he can't do that every time. Just walk to the other side and get ready, Andre. The match will be decided on those few second serves.

He wins the first set, 7–6. I don't break him once. I concentrate on not overreacting, on breathing in, breathing out, remaining patient. When the thought crosses my mind that I'm on the verge of losing my fourth slam final, I casually set that thought aside. In the second set Ivanisevic gives me a few freebies, makes a few mistakes, and I break him. I take the second set. Then the third. Which makes me feel almost worse, because once again I'm a set away from a slam.

Ivanisevic rises up in the fourth set and destroys me. I've made the Croat mad. He loses only a handful of points in the process. Here we go again. I can see tomorrow's headlines as plain as the racket in my hand. As the fifth set begins I run in place to get the blood flowing and tell myself one thing: You want this. You do not want to lose, not this time. The problem in the last three slams was that you didn't want them enough, and therefore you didn't bring it, but this one you want, so this time you need to let Ivanisevic and everyone else in this joint *know* you want it.

At 3–3, I'm serving, break point. I haven't been able to make a first serve this entire set, but now, mercifully, I make one. He returns it to the center of the court, I hit to his backhand, he hits a chip lob. I have to back up two steps. The overhead is one of the easiest shots you can play. It's also the epitome of my struggles at slams, because it's too easy. I don't like things too easy. It's there for the taking—will I take it? I swing, hit a textbook overhead, and win the point. I go on to hold serve.

Now Ivanisevic's serving at 4–5. He double-faults. Twice. He's down love–30. He's cracking under the strain. I haven't broken this guy in the last hour and a half and now he's breaking himself. He misses another first serve. He's coming apart. I know it. I *see* it. No one knows better than I what coming apart looks like. I also know how it feels. I know precisely what's happening inside Ivanisevic's body. His throat is closing. His legs are quivering. But then he quiets his body and hits a second serve to the back of the box, a beam of yellow light that barely nicks the line. A puff of chalk shoots up as if he hit the line with an assault rifle. Then he hits another unreturnable serve. Suddenly it's 30–all.

He misses another first serve, makes the second. I crush a return, he hits a half volley, I run in and pass him and start the long walk back to the baseline. I tell myself, You can win this thing with one swing. *One swing.* You've never been this close. You may never be again.

And that's the problem. What if I get this close and don't win? The ridicule. The condemnation. I pause, try to shift my focus back to Ivanisevic. I need to guess which way he's coming with his serve. OK, a typical lefty, serving to the ad court in a pressure point, hits a bending slider, out wide, that sweeps his opponent off the court. But Ivanisevic isn't typical. His serve in a pressure point is generally a flat bomb up the middle. Why he prefers that serve, God knows. Maybe he shouldn't. But he does. I know this about him. I know he's coming up the middle. Sure enough, here he comes, but he nets the serve. Good thing, because that thing was a comet, right on the line. Even though I guessed right, moved right, I couldn't have put my racket on it.

Now the crowd rises. I call time, to have a talk with myself, aloud, saying: Win this point or I'll never let you hear the end of it, Andre. Don't hope he double-faults, don't hope he misses. *You* control what *you* can control. Return this serve with all your strength, and if you return it hard but miss, you can live with that. You can survive that. One return, no regrets.

Hit *harder.*

He tosses the ball, serves to my backhand. I jump in the air, swing with all my strength, but I'm so tight that the ball to his backhand side has mediocre pace. Somehow he misses the easy volley. His ball smacks the net and just like that, after twenty-two years and twenty-two million swings of a tennis racket, I'm the 1992 Wimbledon champion.

I fall to my knees. I fall on my stomach. I can't believe the emotion pouring out of me. When I stagger to my feet, Ivanisevic appears at my side. He hugs me and says warmly, Congratulations, Wimbledon champ. You deserved it today.

Great fight, Goran.

He pats my shoulder. He smiles, walks to his chair, and wraps his head in a towel. I understand his emotions better than my own. Much of my heart is with him as I sit in my chair, trying to collect myself.

A very British man approaches and tells me to stand. He hands me a large gold loving cup. I don't know how to hold it, or where to go with it. He points and tells me to walk in a circle around the court. Hold the trophy over your head, he says.

I walk around the court holding the trophy above my head. The fans cheer. Another man tries to take the trophy from me. I pull it back. He explains that he's going to have it engraved. With my name.

I look at my box, wave to Nick and Wendi and Philly. They are all clapping, beaming. Philly is hugging Nick. Nick is hugging Wendi. I love you, Wendi. I bow to the royals and walk off the court.

In the locker room I stare at my warped reflection in the trophy. I address the trophy and the warped reflection: All the pain and suffering you've caused me.

I'm unnerved by how giddy I feel. It shouldn't matter this much. It shouldn't feel this good. Waves of emotion continue to wash over me, relief and elation and even a kind of hysterical serenity, because I've finally earned a brief respite from the critics, especially the internal ones.

LATER IN THE AFTERNOON, back at the house we've rented, I phone Gil, who couldn't make the trip, because he needed to be home with his family after the long clay season. He wishes so much that he could have been here. He discusses the match with me, the ins and outs—it's shocking how much he's learned about tennis in such a short time. I phone Perry, and J.P., and then, trembling, I dial my father in Vegas.

Pops? It's me! Can you hear me? What'd you think?

Silence.

Pops?

You had no business losing that fourth set.

Stunned, I wait, not trusting my voice. Then I say, Good thing I won the fifth set, though, right?

He says nothing. Not because he disagrees, or disapproves, but because he's crying. Faintly I hear my father sniffling and wiping away tears, and I know he's proud, just incapable of expressing it. I can't fault the man for not knowing how to say what's in his heart. It's the family curse.

. . .

THE NIGHT OF THE FINAL is the famed Wimbledon Ball. I've heard about it for years, and I'm dying to go, because the men's winner gets to dance with the women's winner, and this year, as in most years, that means Steffi Graf. I've had a crush on Steffi since I first saw her doing an interview on French TV. I was thunderstruck, dazzled by her understated grace, her effortless beauty. She looked, somehow, as if she smelled good. Also, as if she *was* good, fundamentally, essentially, inherently good, brimming with moral rectitude and a kind of dignity that doesn't exist anymore. I thought I saw, for half a second, a halo above her head. I tried to get a message to her after last year's French Open, but she didn't respond. Now, I can't wait to twirl her across a dance floor, never mind that I don't know how to dance.

Wendi knows about my feelings for Steffi, and she's not at all jealous. We have an open relationship, she reminds me. We're both over twenty-one. In fact, on the eve of the final, we both go to Harrods to buy my tuxedo, in case I need it, and Wendi jokes with the salesgirl that I only want to win so that I can dance with Steffi Graf.

And so, wearing black tie for the first time ever, with Wendi on my arm, I walk smartly into the ball. We're instantly set upon by silver-haired British couples. The men have hair in their ears, and the women smell like old liqueur. They seem delighted by my win, but mainly because it means fresh blood in the club. Someone new to talk to at these dreadful, dreadful affairs, someone says. Wendi and I stand with our backs to each other, like scuba divers in a school of sharks. I struggle to decipher some of the thicker British accents. I try to make clear to one older woman who looks like Benny Hill that I'm quite excited about the traditional dance with the women's champion.

Sadly, the woman says, that dance isn't happening this year.

Say what?

The players haven't embraced the dance quite so enthusiastically in years past. So it's been canceled.

She sees my face fall. Wendi turns, sees it too, and laughs.

I don't get to dance with Steffi, but there will be a kind of consolation match: a formal introduction. I look forward to it all night. Then it happens. Shaking her hand, I tell Steffi that I tried to reach her at last year's French Open and I hope she didn't misunderstand my intentions. I say, I'd really love to talk with you some time.

She doesn't respond. She merely smiles, an enigmatic smile, and I can't tell if she's happy about what I've just said, or nervous.

14

I'M SUPPOSED TO BE A DIFFERENT PERSON now that I've won a slam. Everyone says so. No more *Image Is Everything*. Now, sportswriters assert, for Andre Agassi, winning is everything. After two years of calling me a fraud, a choke artist, a rebel without a cause, they lionize me. They declare that I'm a winner, a player of substance, the real deal. They say my victory at Wimbledon forces them to reassess me, to reconsider who I really am.

But I don't feel that Wimbledon has changed me. I feel, in fact, as if I've been let in on a dirty little secret: winning changes nothing. Now that I've won a slam, I know something that very few people on earth are permitted to know. A win doesn't feel as good as a loss feels bad, and the good feeling doesn't last as long as the bad. Not even close.

I do feel happier in the summer of 1992, and more substantive, but the cause isn't Wimbledon. It's Wendi. We've grown closer. We've whispered promises to each other. I've accepted that I'm not meant to be with Steffi. It was a nice fantasy while it lasted, but I've devoted myself to Wendi, and vice versa. She doesn't work, doesn't go to school. She's been to several colleges and none was right. So now she spends all her time with me.

In 1992, however, spending time together suddenly becomes more complicated. Sitting in a movie theater, eating in a restaurant, we're never truly alone. People appear from nowhere, requesting my picture, demanding my autograph, seeking my attention or opinion. Wimbledon has made me famous. I thought I was famous long ago—I signed my first autograph when I was six—but now I discover that I was actually infamous. Wimbledon has legitimized me, broadened and deepened my appeal, at least according to the agents and managers and marketing experts with whom I now regularly meet. People want to get closer to me; they feel they have that right. I understand that there's a tax on everything in America. Now I discover that *this* is the tax on success in sports—fifteen seconds of time for every fan. I can accept this, intellectually. I just wish it didn't mean the loss of privacy with my girl.

Wendi shrugs it off. She's a good sport about every intrusion. She keeps me from taking anything too seriously, including myself. With her help I decide that the best approach to being famous is to forget you're famous. I work hard at putting fame out of my mind.

But fame is a force. It's unstoppable. You shut your windows to fame and it slides under the door. I turn around one day and discover that I have dozens of famous friends, and I don't know how I met half of them. I'm invited to parties and VIP rooms, events and galas where the famous gather, and many ask for my phone number, or press their numbers on me. In the same way that my win at Wimbledon automatically made me a lifetime member of the All England Club, it also admitted me to this nebulous Famous People's Club. My circle of acquaintants now includes Kenny G, Kevin Costner, and Barbra Streisand. I'm invited to spend the night at the White House, to eat dinner with President George Bush before his summit with Mikhail Gorbachev. I sleep in the Lincoln Bedroom.

I find it surreal, then perfectly normal. I'm struck by how fast the surreal becomes the norm. I marvel at how unexciting it is to be famous, how mundane famous people are. They're confused, uncertain, insecure, and often hate what they do. It's something we always hear—like that old adage that money can't buy happiness—but we never believe it until we see it for ourselves. Seeing it in 1992 brings me a new measure of confidence.

I'M SAILING NEAR VANCOUVER ISLAND, vacationing with my new friend David Foster, the music producer. Shortly after Wendi and I board Foster's yacht, Costner comes aboard and invites us to join him on his yacht, anchored fifty yards away. We hit it off immediately. Even though he has a yacht, Costner seems like the classic man's man. Easygoing, funny, cool. He loves sports, follows them avidly, and assumes I do too. I tell him shyly that I don't follow sports. That I don't like them.

How do you mean?

I mean, I don't like sports.

He laughs. You mean besides tennis?

I hate tennis most of all.

Right, right. I guess it's a grind. But you don't actually hate tennis.

I do.

Wendi and I spend much of the boating trip watching Costner's three children. Well mannered, personable, they're also remarkably beautiful. They look as if they tumbled out of one of my mother's Norman Rockwell puzzles. Shortly after meeting me, four-year-old Joe Costner grabs at my pants leg and looks up at me with his big blue eyes. He shouts: Let's play *wrestle*! I pick him up and hold him upside down, and the sound of his giggling is one of the most delicious sounds I've ever heard. Wendi and I tell ourselves we're hopelessly charmed by the little Costners, but in reality we're deliberately playing at being their parents. Now and then I catch Wendi slipping away from the grownups to have another look at the children. I can see that she's going to be a great mother. I imagine being there by her side, through it all, helping her raise three towheads with green eyes. The thought thrills me—and her. I broach the subject of family, the future. She doesn't blink. She wants it too.

Weeks later, Costner invites us to his house in Los Angeles for a preview of his new film, *The Bodyguard*. Wendi and I don't think much of the movie, but we swoon over the theme song, I Will Always Love You.

This will be our song, Wendi says.

Always.

We sing this song to each other, quote it to each other, and when the song comes on the radio we stop whatever we're doing and make goo-goo eyes at each other, which makes everyone around us sick. We couldn't care less.

I tell Philly and Perry that I can imagine spending the rest of my life with Wendi, that I might soon propose. Philly gives me a full nod. Perry gives me the green light.

Wendi is the one, I tell J.P.

What about Steffi Graf?

She blew me off. Forget her. It's Wendi.

I'M SHOWING OFF my new toy for J.P. and Wendi.

J.P. asks, What's this thing called again?

A Hummer. They used it in the Gulf War.

Mine is one of the first to be sold in the U.S. We're driving it all over the desert outside Vegas when we get stuck in the sand. J.P. jokes that they must not have run into any sand during the Gulf War. We hop out and set across the desert. I have a flight this afternoon and a match tomorrow. If I can't get us out of this desert, all kinds of people are going to be angry with me. But as we walk and walk, my match suddenly seems a trivial matter. Survival starts to be a real concern. In every direction, we see nothing, and darkness is coming on.

It feels as though this might become a turning point in our lives, J.P. says. And I don't mean in a good way.

Thanks for the positive thinking.

Finally we come to a shack. An old hermit loans us his shovel. We hike back to the Hummer, and I hurriedly set about digging around the back wheel. Suddenly my shovel hits something hard. Caliche, the cement-like layer of soil under the Nevada desert. I feel something snap deep inside my wrist. I cry out.

What is it? Wendi says.

I don't know.

I look at my wrist.

Rub some dirt on it, J.P. says.

I dig out the Hummer, make my flight, even win my match the next day. Days later, however, I wake in agony. The wrist feels broken. I can barely bend it back and forth. I feel as if several sewing needles and rusty razor blades have been implanted in the joint. This is bad. This is big.

Then the pain goes away. I'm relieved. Then it comes back. I'm scared. Soon the occasional pain becomes constant. It's tolerable in the morning, but by day's end the needle-razor feeling is all I can think about.

A doctor says I have tendinitis. Specifically *dorsal capsulitis*. Tiny rips in the wrist that refuse to heal. The result of overuse, he says. The only possible cures are rest and surgery.

I choose rest. I shut myself down, gentle the wrist. After weeks of carrying the wrist around like a wounded bird, I still can't work out, do a push-up, or open a door without grimacing.

The one upside of the wrist injury is that I get to spend more time with Wendi. Instead of hard-court season, the start of 1993 becomes Wendi Season, and I throw myself into it. She enjoys the extra attention, but she also worries that she's neglecting her studies. She's enrolled in yet another college. Her fifth. Or sixth. I've lost track.

Driving along Rainbow Boulevard, steering with my left hand to avoid engaging my bad right wrist, I roll down the window and turn up the radio. The spring breeze flutters Wendi's hair. She turns down the radio and says how long it's been since she really knew what she wanted.

I nod and turn up the radio.

She turns down the radio and says she's attended all these different colleges, lived in all these different states, she's been searching her whole life for meaning, purpose—nothing ever feels right. She just can't seem to figure out who she is.

Again, I nod. I agree. I know that feeling. Winning Wimbledon has done nothing to salve it. Then I look over at Wendi and realize she's not just idly talking, she's going somewhere with this. She's making a point— about us. She turns in her seat and looks me in the eye. Andre, I've been giving this a lot of thought, and I just don't think I can be happy, really happy, until I figure out who I am and what I'm supposed to do with my life. And I don't see how I can do that if we stay together.

She's crying.

I can't be your traveling companion, she says, your sidekick, your fan, anymore. Well, I'll always be your fan, but you know what I mean.

She needs to find herself, and to do that she needs to be free.

And so do you, she says. We can't realize our separate goals if we stay together.

Even an open relationship is too confining.

I can't argue with her. If that's how she feels, there's nothing I can say. I want her to be happy. Of course at this moment our song comes on the radio. *I will always love you.* I stare at Wendi, try to catch her eye, but she keeps her face turned away. I make a U-turn, drive back to her house, walk her to the door. She gives me one long, last hug.

I drive away and barely make it to the end of the block before pulling over and phoning Perry. When he answers I can't speak. I'm crying too hard. He thinks it's a prank call.

Hello, he says, annoyed. Hel-*lo*?

He hangs up.

I call back, but still can't speak. Again he hangs up.

I GO UNDERGROUND. I hole up in the bachelor pad, boozing, sleeping, eating junk. I feel shooting pains in my chest. I tell Gil. He says it sounds like a typical broken heart. Tiny rips that refuse to heal. The result of overuse.

Then he says, What are we doing about Wimbledon? Time to start thinking about getting ourselves overseas. Time to throw down, Andre. It's on.

I can barely hold the phone, let alone a tennis racket. Still, I want to go. I could use the distraction. I could use some time on the road with Gil, working on a common goal. Also, I'm defending champion. I have no choice. Right before our flight Gil arranges for a doctor in Seattle, who's supposed to be the best, to give me a shot of cortisone. The shot works. I arrive in Europe wiggling the wrist, pain-free.

We go first to Halle, Germany, for a tune-up tournament. Nick meets us there and immediately puts the touch on me for money. He sold the Bollettieri Academy, because he got himself into debt, and it was the biggest mistake of his life. He let it go for too little. Now he needs cash. He's not himself—or maybe he's more himself. He says he's not getting paid what he's worth. He says I've been an unsound investment. He's spent hundreds of thousands of dollars developing me, and he's entitled to hundreds of thousands above the hundreds of thousands I've already given him. I ask if we can please talk about this back home. I have a few things weighing on my mind right now.

Of course, he says. When we get back.

I'm so shaken by the confrontation that in the Halle tournament I fall on my face in my first-round match against Steeb. He beats me in three sets. So much for the tune-up.

I've barely played in the last year, and when I've played, I've played badly, so I'm the lowest-seeded defending champ in Wimbledon history. My first match on center court is against Bernd Karbacher, a German whose thick hair always looks the same, from the beginning of the match to the end, which irks me, for obvious reasons. Everything about Karbacher seems designed to distract. Apart from his enviable locks, he's bowlegged. He walks as if he not only sits on a horse all day, but as if he just dismounted, and it's been a long ride, and his ass is chapped. Befitting his appearance, he plays a very odd game. His backhand is huge, one of the game's best, but he uses it to avoid running. He hates running. Hates moving. At times he doesn't care much for serving, either. He has an aggressive first serve, but not much of a second serve.

With my numbed wrist I have my own serve issues. I'll have to alter my motion, taking only a small backswing, limiting sudden movements. Naturally this causes problems. I fall behind quickly in the first set, 2–5. I'm about to become the first defending champion in decades to get knocked out in the first round. But I collect myself, force myself to make peace with my new serve, and tough out the win. Karbacher hops on his horse and rides away.

British fans are kind. They cheer, they roar, they appreciate the effort it's taken to get my wrist ready. British tabloids, however, are another matter. They're filled with venom. They carry strange stories about, of all things, my chest, which I've recently shaved. Just a bit of innocent manscaping, but you'd think I'd cut off a limb. My wrist is broken, and they talk only about my chest. My news conferences turn into Monty Python skits, every other question about my newly smooth pectorals. British reporters are hair obsessed—if they only knew the truth about the hair on my head. Several tabloids also say I'm fat, and writers take malicious joy in calling me Burger King. Gil tries to blame my appearance on the cortisone injection in my wrist, which can cause bloating, but no one is buying it.

Nothing, however, fascinates the Brits quite like Barbra Streisand. She arrives at Centre Court to watch me play and there is practically a flurry of trumpets. Celebrities attend Wimbledon all the time, but Barbra's appearance causes a stir like none I've seen. Reporters harass her, then later pester me about her, and the tabloids take great pains to dissect and belittle our relationship, which is nothing more than a passionate friendship.

They want to know how we met. I refuse to tell them, because Barbra is the shyest, most private person I know.

It began with Steve Wynn, the casino impresario, whom I'd known since I was a kid. He and I were playing golf one day, and I mentioned that I enjoyed Barbra Streisand's music. He said she was a good friend. Thus began a series of phone calls, during which Barbra and I connected. When I won Wimbledon, she sent a sweet telegram, congratulating me, telling me, sarcastically, it was nice to put a face with the voice.

She invited me weeks later to a small get-together at her ranch in Malibu. David Foster would be there, she said, and a few other friends. Finally we'd meet.

Her ranch was dotted with cottages, one of which was a movie theater. After a luncheon we wandered down there for a sneak preview of *The Joy Luck Club,* a quintessential chick flick, during which I thought I might expire of boredom. Then we all wandered over to another cottage, a music salon, with a grand piano under a window. We stood around eating and talking while David sat at the piano, playing a medley of torch songs. He made several attempts to get Barbra to sing. She wouldn't. He persisted. She refused. He kept after her until it became awkward. I wished he would stop. Barbra's elbows were resting on the piano, and her back was to me. I saw her stiffen. She was clearly petrified about performing in front of other people.

Not five minutes later, however, she let fly a few bars. The sound filled the room from the rafters to the floorboards. Everyone stopped talking. Glasses shook. Flatware rattled. The bones in my ribs and wrist vibrated. I briefly thought someone had put one of Barbra's albums on a Bose sound system and turned the volume up full blast. I couldn't believe that a human being was capable of producing that much sound, that a human voice could pervade every square inch of a room.

From that moment I was even more intrigued by Barbra. The idea that she possessed such a devastating instrument, such a powerful talent, and couldn't use it freely, for pleasure, was fascinating. And familiar. And depressing. We met soon after that day. She invited me to the ranch. We shared a pizza and talked for hours, discovering many things in common. She was a tortured perfectionist who hated doing something at which she excelled. And yet, despite years of semiretirement, despite all her self-doubts and nagging fears, she admitted that she was pondering a come-back to the concert stage. I urged her to do it. I told her it was wrong to deprive the world of that voice, that astonishing voice. Above all, I told her that it would be dangerous to surrender to fear. Fears are like gateway drugs, I said. You give in to a small one, and soon you're giving in to big-ger ones. So what if she didn't want to perform? She had to.

Naturally I felt like a hypocrite every time I said this to Barbra. In my own struggles with fear and perfectionism, I was losing more than I won. I talked to her the way I talked to reporters: I told her things I knew to be true, and things I hoped to be true, most of which I couldn't bring myself to fully believe and act on.

After we'd spent one long spring afternoon playing tennis, I told Bar-bra about a new singer I'd seen in Vegas, a woman with a big voice not unlike Barbra's. I asked, Do you want to hear her?

Sure.

I brought her out to my car and put in a CD by this new sensation, a Canadian named Céline Dion. Barbra listened closely, biting her thumb-nail. I could tell she was thinking: I can do that. She was picturing herself back in the game. Again, I felt helpful, but also like a raging hypocrite.

My sense of hypocrisy reached a crescendo when Barbra finally did push herself to perform. There I was, front row—wearing a black base-ball cap. My hairpiece was malfunctioning again, and I feared what peo-ple would think and say. Beyond being a hypocrite that night, I felt a slave to fear.

More often than not, Barbra and I laugh at the shock and scandal our dates cause. We agree that we're good for each other, and so what if she's twenty-eight years older? We're simpatico, and the public outcry only adds spice to our connection. It makes our friendship feel forbidden, taboo—another piece of my overall rebellion. Dating Barbra Streisand is like wearing Hot Lava.

Still, if I'm fatigued, if I'm not in the right mood, as is the case at Wimbledon, then the public belittling can sting. And Barbra plays into the hands of the belittlers by telling a reporter that I'm a Zen master. Newspapers have a field day with this comment. I begin to hear the Zen master quote constantly; it briefly replaces *Image Is Everything*. I don't understand the reaction, maybe because I don't know what a Zen master is. I can only assume it's a good thing, since Barbra's a friend.

BRUSHING ASIDE THE SUBJECT OF BARBRA, avoiding newspapers and TV, I stay on task at the 1993 Wimbledon. After surviving Karbacher, I beat João Cunha-Silva, from Portugal, Patrick Rafter, from Australia, then Richard Krajicek, from the Netherlands. I'm in the quarters, facing Pete. As always, it's Pete. I wonder how my wrist can possibly hold up against his serve, which he's developed into a force. But Pete's suffering his own aches and pains. His shoulder is sore, his game is a tad off. Or so they say. You'd never know it the way he comes out against me. He wins the first set in less time than I spent getting dressed for the match. He wins the second set just as fast.

Going to be a short day, I tell myself. I look up at my box, and there's Barbra, flashes going off around her. I think: Is this really my life?

As the third set begins, Pete stumbles. I get a second wind. The set falls to me, as does the fourth. The wheel clicks in my direction. I see fear creep into Pete's face. We're tied, two sets apiece, and doubt, unmistakable doubt, is trailing him like the long afternoon shadows on the Wimbledon grass. For once, it's not me but Pete yelling and cursing at himself.

In the fifth set, Pete's wincing, kneading his shoulder. He asks for a trainer. During the delay, while he's being worked on, I tell myself this match is mine. Two Wimbledons in a row—won't that be something? We'll see what the tabloids have to say then. Or what I'll say. *How do you like your Burger King now?*

When we resume play, however, Pete is a different person. Not revived, not reenergized—wholly different. He's done it again, sloughed off that other doubt-ridden Pete as a snake sheds its skin. And now he's in the process of shedding me. Leading 5–4, he starts the tenth game of the set by blasting three straight aces. But not just any aces. They even have a different sound about them. Like Civil War cannons. Triple match point.

Suddenly he's walking toward the net, extending his hand, the victor once again. The handshake physically hurts, and it has nothing to do with my tender wrist.

. . .

BACK AT THE BACHELOR PAD, days after losing to Pete, I have one simple goal. I want to avoid thinking about tennis for seven days. I just need a break. I'm heart sore, wrist sore, bone tired. I need to do nothing for one week—just sit and be quiet. No pain, no drama, no serves, no tabloids, no singers, no match points. I'm sipping my first cup of coffee, flipping through *USA Today,* when a headline catches my eye. Because my name is in it. *Bollettieri Parts Ways with Agassi.* Nick tells the newspaper he's done with me. He wants to spend more time with his family. After ten years, this is how he lets me know. Not even a panda ass-up in my chair.

Minutes later a FedEx envelope arrives with a letter from Nick. It says no more than the newspaper story. I read it a few dozen times before putting it in a shoe box. I go to the mirror. I don't feel all that bad. I don't feel anything. Numb. As if the cortisone has spread from my wrist to engulf my being.

I drive over to Gil's and sit with him in the gym. He listens and feels bad and angry right along with me.

Well, I say, I guess it's Break-Up-With-Andre time. First Wendi, now Nick.

My entourage is thinning faster than my hair.

THOUGH IT MAKES NO SENSE, I'd like to get on the court again. I want the pain that only tennis provides.

But not this much pain. The cortisone has completely worn off, and the needle-razor feeling in my wrist is simply too much. I see a new doctor, who says the wrist needs surgery. I see another doctor, who says more resting might do the trick. I side with the rest doctor. After four weeks of rest, however, I step on a court and realize with one swing that surgery is my only option.

I just don't trust surgeons. I trust very few people, and I especially dislike the notion of trusting one perfect stranger, surrendering all control to one person whom I've only just met. I cringe at the thought of lying on a table, unconscious, while someone slices open the wrist with which I make my living. What if he's distracted that day? What if he's off? I see it happening on the court all the time—half the time it's happening to me. I'm in the top ten, but some days you'd think I was a rank amateur. What if my surgeon is the Andre Agassi of medicine? What if he doesn't have his A game that day? What if he's drunk or on drugs?

I ask Gil to be there in the operating room during my surgery. I want him to act as sentry, monitor, backstop, witness. In other words, I want him to do what he always does. Stand guard. But this time wearing a gown and mask.

He frowns. He shakes his head. He doesn't know.

Gil has several endearingly dainty qualities, like his horror of the sun, but the most endearing is his squeamish streak. He can't abide the sight of needles. He gets the willies when he has to have a flu shot.

For me, however, he'll rally. He says, I'll tough it out.

I owe you, I tell him.

Never, he says. No such thing as debts between us.

On December 19, 1993, Gil and I fly to Santa Barbara and check into the hospital. As nurses flutter about, prepping me, I tell Gil that I feel so nervous, I might pass out.

Then they won't need to give you the gas.

This could be it, Gil, the end of my tennis career.

No.

Then what? What will I do?

They put a mask over my nose and mouth. Breathe deeply, they say. My eyelids are heavy. I fight to keep them open, fight against the loss of control. Don't go away, Gil. Don't leave me. I stare at Gil's black eyes, above his surgical mask, watching, unblinking. Gil is here, I tell myself. Gil's got this. Gil's on duty. Everything's going to be all right. I let my eyes close, let a kind of mist swallow me, and a half second later I'm waking and Gil is leaning over me, saying the wrist was worse than they thought. Much worse. But they cleaned it out, Andre, and we'll hope for the best. That's all we can do, right? Hope for the best.

I TAKE UP RESIDENCE on the green chenille double-stuffed goose-down couch, remote in one hand, phone in the other. The surgeon says I must keep my wrist elevated for several days, so I lie with it propped on a large, hard pillow. Though I'm on powerful pain pills, I still feel wounded, worried, vulnerable. At least I have something to distract me. A woman. A friend of Kenny G's wife, Lyndie.

I met Kenny G through Michael Bolton, whom I met while playing Davis Cup. We were all at the same hotel. Then, out of the blue, Lyndie phoned me and said she'd met the perfect woman.

Well, I like perfect.

I think you two will really hit it off.

Why?

She's beautiful, brilliant, sophisticated, funny.

I don't think so. I'm still trying to get over Wendi. Plus, I don't do setups.

You'll do this setup. Her name is Brooke Shields.

I've heard of her.

What have you got to lose?

Plenty.

Andre.

I'll think about it. What's her number?

You can't phone her. She's in South Africa, doing a film.

She must have a phone.

Nope. She's in the middle of nowhere. She's in a tent, or a hut, in the bush. You can only reach her by fax.

She gave me Brooke's fax number and asked for mine.

I don't have a fax. It's the only gadget I don't have in the house.

I gave her Philly's fax number.

Then, just before my surgery, I got a call from Philly.

You have a fax here at my house—from Brooke Shields?

And so it began. Faxes back and forth, a long-distance correspondence with a woman I'd never met. What began oddly became progressively more odd. The pace of the conversation was outrageously slow, and this suited us both—neither of us was in any hurry. But the enormous geographical distance also led us to quickly let down our guard. We segued within a few faxes from innocent flirting to innermost secrets. Within a few days our faxes took on a tone of fondness, then intimacy. I felt as if I were going steady with this woman I'd never met or spoken to.

I stopped phoning Barbra.

Now, immobilized, my bandaged wrist propped on the pillow, I have nothing to do but obsess about the next fax to Brooke. Gil comes over some days and helps me work through several drafts. I'm intimidated by the fact that Brooke graduated from Princeton with a degree in French literature, whereas I dropped out of ninth grade. Gil brushes aside such talk, pumps up my confidence.

Besides, he says, don't worry about whether she likes you. Worry about whether you like her.

Yeah, I say. *Yeah. You're right.*

So I ask him to rent the collected works of Brooke Shields, and we have a two-man film festival. We make popcorn, dim the lights, and Gil puts in the first movie. *The Blue Lagoon.* Brooke as a prepubescent mermaid, stranded with a boy on an island paradise. A retelling of Adam and Eve. We rewind, fast-forward, freeze-frame, debate if Brooke Shields is my type.

Not bad, Gil says. Not bad at all. She's definitely worth another fax.

The courtship via fax continues for weeks, until Brooke sends a short fax saying she's finished filming her movie and she's coming back to the U.S. She'll be here in two weeks. She lands at LAX. By coincidence I have to be in Los Angeles the day after she arrives. I'm filming an interview with Jim Rome.

WE MEET AT HER HOUSE. I race there straight from the studio, still wearing the heavy TV makeup from my interview with Rome. She throws open the door, looking very much the movie star, wearing a flowing scarfy thing around her neck. And no makeup. (Or at least less than I.) But her hair is chopped short, which gives me a jolt. All this time I've been picturing her with long, flowing hair.

I cut it for a part, she says.

In what? *Bad News Bears*?

Her mother appears from nowhere. We shake hands. She's cordial, but stiff. I get a strange vibe. I know, instinctively, regardless of what happens, this woman and I will never get along.

I drive Brooke to dinner. Along the way I ask, Do you live with your mother?

Yes. Well, no. Not really. It's complicated.

It always is with parents.

We go to Pasta Maria, a little Italian joint on San Vicente. I ask to be seated in a corner of the restaurant, so we can have privacy, and it doesn't take long before I forget about Brooke's mother, her haircut, everything. She has remarkable poise, and charisma, and she's surprisingly funny. We both laugh when the waiter comes to our table and asks, Have you two ladies had a chance to look over the menu?

Might be time for a haircut, I say.

I ask about the movie Brooke just wrapped in Africa. Does she like being an actress? She talks with passion about the adventure of filmmaking, the fun of working with talented actors and directors, and it strikes me that she's the polar opposite of Wendi, who never knew what she wanted. Brooke knows exactly what she wants. She sees her dreams and doesn't falter in describing them, even if she's having trouble figuring out how to make them come true. Five years older than I, she's more worldly, more aware, and yet she also gives off an airy innocence, a neediness, which makes me want to protect her. She brings out the Gil in me, a side I didn't know I had.

We say most of the same things we've said by fax, but now, in person, over plates of pasta, they sound different, more intimate. There is nuance now, subtext, body language, and pheromones. Also, she's making me laugh, a lot, and making herself laugh. She has a lovely laugh. As with my wrist surgery, three hours pass in a millisecond.

She's exceptionally kind and sweet about my wrist, examining the inch-long pink scar, touching it lightly, asking questions. She's also empathetic, because she's facing surgery too, on both her feet. Her toes are damaged from years of dance training, she says, and doctors will need to break them and reset them. I tell her about Gil standing guard in the operating room with me, and she asks, joking, if she can borrow him.

We discover that, despite our outwardly different lives, we share similar starting points. She knows what it's like to grow up with a brash, ambitious, abrasive stage parent. Her mother has been her manager since Brooke was eleven months old. The difference: her mother still manages her. And they're nearly broke, because Brooke's career is slumping. The Africa movie was the first big job she's landed in a while. She does coffee commercials in Europe just to pay the mortgage. She says things like this, startlingly candid, as if we've known each other for decades. It's not only that we've softened the ground with faxes. She's just naturally open, all the time, I can tell. I wish I could be half as open. I can't tell her much about my own inner torments, though I can't avoid admitting that I hate tennis.

She laughs. You don't actually hate tennis.

Yes.

But you don't *hate* hate it.

I do. I hate it.

We talk about our travels, our favorite foods, music, movies. We bond over one recent movie, *Shadowlands,* the story of British writer C. S. Lewis. I tell Brooke that the movie struck a chord with me. There was Lewis's close relationship with his brother. There was his sheltered life, walled off from the world. There was his fear of risk and the pain of love. But then one singularly brave woman makes him see that pain is the price of being human, and well worth it. In the end Lewis tells his students: *Pain is God's megaphone to rouse a deaf world.* He tells them: *We are like blocks of stone . . . [T]he blows of His chisel, which hurt us so much, are what make us perfect.* Perry and I have seen the movie twice, I tell Brooke, and we've memorized half the lines. I'm moved that Brooke too loves *Shadowlands*. I'm slightly awed that she's read several of Lewis's books.

Well after midnight, lingering over empty coffee cups, we can no longer ignore the impatient stares of the waiters and restaurant owner. We need to go. I drive Brooke home, and on the sidewalk outside her house I have a feeling that her mother is watching us through an upstairs curtain. I give Brooke a chaste kiss and ask if I can call her again.

Please do.

As I walk away she notices a hole in my jeans, at the small of my back. She sticks her finger through the hole, scratching my tailbone with her nail. She flashes a sly grin before running inside.

I drive my rental car along Sunset Boulevard. I'd planned to head back to Vegas, never dreaming the date would go so well or last so long, but it's too late to catch a flight. I decide to stop for the night at the next hotel I come to, which turns out to be a Holiday Inn that's seen better days. Ten minutes later I'm lying in a musty room on the second floor, listening to traffic hissing along Sunset and the 405. I try to review the date—and, more importantly, to reach some conclusions about it, about what it means. But my eyelids are heavy. I fight to keep them open, fight as always the loss of control, which feels like the ultimate loss of choice.

15

My third date with Brooke is the night before her foot surgery. We're in Manhattan, in the ground-floor sitting room of her brownstone. We're kissing, on the verge, but first I need to tell her the truth about my hair.

She can sense that I have something on my mind. What's wrong? she asks.

Nothing.

You can tell me.

It's just that I haven't been completely honest with you.

We're lying on a couch. I sit up, punch a pillow, take a breath. Still searching for the right words, I look at the walls. They're decorated with African masks, eyeless faces with no hair. They're eerie. Also, vaguely familiar.

Andre, what is it?

This isn't easy to admit, Brooke. But, look, I've been losing my hair for quite some time and I wear a hairpiece to cover it up.

I reach out, take her hand, put it on my hairpiece.

She smiles. I had a feeling, she says.

You did?

It's no big deal.

You're not just saying that?

It's your eyes I find attractive. And your heart. Not your hair.

I stare at the eyeless, hairless faces and wonder if I'm falling.

I go with Brooke to the hospital and wait for her in the recovery room. I'm there when they wheel her in, her feet bandaged like mine before a match, and I'm there when she wakes up. I feel an enormous surge of protectiveness, and tenderness—which ebbs when she gets a phone call from her close friend, Michael Jackson. I can't fathom her continuing friendship with Jackson, given all the stories and accusations. But Brooke says he's just like us. Another prodigy who didn't have a childhood.

I follow Brooke home and spend days at her bedside while she recuperates. Her mother finds me one morning on the floor beside Brooke's bed. She's scandalized. Sleeping on the floor? It simply isn't done. I tell her that I prefer sleeping on the floor. My back. She walks away in a huff.

I kiss Brooke good morning. Your mother and I are getting off on the wrong foot.

We look down at her feet. Poor choice of words.

I need to leave. I'm due in Scottsdale for my first tournament since the surgery.

See you in a few weeks, I tell her, kissing her again, holding her.

I HAVE AN EASY DRAW IN SCOTTSDALE, but this doesn't make me any less fearful. Here comes the first real test of my wrist—what if it's not healed? What if it's worse? I have a recurring nightmare about being in the middle of a match and my hand falling off. I'm in my hotel room, closing my eyes, trying to visualize the wrist being fine and the match going well, when there's a knock at the door.

Who is it?

Brooke.

With two broken feet, she rallied to be here.

I win the tournament, feeling no pain.

WEEKS LATER, Pete and I agree to do a simultaneous interview with a magazine reporter. Pete comes to my hotel room, where the interview is to take place, and he's shocked to meet Peaches.

What the hell? Pete says.

Pete, meet Peaches. She's an old parrot I rescued from a Vegas pet store that was going out of business.

Nice bird, Pete says mockingly.

She *is* a nice bird, I say. She doesn't bite. She imitates people.

Like who?

Like me. She sneezes like me, talks like me—except she has a better vocabulary. I crack up every time the phone rings. Peaches yells, Telephone! *Tel*-ephone!

I tell Pete that back in Vegas I have a whole menagerie. A cat named King, a rabbit named Buddy, whatever it takes to fend off the loneliness. No man is an island. He shakes his head. Apparently he doesn't find tennis as lonely as I do.

We do the interview, and suddenly I feel as if I'm in the room with two parrots. At least when I bullshit a reporter, I do it with some flair, a little color. Pete sounds more robotic than Peaches.

I don't bother telling Pete, but I consider Peaches an integral part of my team, which is ever growing, ever changing, a constant experiment. I lost Nick and Wendi, but I've added Brooke and Slim, a bright, sweet kid from Vegas. We went to grade school together. We were born a day apart—at the same hospital. Slim is a good guy, if a lost soul, so I put him to work as my personal assistant. He watches my house, lets in the pool guy and the various handymen, sorts the mail, and answers fan requests for photos and autographs.

Now I think I might need to add a manager to the team. I pull Perry aside and ask him to take a look at my current management, see if they're overcharging me. He reviews the contracts and says that indeed I could do better. I put my arms around him, thank him—then get an idea. Why don't *you* be my manager, Perry? I need someone I trust.

I know he's busy. He's in his second year at the University of Arizona Law School, busting his ass. But I ask him to please consider taking this on, at least part-time.

I don't need to ask twice. Perry wants the job, and he wants to start right away. He'll work between classes, he says. Mornings, weekends, whenever. Aside from being a great opportunity, the job will enable him to whittle down what he owes me. I loaned Perry the money for law school because he didn't want to ask his father. He sat before me one night, telling me how his father uses money to control people, especially Perry. I have to break free of my father, Perry said. I've got to break free, Andre, once and for all.

There are few pleas I could find more compelling. I wrote him a check on the spot.

As my new manager, Perry's primary task is finding me a new coach, someone to replace Nick. He draws up a short list of candidates, and at the top of the list is a guy who's just written a book about tennis: *Winning Ugly.*

Perry hands me the book, urges me to read it.

I shoot him a dirty look. Thanks, no thanks. No more school for me.

Besides, I don't need to read the book. I know the author, Brad

Gilbert. I know him well. He's a fellow player. I've faced him many times, including weeks ago. His game is the opposite of mine. He's a junker, meaning he mixes speeds, uses change of pace, misdirection, guile. He has limited skills, and takes a conspicuous pride in this fact. If I'm the classic underachiever, Brad's the consummate overachiever. Rather than overpowering opponents, he frustrates them, preys on their flaws. He's preyed on me plenty. I'm intrigued, but it's not feasible. Brad's still playing. In fact, due to my surgery and my time away from the game, he's ranked higher than I.

No, Perry says, Brad is nearing the end of his career. He's thirty-two, and maybe he's open to the idea of coaching. Perry repeats that he's deeply impressed with Brad's book and thinks it contains the kind of practical wisdom I need.

In March 1994, when we're all in Key Biscayne for the tournament, Perry invites Brad to dinner at an Italian restaurant on Fisher Island. Café Porte Chervo. Right on the water. One of our favorites.

It's early evening. The sun is just disappearing behind the masts and sails of the boats at the dock. Perry and I are early, Brad is right on time. I'd forgotten how distinctive looking he is. Dark, rugged, he's certainly handsome, but not classically so. His features aren't chiseled; they look *molded*. I can't shake the idea that Brad looks like Early Man, that he just jumped from a time machine, slightly out of breath from discovering fire. Maybe it's all his hair that makes me think this. His head, arms, biceps, shoulders, face are covered with black hair. Brad has so much hair, I'm both horrified and jealous. His eyebrows alone are fascinating. I think: I could make a beautiful toupee out of just that left eyebrow.

The maître d', Renato, says we can sit on the terrace overlooking the dock.

I say, Sounds great.

No, Brad says. Uh-uh. We have to sit *inside*.

Why?

Because of Manny.

Excuse me? Who's Manny?

Manny Mosquito. Mosquitoes—yeah, I have a real thing about them, and trust me, Manny is here, Manny is out in force, and Manny likes me. Look at them all! Swarms! Look! No, I need to sit inside. *Far* from Manny!

He explains that mosquitoes are the reason he's wearing jeans instead of shorts, even though it's a hundred degrees and muggy. Manny, he says one last time, with a shudder.

Perry and I look at each other.

OK, Perry says. Inside it is.

Renato puts us at a table by the window. He hands us menus. Brad scans his and frowns.

Problem, he says.

What?

They don't carry my beer. Bud Ice.

Maybe they have—

Got to have Bud Ice. It's the only beer I drink.

He stands and says he's going to the market next door to buy some Bud Ice.

Perry and I order a bottle of red wine and wait. We say nothing while Brad's gone. He returns in five minutes with a six of Bud Ice, which he asks Renato to put on ice. Not the refrigerator, Brad says, because that's not cold enough. On ice, or else in the freezer.

When Brad is finally settled, half a cold Bud Ice down his gullet, Perry starts.

So, listen, Brad, one reason we wanted to meet with you is, we want to get your take on Andre's game.

Say what?

Andre's game. We'd like you to tell us what you think.

What I think?

Yes.

You want to know what I think of his game?

That's right.

You want me to be honest?

Please.

Brutally honest?

Don't hold back.

He takes an enormous swallow of beer and commences a careful, thorough, brutal-as-advertised summary of my flaws as a tennis player.

It's not rocket science, he says. If I were you, with your skills, your talent, your return and footwork, I'd dominate. But you've lost the fire you had when you were sixteen. That kid, taking the ball early, being aggressive, what the hell happened to that kid?

Brad says my overall problem, the problem that threatens to end my career prematurely—the problem that feels like my father's legacy—is perfectionism.

You always try to be perfect, he says, and you always fall short, and it fucks with your head. Your confidence is shot, and perfectionism is the reason. You try to hit a winner on every ball, when just being steady, consistent, meat and potatoes, would be enough to win ninety percent of the time.

He talks a mile a minute, a constant drone, not unlike a mosquito. He builds his argument with sports metaphors, from all sports, indiscriminately. He's an avid sports fan, and an equally avid metaphor fan.

Quit going for the knockout, he says. Stop swinging for the fences. All you have to be is solid. Singles, doubles, move the chains forward. Stop thinking about yourself, and your own game, and remember that the guy on the other side of the net has weaknesses. Attack his weaknesses. You don't have to be the best in the world every time you go out there. You just have to be better than one guy. Instead of you succeeding, make *him* fail. Better yet, *let* him fail. It's all about odds and percentages. You're from Vegas, you should have an appreciation of odds and percentages. The house always wins, right? Why? Because the odds are stacked in the house's favor. So? Be the house! Get the odds in your favor. Right now, by trying for a perfect shot with every ball, you're stacking the odds against yourself. You're assuming too much risk. You don't need to assume so much risk. Fuck that. Just keep the ball moving. Back and forth. Nice and easy. Solid. Be like *gravity*, man, just like motherfucking gravity. When you chase perfection, when you make perfection the ultimate goal, do you know what you're doing? You're chasing something that doesn't exist. You're making everyone around you miserable. You're making yourself miserable. Perfection? There's about five times a year you wake up perfect, when you can't lose to anybody, but it's not those five times a year that make a tennis player. Or a human being, for that matter. It's the other times. It's all about your head, man. With your talent, if you're fifty percent game-wise, but ninety-five percent head-wise, you're going to win. But if you're ninety-five percent game-wise and fifty percent head-wise, you're going to lose, lose, lose. Again, since you're from Vegas, put it this way. It takes twenty-one sets to win a slam. That's all. You need to win just twenty-one sets. Seven matches, best of five. That's twenty-one. In tennis, like cards, twenty-one's a winner. Blackjack! Focus on that number, and you won't go wrong. Simplify, simplify. Every time you win a set, say to yourself, That's one down. That's one in my pocket. At the start of a tournament, count *backward* from twenty-one. That's positive thinking, see? Of course, speaking for myself, when I'm playing blackjack, I'd rather win with sixteen, because *that's* winning ugly. No need to win with twenty-one. No need to be perfect.

He's been speaking for fifteen minutes. Perry and I haven't interrupted, haven't glanced at each other, haven't sipped our wine. At last Brad drains his second beer and announces: Where's the head in this place? I have to take a leak.

The moment he's gone I tell Perry: That's our guy.

Absolutely.

When Brad returns, the waiter comes for our order. Brad asks for penne arrabbiata with grilled chicken and mozzarella.

Perry orders chicken parmesan. Brad looks at Perry with disgust. Bad call, he says.

The waiter stops writing.

What you want to do, Brad says, is order a chicken breast, separate, then order all your mozzarella and sauce on the side. See, that way the chicken breast is fresh, not soggy, plus you can control your chicken-to-cheese-and-sauce ratio.

Perry thanks Brad for the menu coaching, but says he'll stick with his order. The waiter looks to me. I point at Brad and say: I'll have whatever he's having.

Brad smiles.

Perry clears his throat and says, So Brad. Would you have any interest in maybe becoming Andre's coach?

Brad thinks it over. For three seconds. Yeah, he says. I think I'd like that. I think I can help you.

I ask, When can we start?

Tomorrow, Brad says. I'll meet you on the courts at ten in the morning.

Huh. Well. That might a problem. I never play before one.

Andre, he says, we start at ten.

I'M LATE, OF COURSE. Brad looks at his watch.

Thought we said ten?

Man, I don't even know what ten a.m. means.

We start hitting, and Brad starts talking. He doesn't stop, as though the hours between last night's monologue and this morning's workout have been a mere intermission. He's picking apart my game, anticipating and analyzing my shots as I make them. The main point he stresses is the backhand up the line.

The second you get a chance to take a backhand up the line, he says, you've got to do it. That's your money shot. That's your equity shot. You can pay a lot of bills with that shot.

We play a few games, and he stops every other point to come to the net and tell me why I just did the dumbest possible thing.

What'd you do that for? I know it's a killer shot, but every shot doesn't have to be killer. Sometimes the best shot is a holding shot, an OK shot, a shot that gives the other guy a chance to miss. Let the other guy play.

I like the way this feels. I respond to Brad's ideas, his enthusiasm, his energy. I find peace in his claim that perfectionism is voluntary. Perfectionism is something I chose, and it's ruining me, and I can choose something else. I must choose something else. No one has ever said this to me. I've always assumed perfectionism was like my thinning hair or my thickened spinal cord. An inborn part of me.

After a light midday meal I put my feet up, watch TV, read the papers, sit under a shade tree—then go out and win my match against Mark Petchey, a British kid my age. My next match is against Becker, who's now being coached by Nick. After saying publicly that he couldn't imagine coaching any of my rivals, Nick is now coaching one of my archrivals. In fact, Nick's sitting in Becker's box. Becker is serving big, as always, 135 miles an hour, but with Nick in his corner, I'm juiced with adrenaline and able to handle anything he dishes up. And Becker knows it. He stops competing and plays to the crowd. Down a set and a break, he hands his racket to the ballgirl as if to say: Here, you can do as well as I'm doing.

I'm thinking: Yes, let her play, I'll beat the both of you.

After dispatching Becker, I'm in the final. My opponent? Pete. As always, Pete.

The match is slated for national TV. Brad and I are both keyed up as we walk into the locker room, only to find Pete lying on the ground. A doctor and a trainer are leaning over him. The tournament director hovers in the background. Pete brings his knees up to his chest and groans.

Food poisoning, the doctor says.

Brad whispers to me, Guess you just won Key Biscayne.

The director takes Brad and me aside and asks if we'd be willing to give Pete time to recover. I feel Brad stiffen. I know what he wants me to say. But I tell the director, Give Pete all the time he needs.

The director sighs and puts his hand on my arm. Thank you, he says. We've got fourteen thousand people out there. Plus the network.

Brad and I lounge around the locker room, flipping channels on the

TV, making phone calls. I dial Brooke, who's auditioning for *Grease* on Broadway. Otherwise, she'd be here.

Brad shoots me an evil glare.

Relax, I tell him, Pete probably won't get better.

The doctor gives Pete an IV, then props him on his feet. Pete wobbles, a newborn colt. He'll never make it.

The tournament director comes to us.

Pete's ready, he says.

Fucking A, Brad says. So are we.

Should be a short night, I tell Brad.

But Pete does it again. He sends his evil twin onto the court. This is *not* the Pete who was curled in a ball on the locker-room floor. This is not the Pete who was getting an IV and wobbling in circles. This Pete is in the prime of life, serving at warp speed, barely breaking a sweat. He's playing his best tennis, unbeatable, and he jumps out to a 5–1 lead.

Now I'm angry. I feel as if I found a wounded bird, brought it home, and nursed it back to health, only to have it try to peck my eyes out. I fight back and win the set. Surely I've withstood the only attack Pete can mount. He can't possibly have anything left.

But in the second set he's even better. And in the third he's a freak. He wins the best-of-three match.

I burst into the locker room. Brad is waiting for me, seething. He says again that if he'd been in my place, he'd have forced Pete to forfeit. He'd have demanded that the director fork over the winner's check.

That's not me, I tell Brad. I don't want to win like that. Besides, if I can't beat a guy who's poisoned, lying on the ground, I don't *deserve* it.

Brad abruptly stops talking. His eyes get big. He nods. He can't argue with that. He respects my principles, he says, even though he doesn't agree.

We walk out of the stadium together like Bogart and Claude Rains at the end of *Casablanca*. The beginning of a beautiful friendship. A vital new member of the team.

THEN THE TEAM goes on an epic losing streak.

Adopting Brad's concepts is like learning to write with my left hand. He calls his philosophy Bradtennis. I call it Braditude. Whatever the hell it's called, it's hard. I feel as if I'm back in school, not comprehending, longing to be somewhere else. Again and again Brad says I need to be consistent, steady, like gravity. He says this over and over: Be like gravity.

Constant pressure, weighing down your opponent. He tries to sell me on the joy of winning ugly, the virtue of winning ugly, but I only know how to lose ugly. And think ugly. I trust Brad, I know his advice is spot on, I do everything he says—so why am I not winning? I've given up perfectionism—so why am I not perfect?

I go to Osaka, lose again to Pete. Instead of gravity, I'm like flubber.

I go to Monte Carlo and lose to Yevgeny Kafelnikov—in the first round.

To add insult to injury, Kafelnikov is asked at the post-match news conference how it felt to beat me, since so many fans were cheering for me.

Difficult, Kafelnikov says, because Agassi is like Jesus.

I don't know what he means, but I don't think it's a compliment.

I go to Duluth, Georgia, lose to MaliVai Washington. Afterward, in the locker room, I feel crushed. Brad appears, smiling. Good things, he says, are about to happen.

I stare, incredulous.

He says, You have to suffer. You have to lose a shitload of close matches. And then one day you're going to win a close one and the skies are going to part and you're going to break through. You just need that one breakthrough, that one opening, and after that nothing will stop you from being the best in the world.

You're crazy.

You're learning.

You're nuts.

You'll see.

I GO TO THE 1994 FRENCH OPEN and play five vicious sets with Thomas Muster. Down 1–5 in the fifth set, something happens. I always hear Brad's philosophy in my head, but now it's coming from inside, not outside. I've internalized it, the way I once did my father's voice. I claw back and tie the set at 5. Muster breaks me. He's serving for the match. Still, I get the game to 30–40, I have hope. I'm on my toes, ready, but he hits a backhand I can't handle. I reach, hit it wide.

Match, Muster.

At the net he rubs my head, musses my hair. Apart from being condescending, his gesture nearly dislodges my hairpiece.

Good try, he says.

I stare at him with pure hatred. Big mistake, Muster. Don't touch the hair. Don't ever touch the hair. Just for that, I tell him at the net, I'll make you a promise. I'll never lose to you again.

In the locker room Brad congratulates me.

Good things, he says, are about to happen.

What?

He nods. Trust me—good things.

Clearly he doesn't understand the pain that losing causes me. And when someone doesn't understand, there's no point trying to explain.

At the 1994 Wimbledon I reach the fourth round but lose a nail-biter to Todd Martin. I'm wounded, frightened, disappointed. In the locker room Brad smiles and says: Good things.

We go to the Canadian Open. Brad shocks me at the start of the tournament. Good things, he says, are *not* about to happen. On the contrary, he sees a few very bad things on the horizon.

He's looking over my draw. NG, he says.

What the hell does NG mean?

Not Good. You got a terrible draw.

Let me see that.

I snatch the paper from his hands. He's right. My first match is a gimme, against Jakob Hlasek, from Switzerland, but in the second round I'll get David Wheaton, who always gives me a host of problems. Still, I love few things more than low expectations. Just tell me I can't do something. I inform Brad that I'm going to win the whole thing.

And when I do, I add, you have to get an earring.

I don't like jewelry, he says.

He thinks about it.

OK, he says. Done, and done.

THE COURT AT THE CANADIAN OPEN feels impossibly small, which makes the opponent look bigger.

Wheaton is a big guy, but here in Canada he looks ten feet tall. It's an optical illusion, but still, I feel as if he's standing two inches from my face. Distracted, I find myself down two match points in the third-set tiebreak.

Then, wholly out of character, I pull myself together. I shake off all distractions and optical illusions and fight back and win. I do what Brad said I would do. I win a close one. Later I tell Brad, That's the match you said I'd win. That's the match you said would change things.

He smiles as if I just sat down in a restaurant all by myself and ordered the chicken parm with the chicken breast separate from the sauce and cheese. Very good, Grasshopper. Wax on, wax off.

My game speeding up, my mind slowing down, I storm through the rest of the draw and win the Canadian Open.

Brad chooses a diamond stud.

GOING INTO THE 1994 U.S. OPEN, I'm number twenty, therefore unseeded. No unseeded player has won the U.S. Open since the 1960s.

Brad likes it. He says he wants me unseeded. He wants me to be the joker in the deck. You'll play someone tough in the early rounds, he says, and if you beat them, you'll win this tournament.

He's sure of it. So sure, he vows to shave his entire body when I do. I'm always telling Brad he's too hairy. He makes Sasquatch look like Kojak. He needs to trim that chest, those arms—and those eyebrows. Either trim them or name them.

Trust me, I tell him, you shave that chest and you'll feel things you've never felt before.

Win the U.S. Open, he says, and so will you.

Because of my low ranking, I'm under the radar at this U.S. Open. (I'd be more under the radar if Brooke weren't on hand, setting off a photo shoot each time she turns her head.) I'm all business, and I dress the part. I wear a black hat, black shorts, black socks, black-and-white shoes. But at the start of my first-rounder, against Robert Eriksson, I feel the old brittle nerves. I feel sick to my stomach. I fight through it, thinking of Brad, refusing to entertain any thought of perfection. I concentrate on being solid, letting Eriksson lose, and he does. He sends me sailing into the second round.

Then—after nearly choking—I beat Guy Forget, from France. Then I take out Wayne Ferreira, from South Africa, in straight sets.

Up next is Chang. I wake the morning of the match with ferocious diarrhea. By match time I'm weak, depleted, and babbling like Peaches. Gil makes me drink an extra dose of Gil Water. This batch has a thickness, a density, like oil. I force it down, nearly puking several times. As I do, Gil whispers, Thank you for trusting me.

Then I walk into a classic Chang buzz saw. He's that rare phenomenon—an opponent who wants to win exactly as much as I do, no more, no less. We both know from the opening serve that it's going down to the wire. Photo finish. No other way to settle it. But in the fifth set, thinking we're destined for a tiebreak, I catch a rhythm and break him early. I'm making crazy shots, and I feel him losing traction. It's almost not fair, after such a back-and-forth fight, the way I'm sneaking away with this match. I should be having more trouble with him in the final minutes, but it's sinfully easy.

At his news conference, Chang tells reporters about a different match than the one I just played. He says he could have played another two sets. Andre got lucky, he says. Furthermore, Chang expresses a great deal of pride that he exposed holes in my game, and he predicts other players in the tournament will thank him. He says I'm vulnerable now. I'm toast.

Next I face Muster. I make good my vow that I will never lose to him again. It takes every ounce of self-control not to rub his head at the net.

I'm in the semis. I'm due to play Martin on Saturday. Friday afternoon, Gil and I are eating lunch at P. J. Clarke's. We order the same thing we always order at P. J. Clarke's—cheeseburgers on toasted English muffins. We're sitting in the section of our favorite waitress, the one we always agree has a story to tell, if only someone were brave enough to ask her. While we're waiting for the food we riffle through a stack of New York newspapers. I see Lupica's column is about me. I shouldn't read it, but I do. He writes that the U.S. Open is mine to lose, but you can count on the fact that I *will* find a way to lose it.

Agassi, Lupica writes, simply isn't a champion.

I close the paper and feel as if the walls are closing in, as if my vision is narrowing to a pinprick. Lupica sounds so sure, as if he's seen the future. What if he's right? What if this is it, my moment of truth, and I'm revealed to be a fraud? If it doesn't happen now, when will I have another chance to win the U.S. Open? So many things have to fall your way. Finals don't grow on trees. What if I never win this tournament? What if I always look back on this moment with regret? What if hiring Brad was a mistake? What if Brooke is the wrong girl for me? What if my team, so carefully assembled, is the wrong team?

Gil looks up and sees me turning white.

What's wrong?

I read him the column. He doesn't move.

I'd like to meet that Lupica one day, he says.

What if he's right?

Control what you can control.

Yeah.

Control what you can control.

Right.

Here comes our food.

Martin, who just beat me at Wimbledon, is a deadly opponent. He has a nice hold game and a solid break game. He's huge, six foot six, and returns the serve off both wings with precision and conviction. He'll cane a serve that isn't first-rate, which puts enormous pressure on an average server like me. With his own serve he's uncannily accurate. If he misses, it's only by a bee's dick. He hits the line, and he hasn't the vaguest interest in hitting the inside half of the line—he wants to hit that outside half. For some reason, I'm better against big servers who miss by a lot. I like to cheat forward, guess which way the serve is coming, and with players like Martin I tend to guess wrong more often, thus leaving myself less lateral coverage. He's a nasty matchup for a player with my tendencies, and as our semi begins I like his chances, and Lupica's, better than mine.

Still, as the first few games unfold, I realize that several things are in my favor. Martin is better on grass than hard court. This is *my* surface. Also, like me, he's an underachiever. He's a fellow slave to nerves. I understand the man I'm playing, therefore, understand him intimately. Simply knowing your enemy is a powerful advantage.

Above all, Martin has a tic. A tell. Some players, when serving, look at their opponent. Some look at nothing. Martin looks at a particular spot in the service box. If he stares a long time at that spot, he's serving in the opposite direction. If he merely glances, he's serving right at that spot. You might not notice it at 0–0, or 15–love, but on break point, he stares at that spot with psycho eyes, like the killer in a horror movie, or glances and looks away like a beginner at the poker tables.

The match unfolds so easily, however, that I don't need Martin's tell. He seems unsteady, dwarfed by the occasion, whereas I'm playing with uncommon determination. I see him doubt himself—I can almost hear his doubt—and I sympathize. As I walk off the court, the winner in four sets, I think, He's got some maturing to do. Then I catch myself. Did I really just say that—about someone else?

In the final I face Michael Stich, from Germany. He's been to the final at three slams, so he's not like Martin, he's a threat on every surface. He's also a superb athlete with an unreal wingspan. He has a mighty first serve, heavy and fast, and when it's on, which it usually is, he can serve you into next week. He's so accurate, you're shocked when he misses, and you have to overcome your shock to stay in the point. Even when he does miss, however, you're not out of the woods, because then he falls back on his safe serve, a knuckleball that leaves you with your jock on the ground. And just to keep you a bit more off balance, Stich is without any patterns or tendencies. You never know if he's going to serve and volley or stay back at the baseline.

Hoping to seize control, dictate the terms, I come fast out of the blocks, hitting the ball clean, crisp, pretending to feel no fear. I like the sound the ball makes off my racket. I like the sound of the crowd, their oohs and aahs. Stich, meanwhile, comes out skittish. When you lose the first set as quickly as he does, 6–1, your instinct is to panic. I can see in his body language that he's succumbing to that instinct.

He pulls himself together in the second set, however, and gives me a two-fisted battle. I win 7–6, but feel lucky. I know it could have gone either way.

In the third set we both raise the stakes. I feel the finish line pulling, but now he's mentally committed to this fight. There have been times in the past when he's given up against me, when he's taken unnecessary risks because he hasn't believed in himself. Not this time. He's playing smart, proving to me that I'm going to have to rip the trophy from him if I really want it. And I do want it. So I will rip it. We have long rallies off my serve, until he realizes I'm committed, I'm willing to hit with him all day. I catch sight of him grabbing his side, winded. I start picturing how the trophy will look in the bachelor pad back in Vegas.

There are no breaks of serve through the third set. Until 5–all. Finally I break him, and now I'm serving for the match. I hear Brad's voice, as clearly as if he were standing behind me. *Go for his forehand. When in doubt, forehand, forehand.* So I hit to Stich's forehand. Again and again he misses. The outcome feels, to both of us, I think, inevitable.

I fall to my knees. My eyes fill with tears. I look to my box, to Perry and Philly and Gil and especially Brad. You know everything you need to know about people when you see their faces at the moments of your greatest triumph. I've believed in Brad's talent from the beginning, but now, seeing his pure and unrestrained happiness for me, I *believe* unrestrainedly in him.

Reporters tell me I'm the first unseeded player since 1966 to win the U.S. Open. More importantly, the first man who ever did it was Frank Shields, grandfather of the fifth person in my box. Brooke, who's been here for every match, looks every bit as happy as Brad.

My new girlfriend, my new coach, my new manager, my surrogate father.

At last, the team is firmly, irrevocably, in place.

16

I THINK you should get rid of that hairpiece, Brooke says. And that ponytail. Shave your hair short, short, and be done with it.

Impossible. I'd feel naked.

You'd feel liberated.

I'd feel exposed.

It's as though she's suggesting I have all my teeth pulled. I tell her to forget it. Then I go away and think about it for a few days. I think about the pain my hair has caused me, the inconvenience of the hairpieces, the hypocrisy and the pretending and the lying. Maybe it isn't crazy after all. Maybe it's the first step toward sanity.

I stand before Brooke one morning and say, Let's do it.

Do what?

Cut it off. Let's cut it *all* off.

We schedule the ceremonial shearing for late at night, at an hour normally reserved for séances and raves. It's to be in the kitchen of Brooke's brownstone, after she returns from the theater. (She got the part in *Grease.*) We'll make a party of it, she says, invite some friends.

Perry is there. And, despite our breakup, Wendi. Brooke is openly irritated by the presence of Wendi, and vice versa. Perry is baffled by it. I explain to Brooke and Perry that despite our romantic history, Wendi is still a close friend, a lifelong friend. Being shorn is a dramatic step, and I need friends in the room for moral support, just as I needed Gil there when I had my wrist surgery. In fact, it crosses my mind that for this surgery I should also be sedated. We send out for wine.

Brooke's hairdresser, Matthew, puts my head over the sink, washes my hair, then pulls it all tight.

Andre—are you sure?

No.

Are you ready?

No.

Do you want to do this in front of a mirror?

No. I don't want to watch.

He puts me in a wooden chair and then—snip. There goes the pony-tail.

Everyone applauds.

He begins cutting the hair on the sides of my head, tight, close to the skull. I think of the mohawk at the Bradenton Mall. I close my eyes, feel my heart pound, as if I'm about to play a final. This was a mistake. Maybe the defining mistake of my life. J.P. warned me not to do this. J.P. said that whenever he attends one of my matches, he hears people talking about my hair. Women love me for it, men hate me for it. Now that J.P. has quit pastoring, devoted himself to music, he's been doing some work in advertising, writing jingles for radio and TV commercials, so he spoke with some authority when he proclaimed: As far as the corporate world is concerned, Andre Agassi *is* his hair. And when Andre Agassi's hair is gone, corporate sponsors will be gone.

He also suggested pointedly that I reread the Bible story about Sam-son and Delilah.

As Matthew cuts and cuts, *and cuts,* I realize I should have listened to J.P. When has J.P. ever steered me wrong? With clumps of my hair falling to the floor, I feel clumps of me falling away.

It takes eleven minutes. Then Matthew whisks away the smock and says, *Ta-dah!*

I walk to the mirror. I see a person I don't recognize. Before me stands a total stranger. My reflection isn't different, it's simply not me. But, really, what the hell have I lost? Maybe I'll have an easier time being *this* guy. All this time with Brad, trying to fix what's *in* my head, it never occurred to me to fix what's *on* my head. I smile at my reflection, run a hand over my scalp. Hello. Nice to meet you.

As night turns to morning, as we work our way through several bot-tles of wine, I feel exhilarated, and heavily indebted to Brooke. You were right, I tell her. My hairpiece was a shackle, and my natural hair, grown to absurd lengths, dyed three different colors, was a weight as well, holding me down. It seems so trivial—hair. But hair has been the crux of my pub-lic image, and my self-image, and it's been a sham.

Now the sham is lying on Brooke's floor in tiny haystacks. I feel well rid of it. I feel true. I feel free.

And I play like it. At the 1995 Australian Open I come out like the Incredible Hulk. I don't drop one set in a take-no-prisoners blitz to the final. This is the first time I've played in Australia, and I can't imagine why I've waited so long. I like the surface, the venue—the heat. Having grown up in Vegas, I don't feel the heat the way other players do, and the defining characteristic of the Australian Open is the unholy temperature. Just as cigar and pipe smoke lingers in the memory after playing Roland Garros, the hazy memory of playing in a giant kiln stays with you for weeks after you leave Melbourne.

I also enjoy the Australian people, and they apparently enjoy me, even though I'm not me, I'm this new bald guy in a bandana and a goatee and a hoop earring. Newspapers go to town with my new look. Everyone has an opinion. Fans who rooted for me are disoriented. Fans who rooted against me have a new reason to dislike me. I read and hear a remarkable succession of pirate jokes. I never knew there could be so many pirate jokes. But I don't care. I tell myself that everyone is going to have to deal with this pirate, accept this pirate, when I hoist that trophy.

In the final I run smack into Pete. I lose the first set in nothing flat. I lose it gutlessly, on a double fault. Here we go again.

I take time before the second set to collect myself. I glance toward my box. Brad looks frustrated. He's never believed that Pete is the better player. His face says, *You're* the better player, Andre. Don't respect him so much.

Pete is serving live grenades, one after another, a typical Pete fusillade. But in the middle of the second set, I feel him tiring. His grenades still have the pins in them. He's wearing down physically, and emotionally, because he's been through hell these last few days. His longtime coach, Tim Gullickson, suffered two strokes, and then they discovered a tumor in his brain. Pete is traumatized. As the match turns my way, I feel guilty. I'd be willing to stop, let Pete go into the locker room, get an IV, and come back as that other Pete who likes to kick my ass at slams.

I break him twice. He slumps his shoulders, concedes the set.

The third set comes down to a jittery tiebreak. I grab a 3–0 lead and then Pete wins the next four points. Suddenly he's up 6–4, serving for the set. I let out a caveman scream, as if I'm in the weight room with Gil, and put everything I've got into a return that nicks the net and stays inside the line. Pete stares at the ball, then me.

On the next point he hits a forehand that sails long. We're deadlocked at 6. A furious rally ends when I shock him by coming to the net and hitting a soft backhand drop volley. It works so well, I do it again. Set, Agassi. Momentum, ditto.

The fourth set is a foregone conclusion. I keep my foot on the gas and win, 6–4. Pete looks resolved. Too much hill to climb. In fact, he's maddeningly unruffled as he comes to the net.

It's my second slam in a row, my third overall. Everyone says it's my best slam yet, because it's my first victory over Pete in a slam final. But I think twenty years from now I'll remember it as my first bald slam.

THE TALK TURNS IMMEDIATELY to my reaching number one. Pete's been number one for seventy weeks, and everyone on my team says I'm destined to kick him off the top of that vaunted mountain. I tell them that tennis has nothing to do with destiny. Destiny has better things to do than count ATP points.

Still, I make it my goal to be number one, because my team wants it.

I cloister myself in Gil's gym and train with fury. I tell him about the goal, and he draws up a battle plan. First, he designs a course of study. He sets about collecting a master list of phone numbers and addresses for the world's most acclaimed sports doctors and nutritionists, and reaches out to all of them, turns them into his private consultants. He huddles with experts at the U.S. Olympic Training Center in Colorado Springs. He flies coast to coast, interviewing the best and brightest, famed researchers on health and wellness, recording every word they tell him in his da Vinci notebooks. He reads everything, from muscle magazines to obscure medical studies and dry reports. He subscribes to the *New England Journal of Medicine*. In no time he makes himself a portable university, with one professor and one subject. The student body: me.

Then he determines my physical limit, and pushes me right up to it. He soon has me bench-pressing almost twice my weight, five to seven sets of more than three hundred pounds. He has me lifting fifty-pound dumbbells in excruciating sets of three-ways: back-to-back-to-back flexes that burn three different muscles in my shoulders. Then we work on biceps and triceps. We burn my muscles to ashes. I like when Gil talks about burning muscles, setting them afire. I like being able to put my pyromania to constructive use.

Next we concentrate on my midsection, beginning with a special machine Gil designed and built. As with all his machines, he chopped it, cut it, re-welded it. (The blueprints in his da Vinci notebooks are stunning.) It's the only machine of its kind in the world, he says, because it allows me to work my abs without engaging my fragile back. We're going to stack heavy on your abs, he says, work them until they're on fire, and then we're going to do Russian Twists: you'll hold a forty-five-pound iron plate, a big wheel, and rotate left, right, left, right. That will burn down your sides and obliques.

Last, we move to Gil's homemade lat machine. Unlike every lat machine in every gym the world over, Gil's doesn't compromise my back or neck. The bar I pull to work my lats is slightly in front of me. I'm never awkwardly positioned.

While I'm lifting, Gil also feeds me constantly, every twenty minutes. He wants me taking in four parts carbs to one part protein, and he times my intake to the nanosecond. *When* you eat, he says, and *how* you eat, that's the thing. Every time I turn around he's shoving a bowl of high-protein oatmeal at me, or a bacon sandwich, or a bagel with peanut butter and honey.

Finally, my upper body and gut pleading for mercy, we go outside and run up and down the hill behind Gil's house. Gil Hill. Quick bursts of power and speed, up and down, up and down, I run until my mind begs me to stop, and then I run some more, ignoring my mind.

Easing into my car at dusk, I often don't know that I'll be able to drive home. Sometimes I don't try. If I don't have the strength to turn the key in the ignition, I go back inside and curl up on one of Gil's benches and fall asleep.

After my mini boot camp with Gil, I look as if I've traded in my old body, upgraded to the newest model. Still, there's room for improvement. I could be better about what I eat outside the gym. Gil, however, doesn't crack the whip about my lapses. He certainly doesn't like the way I eat when I'm not with him—Taco Bell, Burger King—but he says I need comfort food now and then. My psyche, he says, is more fragile than my back, and he doesn't want to overstress it. Besides, a man needs one or two vices.

Gil is a paradox, and we both know it. He can lecture me about nutrition while watching me sip a milkshake. He doesn't slap the milkshake from my hand. On the contrary, he might even take a sip. I like people with contradictions, of course. I also like that Gil's not a taskmaster. I've had enough taskmasters to last me a lifetime. Gil understands me, coddles me, and occasionally—just occasionally—indulges my taste for junk, maybe because he shares it.

At Indian Wells, I face Pete again. If I can beat him I'll be within an inch of the top spot. I'm in peak condition, but we play a sloppy match, filled with unforced errors. Each of us is distracted. Pete is still distressed about his coach. I'm worried about my father, who's having open-heart surgery in a few days. This time, Pete manages to rise above his turmoil, while I let mine consume me. I lose in three sets.

I race to the UCLA Medical Center and find my father strapped to machines with long tubes. They remind me of the ball machine of my youth. *You can't beat the dragon.* My mother hugs me. He watched you play yesterday, she says. He watched you lose to Pete.

I'm sorry, Pops.

He's on his back, drugged, helpless. His eyelids flutter open. He sees me and gestures with his hand. Come closer.

I lean in. He can't speak. He has a tube in his mouth and down his throat. He mumbles something.

I don't understand, Pops.

More gestures. I don't know what he's trying to tell me. Now he's getting angry. If he had the strength he'd get out of this bed and knock me out.

He motions for a pad and pen.

Tell me later, Pops.

No, no. He shakes his head. He *must* tell me now.

The nurses hand him a pad and pen. He scrawls a few words, then makes a brushing gesture. Like an artist, gently brushing. At last I understand.

Backhand, he's trying to say. Hit to Pete's backhand. *You should have hit more to Pete's backhand.*

Vork your wolleys. Hit *harder.*

I stand and feel an overpowering urge to forgive, because I realize that my father can't help himself, that he never could help himself, any more than he could understand himself. My father is what he is, and always will be, and though he can't help himself, though he can't tell the difference between loving me and loving tennis, it's love all the same. Few of us are granted the grace to know ourselves, and until we do, maybe the best we can do is be consistent. My father is nothing if not consistent.

I put my father's hand at his side, force him to stop gesturing, tell him that I understand. Yes, yes, to the backhand. I'll hit to Pete's backhand next week in Key Biscayne. And I'll beat his ass. Don't worry, Pops. I'll beat him. Now rest.

He nods. His hand still flapping against his side, he closes his eyes and falls asleep.

The next week I beat Pete in the final of Key Biscayne.

After the match we fly together to New York, where we're due to catch a flight to Europe for the Davis Cup. But first, upon landing, I drag Pete to the Eugene O'Neill Theater to see Brooke as Rizzo in *Grease*. It's the first time Pete has seen a Broadway show, I think, but it's my fiftieth time seeing *Grease*. I can recite every word of We Go Together, a trick I've performed, deadpan, to much laughter on the *Late Show with David Letterman*.

I like Broadway. I find the ethos of the theater familiar. The work of a Broadway actor is physical, strenuous, demanding, and the nightly pressure is intense. The best Broadway actors remind me of athletes. If they don't give their best, they know it, and if they don't know it, the crowd lets them know it. All this is lost on Pete, however. From the opening number he's yawning, fidgeting, checking his watch. He doesn't like the theater, and he doesn't get actors, since he's never pretended anything in his life. In the quasi-darkness of the footlights, I smile at his discomfort. Somehow, forcing him to sit through *Grease* feels more satisfying than beating him in Key Biscayne. We go together, like rama lama lama . . .

IN THE MORNING we catch the Concorde to Paris, then a private plane to Palermo. I'm barely settled into my hotel room when the phone rings.

Perry.

In my hand, he says, I hold the latest rankings.

Hit me with it.

You—are number one.

I've knocked Pete off the mountaintop. After eighty-two weeks at number one, Pete's looking up at me. I'm the twelfth tennis player to be number one in the two decades since they started keeping computer rankings. The next person who phones is a reporter. I tell him that I'm happy about the ranking, that it feels good to be the best that I can be.

It's a lie. This isn't at all what I feel. It's what I want to feel. It's what I expected to feel, what I tell myself to feel. But in fact I feel nothing.

17

I SPEND MANY HOURS ROAMING the streets of Palermo, drinking strong black coffee, wondering what the hell is wrong with me. I did it— I'm the number one tennis player on earth, and yet I feel empty. If being number one feels empty, unsatisfying, what's the point? Why not just retire?

I picture myself announcing that I'm done. I choose the words I'll speak at the news conference. Several images then come to mind. Brad, Perry, my father, each disappointed, aghast. Also, I tell myself that retiring won't solve my essential problem, it won't help me figure out what I want to do with my life. I'll be a twenty-five-year-old retiree, which sounds a lot like a ninth-grade dropout.

No, what I need is a new goal. The problem, all this time, is that I've had the wrong goals. I never really wanted to be number one, that was just something others wanted for me. So I'm number one. So a computer loves me. So what? What I think I've always wanted, since I was a boy, and what I want now, is far more difficult, far more substantial. I want to win the French Open. Then I'll have all four slams to my credit. The complete set. I'll be only the fifth man to accomplish such a feat in the open era— and the first American.

I've never cared about computer rankings, and I've never cared about the number of slams I won. Roy Emerson has the most slams (twelve), and nobody thinks he's better than Rod Laver. Nobody. My fellow players, along with any tennis expert or historian I respect, agree that Laver was the best, the king, because he won all four. More, he did it in the same year—twice. Granted, there were only two surfaces back then, grass and clay, but still, that's godlike. That's inimitable.

I think about the greats from past eras, how they all chased Laver, how they dreamed of winning all four slams. They all skipped certain slams, because they didn't give a damn about quantity. They cared about versatility. They all feared that they wouldn't be considered truly great if their resumes were incomplete, if one or two of the game's four prizes could elude them.

The more I think about winning all four slams, the more excited I become. It's a sudden and shocking insight into myself. I realize this is what I've long wanted. I've simply repressed the desire because it didn't seem possible, especially after reaching the final of the French Open two years in a row and losing. Also, I've allowed myself to get sidetracked by sportswriters and fans who don't understand, who count the number of slams a player won and use that bogus number to gauge his legacy. Winning all four is the true Holy Grail. So, in 1995, in Palermo, I decide that I will chase this Grail, full speed ahead.

Brooke, meanwhile, never wavers in pursuit of her own personal Grail. Her run on Broadway is deemed a great success, and she doesn't feel empty. She feels hungry. She wants more. She looks to the next big thing. Offers are slow to come in, however. I try to help. I tell her that the public doesn't know her. They think they do, but they don't. A problem with which I have some experience. Some people think she's a model, some think she's an actress. She needs to hone her image. I ask Perry to step in, have a look at Brooke's career.

It doesn't take him long to form an opinion and a plan. He says what Brooke needs now is a TV show. Her future, he says, lies in TV. So she immediately begins searching for scripts and pilots in which she can shine.

Just before the start of the 1995 French Open, Brooke and I go to Fisher Island for a few days. We both need rest and sleep. I can't get either, though. I can't stop thinking about Paris. I lie in bed at night, taut as a wire, playing matches on the ceiling.

I continue to obsess on the plane to Paris, even though Brooke is with me. She's not working just now, so she's able to get away.

Our first time in Paris together, she says, kissing me.

Yes, I say, stroking her hand.

How to tell her that this is not, even partially, a vacation? That this trip isn't remotely about us?

We stay at the Hôtel Raphael, just around the corner from the Arc de Triomphe. Brooke likes the creaky old elevator with the iron door that manually closes. I like the small candlelit bar off the lobby. The rooms are small too, and they have no TVs, which appalls Brad. He can't take it, in fact. He checks out a few minutes after checking in, switching to a more modern hotel.

Brooke speaks French, so she's able to show me Paris through a new, wider lens. I feel comfortable exploring the city, because there's no fear of getting lost, and she can translate. I tell her about the first time I was here, with Philly. I tell her about the Louvre, the painting that freaked us both out. She's fascinated and wants me to take her to see it.

Another time, I say.

We eat at fancy restaurants, visit out-of-the-way neighborhoods I'd never venture into on my own. Some of it charms me, but most leaves me cold, because I'm loath to break my concentration. The owner of one café invites us down to his ancient wine cellar, a musty, medieval tomb filled with dust-covered bottles. He hands one to Brooke. She peers at the date on the label: 1787. She cradles the bottle like a baby, then holds it up to me, incredulous.

I don't get it, I whisper. It's a bottle. It has dust on it.

She glares, as if she'd like to break the bottle over my head.

Late one night we go for a walk along the Seine. It's her thirtieth birthday. We stop near a flight of stone steps leading down to the river, and I present her with a diamond tennis bracelet. She laughs as I put it around her wrist and fiddle with the clasp. We both admire the way it catches the moonlight. Then, just beyond Brooke's shoulder, standing on the stone steps, a drunken Frenchman staggers into view and sends a high, looping arc of urine into the Seine. I don't believe in omens, as a rule, but this seems ominous. I just can't tell if it portends something for the French Open or my relationship with Brooke.

At last the tournament begins. I win my first four matches without dropping a set. It's evident to reporters and commentators that I'm a different player. Stronger and more focused. On a mission. No one sees this more clearly than my fellow players. I've always noticed the way players silently anoint the alpha dog in their midst, the way they single out the one player who's feeling it, who's likeliest to win. At this tournament, for the first time, I'm that player. I feel them all watching me in the locker room. I feel them noting my every move, the little things I do, even studying how I organize my bag. They're quicker to step aside when I walk by, eager to give up the training table. A new degree of respect is directed toward me, and while I try not to take it seriously, I can't help but enjoy it. Better me getting this treatment than someone else.

Brooke, however, doesn't seem to notice any difference in me, doesn't treat me any differently. At night I sit in the hotel room, staring out the window at Paris, an eagle on a cliff, but she talks to me of this and that, *Grease* and Paris and what so-and-so said about such-and-such. She doesn't understand the work I did in Gil's gym, the trials and sacrifices and concentration that have led to this new confidence—or the huge task that lies ahead. And she doesn't try to understand. She's more interested in where we're going to eat next, which wine cellar we're going to explore. She takes it for granted that I'm going to win, and she wishes I'd hurry up and do it, so we can have fun. It's not selfishness on her part, just a mistaken impression that winning is normal, losing is abnormal.

In the quarters I face Kafelnikov, the Russian who likened me to Jesus. I sneer at him across the net as the match begins: Jesus is about to whip you with a car antenna. I know I can beat Kafelnikov. He knows it too. It's written all over his face. But early in the first set, I lunge for a ball and feel something snap. My hip flexor. I ignore it, pretend it didn't happen, pretend I don't have a hip, but the hip sends lines of pain up and down my leg.

I can't bend. I can't move. I ask for the trainer, who gives me two aspirin and tells me there's nothing he can do. His eyes are the size of poker chips when he tells me.

I lose the first set. Then the second. In the third I rally. I'm up 4–1, the crowd urging me onward. *Allez, Agassi!* But I grow less mobile with every minute. Kafelnikov, moving well, ties the set, and I feel my limbs go slack. It's another Russian crucifixion. Au revoir, Grail. I walk off the court without collecting my rackets.

The real test wasn't supposed to be Kafelnikov. It was supposed to be Muster, the hair-musser who's been dominating on clay. So even if I'd gotten by Kafelnikov I don't know how hobbled I would have been against Muster. But I promised Muster I'd never lose to him again, and I meant it, and I liked my chances. I think no matter who was on the other side of that net, I could have done something great. As I leave Paris I don't feel defeated; I feel cheated. This was it, I just know. My last chance. Never again will I be in Paris feeling so strong, so young. Never again will I inspire such fear in the locker room.

My golden opportunity to win all four slams is gone.

Brooke has already flown home ahead of me, so it's just Gil and me on the flight, Gil talking softly about how we're going to treat the flexor, how we're going to adjust after what we've just put ourselves through, and get ready for what's coming—grass. We spend a week in Vegas, doing nothing but watching movies and waiting for my hip to mend. An MRI tells us the damage isn't permanent. Cold comfort.

We fly to England. I'm the number one seed at the 1995 Wimbledon, because I'm still ranked number one in the world. Fans greet me with an enthusiasm and glee that clash sharply with my mood. Nike has been here ahead of time, priming the pump, handing out Agassi Kits—adhesive sideburns, Fu Manchu mustaches, and bandanas. This is my new look. I've morphed from pirate to bandit. It's surreal, as always, to see guys trying to look like me, and as always it's even a bit more surreal to see girls trying. Girls with Fu Manchus and sideburns—it almost makes me crack a smile. Almost.

It rains every day, but still the fans mob Wimbledon. They brave the rain, the cold, they line up all the way down Church Road, for the love of tennis. I want to go out there and stand with them, question them, find out what makes them love it so much. I wonder what it would be like to feel such passion for the game. I wonder if the fake Fu Manchus stay on in the rain, or if they disintegrate like my old hairpieces.

I win my first two matches easily, and then beat Wheaton in four sets. The big news of that day, however, is Tarango, who lost, then fought with an umpire before leaving the court. Then Tarango's wife slapped the umpire. One of the great scandals in Wimbledon history. Instead of facing Tarango, therefore, I'll face Alexander Mronz, from Germany. Reporters ask me which opponent I would have preferred, and I badly want to tell the story of Tarango cheating when I was eight. I don't, however. I don't want to get in a public spat with Tarango, and I fear making an enemy of his wife. I say the diplomatic thing, that it doesn't matter whom I play, even though Tarango was the more dangerous threat.

I beat Mronz in three easy sets.

In the semis I face Becker. I've beaten him the last eight times we've played. Pete has already moved on to the final and he's awaiting the winner of Agassi-Becker, which is to say he's awaiting me, because every slam final is beginning to feel like a standing date between me and Pete.

I take the first set from Becker, no problem. In the second set I jump out to a 4–1 lead. Here I come, Pete. Get ready, Pete. Then, just like that, Becker begins to play a rougher, brawnier game. He wins several scrappy points. After chipping at my confidence with a tiny nail he now pulls out a sledgehammer. He plays from the baseline, an unusual tactic for him, and flat outmuscles me. He breaks me, and though I'm still up 4–2, I feel something snap. Not my hip—my mind. I'm suddenly unable to control my thoughts. I'm thinking of Pete, waiting. I'm thinking of my sister Rita, whose husband, Pancho, just lost a long bout with stomach cancer. I'm thinking of Becker, still working with Nick, who, tanner than ever, the color of prime rib, sits above us in Becker's box. I wonder if Nick has told Becker my secrets—for instance, the way I've figured out Becker's serve.

(Just before he tosses the ball, Becker sticks out his tongue and it points like a tiny red arrow to where he's aiming.) I'm thinking of Brooke, who's been shopping at Harrods this week with Pete's girlfriend, a law student named DeLaina Mulcahy. All these thoughts go crashing through my mind, making me feel scattered, fractured, and this allows Becker to capture the momentum. He never gives it back. He wins in four sets.

The loss is one of the most devastating of my life. Afterward, I don't say a word to anyone. Gil, Brad, Brooke—I don't speak to them because I can't. I am broken, gut-shot.

BROOKE AND I ARE DUE TO FLY AWAY on a vacation. We've been planning it for weeks. We wanted someplace remote, with no phones, no other people, so we booked Indigo Island, 150 miles from Nassau. After the Wimbledon debacle, I want to cancel, but Brooke reminds me we've secured the entire island, our deposit is nonrefundable.

Besides, it's supposed to be paradise, she says. It will be good for us.

I frown.

Just as I feared, from the moment we arrive, paradise feels like Supermax. On the entire island there is one house, and it's not big enough for the three of us—Brooke, me, and my black mood.

Brooke lies in the sun and waits for me to speak. She's not frightened by my silence, but she doesn't understand it, either. In her world, everyone pretends, whereas in mine some things can't be pretended away.

After two days of silence I thank her for being so patient, and tell her I'm back.

I'm going to go for a jog on the beach, I say.

I start at a leisurely pace, then find myself running hundred-meter sprints. I'm already thinking about getting in shape, reloading for the hard courts of summer.

I GO TO WASHINGTON, D.C. The Legg Mason Tennis Classic. The weather is obscenely hot. Brad and I try to get acclimated to the heat by practicing in the middle of the afternoon. When we're done, fans gather and shout questions. Few of the other players hang around talking to fans, but I do. I like it. For me, fans are always preferable to reporters.

After we've signed the last autograph and answered the last question, Brad says he needs a beer. He looks sly. Something's up. I take him to the Tombs, the place Perry and I frequented when I visited him during his

Georgetown days. The bar has a miniature street door, then a narrow staircase down into damp darkness and a smell of unclean bathrooms. It also has one of those open kitchens, so you can watch the cooks, and while that's a good thing at some places, it's not a plus at the Tombs. We find a booth and order drinks. Brad is put out because they don't have Bud Ice. He settles for Bud. I feel tremendous after the workout, relaxed, fit. I haven't thought of Becker in almost twenty minutes. Brad puts a stop to that. From the inside pocket of his black cashmere pullover he removes a wad of papers, and in an agitated way he drops them on the table.

Becker, he says.

What?

This is what he said after beating you at Wimbledon.

What do I care?

He's talking shit.

What kind of shit?

He reads.

Becker used his post-match news conference to complain that Wimbledon promotes me over other players. He complained that Wimbledon officials unfairly bend over backward to schedule my matches on Centre Court. He complained that all major tournaments kiss my ass. Then he got personal. He called me an elitist. He said that I don't associate with other players. He said that I'm not well liked on the tour. He said I'm not open, and if I were open, maybe other players wouldn't fear me so much.

In short, he issued a declaration of war.

Brad has never cared for Becker. Brad has always called him B. B. Socrates, because he thinks Becker tries to come off as an intellectual, when he's just an overgrown farmboy. But Brad is now so incensed that he can't sit still in our booth at the Tombs.

Andre, he says, it is so fucking *on*. Mark my words. We're going to run into this motherfucker again. We're going to run into him at the U.S. Open. And until then, we're going to prepare, train, plot revenge.

I read Becker's quotes again. I can't believe it. I knew the guy didn't like me, but *this*. I look down and find that I'm clenching and unclenching my fist.

Brad says, Do you hear? I want you to *take—this—fucker—OUT*.

Consider it done.

We clink our beer bottles, swear an oath.

What's more, I tell myself, after Becker I'm going to keep on winning. I'm simply not going to lose anymore. At least not until the frost is on the pumpkin. I'm sick of losing, sick of being disappointed, sick and tired of guys disrespecting my game as much as I do.

AND SO THE SUMMER OF 1995 becomes the Summer of Revenge. Running on pure animosity I steamroll through the D.C. tournament. In the final I face Edberg. I'm the better player, but it's well over one hundred degrees, and such extreme heat is a great equalizer. In this heat, all men are the same. At the start of our match I can't think, can't find a groove. Luckily, Edberg can't either. I win the first set, he wins the second, and in the third set I go up 5–2. The fans cheer—those fans who aren't suffering heatstroke. The match is stopped several times so that someone in the stands can receive medical attention.

I'm serving for the match. At least that's what they tell me. I'm also hallucinating. I don't know what game I'm playing. Is this Nerf ping pong? I'm supposed to hit this fuzzy yellow ball back and forth? To whom? My teeth are chattering. I see three balls come across the net, and I hit the middle one.

My only hope is that Edberg is hallucinating too. Maybe he'll black out before I do and I'll win in a forfeit. I wait, watch him closely, but then I take a turn for the worse. My stomach clinches. He breaks me.

Now he's serving. I call time, step away, and toss my breakfast onto a decorative planter at the back of the court. When I resume my position, Edberg has no trouble holding serve.

I'm serving again for the match. We rally, weakly, each of us hitting timid shots in the center of the court, like ten-year-old girls playing badminton. He breaks me—again.

Five–all. I drop my racket and stumble off the court.

There's an unwritten rule, or maybe it's actually written, that if you leave the court with your racket, you forfeit. So I drop the racket, to let people know I'm coming back. In my delirious state, I still care about the rules of tennis, but I also care about the rules of physics. What goes down, in this heat, must come up, and soon. I vomit several times on my way to the locker room. I run to the toilet and bring up a meal I had days ago. Maybe years ago. I feel as if I'm going into shock. At last the locker room's air-conditioning, plus the total purge of my stomach, starts to revive me.

The referee knocks at the door.

Andre! You're going to lose points if you don't return to the court right now.

Stomach empty, head spinning, I return. I break Edberg. I have no idea how. Then I hold on for the match.

I stumble to the net, where Edberg is leaning, close to fainting. We both have a hard time staying on court for the ceremony. When they hand me the trophy I think about vomiting into it. They hand me a microphone, to say a few words, and I think about vomiting on it too. I apologize for my behavior, especially to the people sitting by the ill-used flowerpot. I want to publicly suggest that officials consider relocating this tournament to Iceland, but I need to vomit again. I drop the microphone and run.

Brooke asks why I didn't just quit.

Because it's the Summer of Revenge.

After the match Tarango publicly objects to my behavior. He demands an explanation for why I left the court. He says that he was waiting to get on to play his doubles match, and I delayed him. He's annoyed. I'm delighted. I want to go back to the court, find the flowerpot, have it gift-wrapped and sent to Tarango, with a note that says, Call *this* out, cheater.

I never forget. Something Becker is about to learn the hard way.

From D.C. I go to Montreal, where it's blessedly cooler. I beat Pete in the final. Three hard-fought sets. Beating Pete always feels good, but this time it barely registers. I want Becker. I beat Chang in the final at Cincinnati, praise God, and then go to New Haven, back into the blast furnace of the Northeast summer. I reach the final and face Krajicek. He's big, six foot five at least, and burly, and yet surprisingly light on his feet. Two strides and he's there at the net, snarling, ready to snack on your heart. Also, his serve is monstrous. I don't want to spend three hours coping with that serve. After winning three tournaments in quick succession, I have very little left. Brad, however, won't tolerate such talk.

You're in training, remember? The grudge match to end all grudge matches? Let it fly, he says.

So I let it fly. The problem is, Krajicek does too. He beats me in the first set, 6–3. In the second set he has match point twice. But I don't yield. I tie the set, win the tiebreak, and win the third set going away. It's my twentieth straight match victory, my fourth straight tournament victory. I've won sixty-three of seventy matches this year, forty-four of forty-six on hard court. Reporters ask if I feel invincible, and I say no. They think I'm being modest, but I'm telling the truth. It's how I feel. It's the only way I can allow myself to feel in the Summer of Revenge. Pride is bad, stress is good. I don't want to feel confident. I want to feel rage. Endless, all-consuming rage.

ALL THE TALK ON THE TOUR is about my rivalry with Pete, largely because of a new Nike ad campaign, including a popular TV commercial in which we hop out of a cab in the middle of San Francisco, set up a net, and go at it. The *New York Times Sunday Magazine* publishes a long profile about the rivalry and the chasm between our personalities. It describes Pete's absorption in tennis, his love of the game. I wonder what the writer would have made of the chasm if he'd known my true feelings about tennis. If only I'd told him.

I set the story aside. I pick it up again. I don't want to read it. I must. It feels odd, unnerving, because Pete isn't uppermost in my thoughts right now. Day and night, I think of Becker, only Becker. And yet, skimming the article, I wince when Pete is asked what he likes about me.

He can't think of anything.

Finally he says: I like the way he travels.

AT LAST, AUGUST COMES. Gil and Brad and I drive to New York for the 1995 U.S. Open. On our first morning at Louis Armstrong Stadium I see Brad in the locker room, holding the draw in his hands.

It's good, he says, smiling. Oh it's so good. AG. All Good.

I'm on Becker's side of the draw. If everything goes according to Brad's plan, I'll face Becker in the semis. Then, Pete. I think: If only, when we're born, we could look over our draw in life, project our path to the final.

In the early rounds I'm on autopilot. I know what I want, I see what I want, just ahead, and opponents are mere road cones. Edberg. Alex Corretja. Petr Korda. I need to get past them to reach my target, so I do. After each win Brad isn't his typical ebullient self. He doesn't smile. He doesn't celebrate. He's preoccupied by Becker. He's monitoring Becker's progress, charting his matches. He wants Becker to win every match, every point.

As I walk off the court with another victory, Brad says drily, Another good day.

Thanks. Yeah, felt good.

No. I mean B. B. Socrates. He won.

Pete handles his business. He reaches the final on his side of the draw and now awaits the winner of Agassi-Becker. It's Wimbledon all over again, Part II. But this time I'm not thinking of Pete. I'm not looking ahead. I've been gunning for Becker, and now the moment is here, and my concentration is so intense, it frightens me.

A friend asks if I don't feel even the slightest impulse, when it's personal with an opponent, to drop the racket and go for his throat. When it's a grudge match, when there's bad blood, wouldn't I rather settle it with a few rounds of old-fashioned boxing? I tell my friend that tennis *is* boxing. Every tennis player, sooner or later, compares himself to a boxer, because tennis is noncontact pugilism. It's violent, *mano a mano,* and the choice is as brutally simple as it is in any ring. Kill or be killed. Beat or take your beat-down. Tennis beatings are just deeper below the skin. They remind me of the old Vegas loan shark method of beating someone with a bag of oranges, because it leaves no outer bruises.

And yet, having said that, I'm only human. So before we take the court, as Becker and I stand in the tunnel, I tell the security guard, James: Keep us apart. I don't want this fucking German in my sight. Trust me, James, you don't want me to see him.

Becker feels the same way. He knows what he said, and he knows I've read it fifty times and memorized it. He knows I've been stewing in his remarks all summer, and he knows I want blood. He does too. He's never liked me, and for him this also has been the Summer of Revenge. We walk onto the court, avoiding eye contact, refusing to acknowledge the crowd, focused on our gear, our tennis bags, and the nasty job at hand.

From the opening bell, it's what I thought it would be. We're sneering, snorting, cursing in two different languages. I win the first set, 7–6. Becker looks infuriatingly unfazed. Why shouldn't he? This is how our match at Wimbledon started. He doesn't worry about falling behind— he's proved that he can take my best punch and come back.

I win the second set, 7–6. Now he starts to squirm, to look for an edge. He tries to play with my mind. He's seen me lose my cool before, so he does what he thinks will make me lose my cool again, the most emasculating thing one tennis player can do to another: He blows kisses at my box. At Brooke.

It works. I'm so angry that I momentarily lose focus. In the third set, with me ahead, 4–2, Becker dives for a ball that he has no business reaching. He gets there, wins the point, then breaks me, then wins the set. The crowd is now wild. They seem to have figured it out, that this is personal, that these two guys don't like each other, that we're settling old scores.

They appreciate the drama, and they want it to go the distance, and now it really feels like Wimbledon all over again. Becker feeds on their energy. He blows more kisses at Brooke, smiling wolfishly. It worked once, why not do it again? I look at Brad, next to Brooke, and he gives me a steely glare, the vintage Brad look that says: *Come on! Let's go!*

The fourth set is nip and tuck. We're each holding serve, looking for an opening to break. I glance at the clock. Nine thirty. No one here is going home. Lock the doors, send out for sandwiches, we're not leaving until this fucking thing is settled. The intensity is palpable. I've never wanted a match so much. I never wanted *anything* so much. I hold serve to go up 6–5 and now Becker's serving to stay in the match.

He sticks his tongue to my right, serves right. I guess right and cold-cock it. Winner. I crush his next two serves. Now he's serving at love–40, triple match point.

Perry is barking at him. Brooke is raining bloodcurdling screams down on him. Becker is smiling, waving at them both, as if he's Miss America. He misfires his first serve. I know he's going to get aggressive with his second. He's a champion, he's going to bring it like a champion. Also, his tongue is in the middle of his mouth. Sure enough he brings a faster-paced second serve straight up the gut. Normally you have to worry about the high bounce and kick, so you move in, try to catch it early before it bounces above your shoulder, but I gamble, hold my ground, and the gamble pays off. Here is the ball, in my wheelhouse. I slide my hips out of the way, put myself in place to hit the coldie of a life-time. The serve is a click faster than I anticipated but I adjust. I'm on my toes, feeling like Wyatt Earp and Spider-Man and Spartacus. I swing. Every hair on my body is standing up. As the ball leaves my racket a sound leaves my mouth that's pure animal. I know that I won't ever make this sound again, and I won't ever hit a tennis ball any harder, or any more perfect. Hitting a ball dead perfect—the only peace. As it lands on Becker's side of the court the sound is still coming from me.

AAAAGHHHHHHHHH.

The ball blazes past Becker. Match, Agassi.

Becker walks to the net. Let him stand there. The fans are on their feet, swaying, ecstatic. I'm gazing at Brooke and Gil and Perry and Brad, especially Brad. Come on! I keep gazing. Becker is still at the net. I don't care. I leave him standing there like a Jehovah's Witness on my doorstep. Finally, *finally,* I strip off my wristbands and go to the net and stick my hand in his general vicinity, without looking. He gives my hand a shake, and I snatch it away.

216

A TV reporter rushes onto the court and asks me a few questions. I answer without thinking. Then I look into the camera with a smile and say, Pete! I'm coming!

I run into the tunnel, into the training room. Gil is there, worried. He knows what that victory must have cost me physically.

I'm in bad shape, Gil.

Lie down, man.

My head is ringing. I'm sopping wet. It's ten at night, and I've got to play in the final in less than eighteen hours. Between now and tomorrow I've got to come down from this near-psychotic state, get home, eat a good hot meal, drink a gallon of Gil Water until I piss a kidney, and then get some sleep.

Gil drives me back to Brooke's brownstone. We eat dinner, and then I sit in the shower for an hour. It's one of those showers that makes you think you should write a check to several environmental groups and maybe plant a tree. At two in the morning I lie down beside Brooke and black out.

I OPEN MY EYES FIVE HOURS LATER, no idea where I am. I sit up and let out a scream, a compacted version of my final scream against Becker. I can't move.

At first I think it's a stomach cramp. Then I realize it's much more serious. I roll off the bed, onto my hands and knees. I know what this is. I've had this before. Torn cartilage between the ribs. I have a pretty good idea which shot tore it. But this tear must be particularly severe, because I can't expand my rib cage. I can barely breathe.

I remember vaguely that it takes three weeks for this injury to heal. But I've got nine hours before I face Pete. It's seven in the morning, the match is at four. I call for Brooke. She must be out. I'm lying on my side, saying aloud, This can't be happening. Please don't let this be happening.

I close my eyes and pray that I'll be able to walk onto the court. Even asking for this much seems ridiculous, because I can't stand. Hard as I try, I can't get to my feet.

God, please. I can't not show up for the final of the U.S. Open.

I crawl to the phone and dial Gil.

Gilly, I can't stand up. I literally can't stand up.

I'll be right over.

By the time he arrives, I'm standing, but still having trouble breathing. I tell him what I think it must be, and he concurs. He watches me drink a cup of coffee, then says: It's time. We need to go.

We look at the clock and both do the only thing we can do in such a moment—we laugh.

Gil drives me to the stadium. On the practice court I hit one ball and the ribs grab me. I hit another. I yell in pain. I hit a third. It still hurts, but I can put some mustard on it. I can breathe.

How do you feel?

Better. I'm about thirty-eight percent.

We stare at each other. Maybe that will be enough.

But Pete is pushing 100 percent. He comes out prepared, braced for a dose of what he saw me give Becker. I lose the first set, 6–4. I lose the second set, 6–3.

I win the third set, however. I'm learning what I can get away with. I'm finding shortcuts, compromises, back doors. I see a few chances to turn this thing into a miracle. I just can't exploit them. I lose the fourth set, 7–5.

Reporters ask how it feels to win twenty-six matches in a row, to win all summer long, only to run into the giant net that is Pete. I think: How do you think it feels? I say: Next summer I'm going to lose a little bit. I'm 26–1, and I'd give up all those wins for this one.

On the drive back to the brownstone, I'm holding my ribs, staring out the window, reliving every shot of the Summer of Revenge. All that work and anger and winning and training and hoping and sweating, and it leads to the same empty disappointed feeling. No matter how much you win, if you're not the last one to win, you're a loser. And in the end I always lose, because there is always Pete. As always, Pete.

Brooke steers clear. She gives me kind looks and sympathetic frowns, but it doesn't feel real, because she doesn't understand. She's waiting for me to feel better, for this to pass, for things to get back to normal. Losing is abnormal.

Brooke has told me that she has a ritual when I lose, a way of killing time until normalcy is restored. While I'm mutely grieving, she goes through her closets and pulls out everything she hasn't worn in months. She folds sweaters and T-shirts, reorganizes socks and stockings and shoes into drawers and boxes. The night I lose to Pete, I peer into Brooke's closet.

Neat as a pin.

In our brief relationship, she's had lots of time to kill.

18

WHILE FACING WILANDER IN DAVIS CUP, I alter my movements to protect my torn rib cartilage, but when you protect one thing you often damage another. I hit an odd forehand and feel a chest muscle pull. It stays warm during the match, but when I wake the next morning I can't move.

The doctors shut me down for weeks. Brad is suicidal.

A layoff will cost you the number one rank, he says.

I couldn't care less. Pete is number one, no matter what some computer says. Pete won two slams this year, and he won our showdown in New York. Besides, I still don't give a rat's ass about being number one. Would have been nice; wasn't my goal. Then again, beating Pete wasn't my goal either, but losing to him has caused me to plummet into a bottomless gloom.

I've always had trouble shaking off hard losses, but this loss to Pete is different. This is the ultimate loss, the über-loss, the alpha-omega loss that eclipses all others. Previous losses to Pete, the loss to Courier, the loss to Gómez—they were flesh wounds compared to this, which feels like a spear through the heart. Every day this loss feels new. Every day I tell myself to stop thinking about it, and every day I can't. The only respite is fantasizing about retirement.

Brooke, meanwhile, is working nonstop. Her acting career is taking off. As per Perry's advice, she's bought a house in Los Angeles and she's been pursuing roles on TV. Now she's landed a plum, a small guest spot in an episode of the sitcom *Friends*.

It's the number one show in the world, she says. Number one!

I wince. That phrase again. She doesn't notice.

The producers of *Friends* have asked Brooke to play a stalker. I cringe, thinking of the nightmare she's endured with stalkers and overly enthusiastic fans. But Brooke thinks her experience with so many stalkers will be good preparation for this part. She says she understands the stalker mind-set.

Plus, Andre, it's *Friends*. The number one show on TV. It might lead to a recurring role on the show. And besides the fact that *Friends* is number one, my episode is going to air right after the Super Bowl—fifty million people will see it. This is like *my* U.S. Open.

A tennis analogy. The surest way to make me disconnect from her desire. But I pretend to be pleased, and say the right things. If you're happy, I say, I'm happy. She believes me. Or acts as if she does. Which often feels like the same thing.

We agree that Perry and I will go with her to Hollywood and watch her shoot the episode. We'll be in her box, as she's always been in mine.

Won't that be fun? she says.

No, I think.

Yes, I say. Fun.

I don't want to go. But I also don't want to lie around the house anymore, talking to myself. Sore chest, wounded ego—even I don't want to be alone with me.

In the days leading up to the taping of *Friends* we barricade ourselves in Brooke's house in Los Angeles. She has a fellow actor come over every day to help run lines. I watch them. Brooke is keyed up, feeling pressure, training hard, a process that's familiar to me. I'm proud of her. I tell her she's going to be a star. Good things are about to happen.

WE ARRIVE AT THE STUDIO late in the afternoon. A half-dozen actors greet us warmly. They're the cast, I assume, the eponymous Friends, but for all I know they could be six unemployed actors from West Covina. I've never seen the show. Brooke hugs them, flushes, stammers, even though she's already spent days rehearsing with them. I've never seen her this starstruck. I introduced her to Barbra Streisand and she didn't react this way.

I stay a few steps behind Brooke, in the shadows. I don't want to take any of her limelight, and besides, I'm not feeling sociable. But the actors are tennis fans and they keep drawing me into the conversation. They ask about my injury, congratulate me on a successful year. The year feels anything but successful, but I thank them as politely as I can and step back again.

They persist. They ask about the U.S. Open. The rivalry with Pete. What's that like? You guys are great for tennis.

Yes, well.

Are you guys friends?

Friends? Did they really just ask me that? Are they asking because they're the Friends? I'd never thought of it before, but yes, I guess Pete and I are friends.

I turn to Perry for support. But he's like Brooke, weirdly starstruck. In fact he's going a little native. He's talking showbiz with the actors, dropping names, playing the insider.

Mercifully, Brooke is summoned to her trailer. Perry and I follow and sit with her while a team of people blows out and combs her hair, and another team tends to her makeup and wardrobe. I watch Brooke as she watches herself in the mirror. She's so happy, so hyper, like a girl primping for her sweet sixteen party, and I'm so out of place. I feel myself shutting down. I say the appropriate things, I smile and mouth encouragements, but on the inside I feel something like a valve shut. I wonder if what I feel is the same thing Brooke feels when I'm tense before a tournament, or grieving a loss afterward. My feigned interest, my canned answers, my fundamental lack of interest—is this what I reduce her to half the time?

We walk to the set, a purple apartment with secondhand furniture. We stand around, killing time, while large men fuss with lights and the director confers with writers. Someone is telling jokes, trying to warm up the crowd. I find a seat in the front row, close to a fake door Brooke is supposed to enter. The crowd is buzzing, as is the crew. There is a sense of building anticipation. I can't stop yawning. I feel like Pete, forced to watch *Grease*. I wonder why I have so much respect for Broadway, and such disdain for this.

Someone yells: Quiet! Someone else yells: Action! Brooke steps forward and knocks at the fake door. It swings open, and Brooke delivers her first line. The audience laughs and cheers. The director yells, Cut! A woman several rows behind me yells: You're doing great, Brooke!

The director praises Brooke. She listens to the praise, nodding. Thank you, she says, but I can do it better. She wants to do it again, she wants another chance. OK, the director says.

While they set up for the next take, Perry gives Brooke pointers. He doesn't know the first thing about acting, but Brooke is feeling so insecure that she'd take notes from anyone right now. She listens and nods. They're standing just below me, and he's lecturing her as if he's the head of the Actors Studio.

Places, please!

Brooke thanks Perry and runs to the door.

Quiet, everybody!

Brooke closes her eyes.

Action!

She knocks at the fake door, does the scene exactly the same way.

Cut!

Fantastic, the director tells Brooke.

She hurries over to me and asks what I thought. Terrific, I say, and I'm not lying. She was. Even if TV annoys me, even if the atmosphere and the fakery turn me off, I respect hard work. I admire her dedication. She's giving her all. I kiss her and tell her I'm proud.

Are you finished?

No, I have another scene.

Oh.

We move to a different set, a restaurant. Brooke's stalker character is on a date with the object of her affection, Joey. She's seated at a table across from the actor playing Joey. Another interminable wait. More notes from Perry. At last the director yells, Action!

The actor playing Joey seems like a nice enough guy. When the scene starts, however, I realize I'm going to have to kick his ass. Apparently the script calls for Brooke to grab Joey's hand and lick it. But she takes it one step further, devouring his hand like an ice cream cone. Cut! That was great, the director says. But let's try it once more. Brooke is laughing. Joey is laughing—wiping his hand on a napkin. I'm staring, wide-eyed. Brooke didn't mention anything about hand licking. She knew what my reaction would be.

This is not my life, this cannot be my life. I'm not really here, I'm not really sitting with two hundred people and watching my girlfriend lick another man's hand.

I look up at the ceiling, directly into the lights.

They're going to do it again.

Quiet, please!

Action!

Brooke takes Joey's hand and puts it in her mouth, up to the knuckles. This time she rolls her eyes back and runs her tongue along—

I jump out of my seat, run downstairs, push through a side door. It's dark. How did it get dark so fast? Right outside the door is my rented Lincoln. Behind me come Perry and Brooke. Perry's mystified. Brooke's frantic. She grabs my arm and asks, Where are you going? You can't be going!

Perry says, What's wrong? What's the matter?

You know. You both know.

Brooke is begging me to stay. So is Perry. I tell them there's no chance, I don't want to watch her lick that man's hand.

Don't do this, Brooke says.

Me? *Me?* I'm not doing anything. Go back and enjoy yourselves. Break a leg. Have some more hand. I'm out of here.

I'M DRIVING FAST ON THE FREEWAY, weaving in and out of traffic. I'm not sure where I'm going, except that I'm not going back to Brooke's. Fuck that. Suddenly I realize that I'm going all the way to Vegas, and I'm not stopping until I get there, and I feel great about this decision. I open up the engine and roar past the city limits, on into the desert, nothing between me and my bed but a stretch of wasteland and a swirl of stars.

When the radio turns to static, I try to tune in my emotions. I felt jealous, yes, but also dislocated, out of touch with myself. Like Brooke, I was playing a part, the role of the Dopey Boyfriend, and I thought I was pulling it off. But when the hand licking started I couldn't stay in character any longer. Of course, I've watched Brooke kiss men onstage before. I've also had the experience of meeting a perv who couldn't wait to tell me about making out with my girlfriend on a movie set when she was fifteen. This is different. This is over the line. I don't pretend to know where the line is, but hand licking is definitely over it.

I pull up to the bachelor pad at two a.m. The driving has tired me, taken the edge off my anger. I'm still angry, but also contrite. I dial Brooke.

I'm sorry. I just—I needed to get out of there.

She says everyone asked where I was. She says I humiliated her, jeopardized her big break. She says everyone told her how good she was, but she couldn't enjoy a minute of her success, because the only person she wanted to share it with was gone.

You were a major distraction, she says, raising her voice. I had to block you out of my mind so that I could concentrate on my lines, which made everything harder. If I ever did anything like that to you, at a match, you'd be incensed.

I couldn't watch you lick that guy's hand.

I was acting, Andre. *Acting.* Did you forget that I'm an *actor,* that acting is what I do for a living, that it's all pretend? Make-believe?

If only I *could* forget.

I start to defend myself, but Brooke says she doesn't want to hear it. She hangs up.

I stand in the middle of my living room and feel the floor shaking. I briefly consider the possibility that Vegas is being struck by an earthquake. I don't know what to do, where to stand. I walk to the shelf that holds my tennis trophies and pick one up. I hurl it through the living room, through the kitchen. It breaks in several pieces. I pick up another and hurl it against the wall. One by one I do this with all my trophies. Davis Cup? Smash. U.S. Open? Smash. Wimbledon? Smash, smash. I pull the rackets out of my tennis bag and try to smash the glass coffee table, but only the rackets shatter. I pick up the broken trophies and smash them against the walls and then against other things in the house. When the trophies can't be smashed anymore, I fling myself on the couch, which is covered with plaster from the gouged walls.

Hours later I open my eyes. I survey the damage as if someone else is responsible—and it's true. It was someone else. The someone who does half the shit I do.

My phone rings. Brooke. I apologize again, tell her about breaking my trophies. Her tone softens. She's concerned. She hates that I was so upset, that I got jealous, that I'm in pain. I tell her I love her.

ONE MONTH LATER I'm in Stuttgart for the start of the indoor season. If I were to list all the places in the world where I don't want to be, all the continents and countries, the cities and towns, the villages and hamlets and burgs, Stuttgart would be at the top of my list. If I live to be a thousand years old, I think, nothing good is ever going to happen to me in Stuttgart. Nothing against Stuttgart. I just don't want to be here, now, playing tennis.

Nevertheless, here I am, and it's an important match. If I win, I will consolidate my number one ranking, which Brad badly wants. I'm playing MaliVai Washington, whom I know well. I played him all through juniors. Good athlete, covers the court like a tarp, always makes me beat him. His legs are pure bronze, so I can't attack them. I can't tire him out like a typical opponent. I have to outthink him. And so I do. I'm up a set, rolling along, when suddenly I feel as if I've stepped in a mousetrap. I look down. The bottom of my shoe has fallen off. Peeled away.

I didn't bring an extra pair of tennis shoes.

I halt the match, tell officials that I need new shoes. An announcement is made over the loudspeaker, in urgent staccato German. Can someone lend a shoe to Mr. Agassi? Size ten and a half?

It has to be a Nike, I add—because of my contract.

A man in the upper bleachers rises and waves his shoe. He would be happy, he says, to loan me his *Schuh*. Brad goes up to the stands and retrieves it. Though the man is a size nine, I force his shoe on my foot, like some half-wit Cinderella, and resume play.

Is this my life?

This can't be my life.

I'm playing a match for the number one ranking in the world, wearing a shoe borrowed from a stranger in Stuttgart. I think of my father using tennis balls to mend our shoes when we were kids. This feels more awkward, more ridiculous. I'm emotionally exhausted, and I wonder why I don't just stop. Walk off. Leave. What keeps me going? How am I managing to select shots and hold serve and break serve? Mentally I leave the arena. I go to the mountains, rent a ski cabin, make myself an omelet, put my feet up, breathe in the snowy smell of the forest.

I tell myself: If I win this match, I'll retire. And if I lose this match, I'll retire.

I lose.

I don't retire. Instead, I do the opposite of retiring: I get on a plane to Australia to play in a slam. The 1996 Australian Open is only days away, and I'm the defending champ. I'm in no frame of mind. I look deranged. My eyes are bloodshot, my face is gaunt. The flight attendant should kick me off. I almost kick myself off. Minutes after Brad and I board, I nearly jump out of my seat and run for it. Brad, seeing my expression, takes my arm.

Come on, he says. Relax. You never know. Maybe something good will happen.

I swallow a sleeping pill and down a vodka, and when I open my eyes the plane is taxiing to the gate in Melbourne. Brad drives us to the hotel, the Como. My head is in a fog as thick as mashed potatoes. A bellboy shows me to my room, which has a piano and a spiral staircase with shiny wood steps in the center. I tap a few keys on the piano, stagger up the steps to bed. I fall backward. My knee hits the sharp edge of a metal balustrade and tears open. I tumble down the stairs. Blood is everywhere.

I call Gil. He's there in two minutes. He says it's the patella, the kneecap. Bad cut, he says. Bad bruise. He bandages me, puts me on the couch. In the morning he shuts me down. He doesn't let me practice. We have to be careful with that patella, he says. It'll be a miracle if the thing holds up for seven matches.

Limping noticeably, I play the first round with a bandage on my knee and a film over my eyes. It's plain to fans, sportswriters, commentators, that I'm not the player I was a year ago. I drop the first set and quickly fall behind two breaks in the second. I'm going to be the first defending champion since Roscoe Tanner to lose a first-round match in a slam.

I'm playing Gastón Etlis, from Argentina, whoever that is. He doesn't even look like a tennis player. He looks like a substitute schoolteacher. He has sweaty ringlets and a sinister five-o'clock shadow. He's a doubles guy, only playing singles because by some miracle he qualified. He looks astonished to be here. A guy like this, I normally beat him in the locker room with one hard stare, but he's up a set on me and leading in the second set. Jesus. And he's the one suffering. If I look pained, he looks panicked. He looks as if he has a ninety-pound bullfrog lodged in his throat. I hope he has the balls to close me out, to finish me off, because I'm better off right now with a loss and an early exit.

But Etlis gags, freezes, makes shockingly bad decisions.

I start to feel weak. I shaved my head this morning, full-on, bare-scalp bald, because I wanted to punish myself. Why? Because it still rankles that I ruined Brooke's cameo on *Friends,* because I broke all my trophies, because I came to a slam without putting in the work—and because I lost to Pete at the U.S. Fucking Open. You can't fool the man in the mirror, Gil always says, so I'm going to make that man pay. My nickname on the tour is The Punisher, because of the way I run guys back and forth. Now I'm hell-bent on punishing my most intractable opponent, myself, by burning his head.

Mission accomplished. The Australian sun is flame-broiling my skin. I scold myself, then forgive myself, then press reset and find a way to tie the second set. Then I win the tiebreak.

My mind is chattering. What else can I do with my life? Should I break up with Brooke? Should I marry her? I lose the third set. Again Etlis can't stand prosperity. I win the fourth set in another tiebreak. In the fifth set Etlis wears out, gives up. I'm neither proud nor relieved. I'm embarrassed. My head looks like a blood blister. *Put a blister on his brain.*

Later, reporters ask if I worry about sunburn. I laugh. Honestly, I tell them, sunburn is the least of my worries. I want to add: I'm already mentally fried. But I don't.

In the quarters I play Courier. He's beaten me six straight times. We've had terrific battles, on the court and in the newspapers. After he beat me at the 1989 French Open, he complained about all the attention I get. He said he felt as if he forever plays second fiddle to me.

Sounds like an insecurity problem, I told reporters.

To which Courier shot back: *I'm* insecure?

He's also been chippy about my ever-changing appearance and psyche. Asked what he thought of the new Agassi, he once said: You mean the new Agassi, or the new *new* Agassi? We've patched things up since then. I've told Courier that I root for his success, that I consider him a friend, and he's said the same. But there's still a curtain of tension between us, and there may always be, at least until one of us retires, since our rivalry dates back to puberty, back to Nick.

The match starts late, delayed by the women's quarters. We get on the court close to midnight and play nine games on serve. So this is how it's going to be. Then the rain falls. Officials could close the roof, but it would take forty minutes. They ask if we'd rather come back tomorrow. We both say yes.

Sleep helps. I wake refreshed, wanting to beat Courier. But it's not Courier on the other side of the net—it's a pale facsimile. Despite being up two sets to love, he looks tentative, burned out. I recognize that look. I've seen it in the mirror many times. I swoop in for the kill. I win the match, beating Courier for the first time in years.

When reporters ask about Courier's game I say: He's not where he wants to be.

I want to say: There's a lot of that going around.

The win helps me regain the number one rank. Once again I've dethroned Pete, but it's just another reminder of when I didn't, couldn't, beat him.

In the semis I face Chang. I know I can win, but I also know that I will lose. In fact I want to lose, I must lose, because Becker is waiting in the final. The last thing I need right now is another holy war with Becker. I couldn't handle that. I wouldn't have the stomach for it, which means I'd lose. Given a choice between Becker and Chang, I'd rather lose to Chang. Besides, it's always easier psychologically to lose in the semis than in the final.

So I'll lose today. Congratulations, Chang. I hope you and your Messiah will be very happy.

But losing on purpose isn't easy. It's almost harder than winning. You have to lose in such a way that the crowd can't tell, and in a way that *you* can't tell—because of course you're not wholly conscious of losing on purpose. You're not even half conscious. Your mind is tanking, but your body is fighting on. Muscle memory. It's not even all of your mind that purposely loses, but a breakaway faction, a splinter group. The deliberately bad decisions are made in a dark place, far below the surface. You don't do those tiny things you need to do. You don't run the extra few feet, you don't lunge. You're slow to come out of stops. You hesitate to bend or dig. You get handsy, not using your legs and hips. You make a careless error, compensate for the error with a spectacular shot, then make two more errors, and slowly but surely you slide backward. You never actually think, I'm going to net this ball. It's more complicated, more insidious.

At the post-match news conference Brad tells reporters: Today, Andre hit the wall.

True, I think. So very true. But I don't tell Brad that I hit the wall every day. It would crush him to know that today the wall felt good, that I kissed the wall, that I'm glad I lost, that I'd rather be on that plane back to Los Angeles than lacing them up for a rematch with our old friend B. B. Socrates. I'd rather be anywhere but here—even Hollywood, my next stop. Since I lost, I'll get home just in time to watch the Super Bowl, followed by the special hour-long episode of *Friends,* featuring Brooke Shields.

19

PERRY GRINDS ME EVERY DAY, asking what's wrong, what's the matter. I can't tell him. I don't know. More accurately, I don't want to know. I don't want to admit to Perry or myself that a loss to Pete can have this kind of lingering effect. For once I don't want to sit with Perry and try to unravel the skeins of my subconscious. I've given up on understanding myself. I have no interest in self-analysis. In the long, losing struggle with myself, I'm tanking.

I go to San Jose and get annihilated by Pete. Definitely not what the doctor ordered. I lose my temper several times during the match, cursing at my racket, screaming at myself. Pete looks bemused. The umpire penalizes me for swearing.

Oh, you like that? Here, take this.

I serve a ball into the upper deck.

I go to Indian Wells, lose to Chang in the quarters. I can't face the post-match press conference. I skip out, pay a hefty fine. I go to Monte Carlo. I lose to Alberto Costa of Spain in fifty-four minutes. As I walk off the court I hear whistles, catcalls. They may as well be coming from inside my heart. I want to yell at the crowd: I agree!

Gil asks me, What is it?

I tell him. I come right out with it. Since losing to Pete at the U.S. Open, I've lost the will.

Then let's not do this, Gil says. We've got to be clear on what we're doing.

I want to quit, I say, but I don't know how—or when.

At the 1996 French Open I'm coming unglued. I'm screaming at myself all through my first-round match. I receive an official warning. I scream louder. I'm penalized a point. I'm one *motherfucking cocksucker* away from getting DQ'd for the tournament. Rain starts to fall, and during the delay I sit in the locker room and stare straight ahead as if hypnotized. When play resumes I outlast my opponent, Jacobo Díaz, whom I can't see. He's as blurry and watery as the reflections in the rain puddles along the alleys of the court.

Beating Díaz merely delays the inevitable. In the next round I lose to Chris Woodruff, from Tennessee. He always reminds me of a country-western singer, and plays as if he'd rather be performing at a rodeo. He's even more awkward on clay, and to compensate he gets aggressive, especially on his backhand. I can't counter his aggression. I make sixty-three unforced errors. He reacts with unbridled joy, and I gaze at him, coveting not his victory but his enthusiasm.

Sportswriters accuse me of tanking, not going for every ball. They never get it right. When I tank, they say I'm not good enough; when I'm not good enough, they say I tank. I nearly tell them I wasn't tanking, that I was torturing myself for not being good enough. Whenever I know that I don't deserve to win, that I'm unworthy of winning, I torture myself. You could look it up.

But I don't say anything. Once again I leave the stadium without sitting for the obligatory news conference. Once again I happily pay the fine. Money well spent.

BROOKE TAKES ME TO A JOINT in Manhattan where the front room is smaller than a phone booth but the main dining room is big and warm and mustard yellow. Campagnola—I like the way she says it, I like the way it smells, I like the way we both feel as we walk in off the street. I like the autographed photo of Sinatra next to the coat room.

This is my *favorite* place in New York, Brooke says, so I christen it my favorite too. We sit in a corner, eating a light meal in that hazy twilight hour between the lunch crowd and the dinner rush. They don't normally serve food at this hour, but the manager says in our case they'll make an exception.

Campagnola quickly becomes an extension of our kitchen, and then of our entire relationship. Brooke and I go there to remind ourselves of the reasons we're good together. We go there on special occasions, and we go there to make humdrum weekdays feel like special occasions. We go there so often and so automatically after every match at the U.S. Open that the chefs and waiters begin to set their watches by us. In a fifth set I sometimes find myself thinking of the gang at Campagnola, knowing that they're keeping one eye on the TV while prepping the mozzarella, tomatoes, and prosciutto. I know, as I'm bouncing the ball, just about to serve, that I'll soon be seated at the corner table, eating buttery fried shrimp with white wine sauce and lemon, plus a side of raviolis so soft and sweet they should count as dessert. I know that when Brooke and I walk in the door, win or lose, the place will erupt with applause.

Campagnola's manager, Frankie, is always dressed razor sharp, Gil sharp. Italian suit, flowered tie, silk handkerchief. He always greets us with a gap-toothed smile and a fresh batch of funny stories. He's a second father to me, Brooke says when she introduces us, and those are magic words. Surrogate father is a role for which I have the greatest respect, so I like Frankie right away. Then he buys us a bottle of red, tells us about the celebs and grifters and bankers and mobsters who hang out in his joint, makes Brooke laugh until her cheeks are pink, and now I like him for my own reasons.

Frank says, John Gotti? You want to know about Gotti? He always sits right over there, corner table, facing out. If anybody's going to take him down, he wants to see it coming.

I feel the same way, I say.

Frankie laughs darkly, then nods. I know, right?

Frankie is honest, hardworking, sincere, my kind of people. I find myself looking for his face the moment we walk through the door. I feel better, my aches and anxieties fade, when Frankie throws out his arms and smiles and whisks us to our table. Sometimes he kicks out other customers, and Brooke and I pretend not to notice their frowning and complaining.

Frankie's chief virtue, in my book, is the way he talks about his kids. He loves them, brags about them, pulls out photos of them at the drop of a hat. But clearly he worries about their future. Running a hand over his tired face one night, he tells me his kids are only in grade school, but he's already stressed about college. He groans about the cost of higher education. He doesn't know how he's going to make it.

Days later I talk to Perry and ask him to put aside a nest egg of Nike stock in Frankie's name. When Brooke and I next drop into Campagnola, I tell Frankie about it. The shares can't be touched for ten years, I say, but by then they should be worth enough to significantly lighten that tuition burden.

Frankie's bottom lip trembles. Andre, he says, I can't believe you'd do that for me.

The look on his face is a complete shock. I didn't understand the meaning and value of education, the hardship and stress it causes most parents and children. I've never thought of education like that. School was always a place I managed to escape, not a thing to be treasured. Setting aside the stock was merely something I did because Frankie specifically mentioned college and I wanted to help. When I saw what it meant to him, however, I was the one who got educated.

Helping Frankie provides more satisfaction and makes me feel more connected and alive and *myself* than anything else that happens in 1996. I tell myself: Remember this. Hold on to this. This is the only perfection there is, the perfection of helping others. This is the only thing we can do that has any lasting value or meaning. This is why we're here. To make each other feel safe.

And as 1996 wears on, safety seems like an especially precious commodity. Brooke is regularly receiving letters from stalkers, threatening her—and sometimes me—with death and unspeakable horrors. The letters are detailed, grisly, sick. We forward them to the FBI. We also ask Gil to work with the agents, monitor their progress. Several times, when a letter is traceable, Gil goes rogue. He boards a plane and pays the stalker a visit. He usually appears early in the morning, just after dawn, at the stalker's house or workplace. He holds up the letter and says very softly, I know who you are and where you live. Now take a good look at me, because if you ever bother Brooke and Andre again, you will see me again, and you don't want that, because then it will be *on*.

The scariest letters can't be traced. When they rise above a certain gruesome threshold, when they threaten that something is going to happen on a specific date, Gil will stand outside Brooke's brownstone while we sleep. By stand I mean *stand*. On the stoop. Arms folded. He stations himself there, looking left, then right, and he stays that way all night.

Night after night.

The strain, the sordidness, exact a heavy toll on Gil. He worries constantly that he's not doing enough, that he may have missed something, that he'll blink or look away one time and some creep will slither past. He becomes obsessed. He falls into a nearly debilitating depression, and I fall with him, because I'm the cause. I brought this on Gil. I feel deep guilt, and I'm beset by premonitions of doom.

I try to talk myself out of it. I tell myself that you can't be unhappy when you have money in the bank and own your own plane. But I can't help it, I feel listless, hopeless, trapped in a life I didn't choose, hounded by people I can't see. And I can't discuss any of it with Brooke, because I can't admit to such weakness. Feeling depressed after a loss is one thing, but feeling depressed about nothing, about life in general, is another thing altogether. I can't feel this way. I refuse to admit that I feel this way.

Even if I wanted to discuss it with Brooke, we're not communicating well these days. We're not on the same frequency. We don't have the same bandwidth. For instance, when I try to talk with her about Frankie, about the satisfaction of helping him, she doesn't seem to hear. After the initial fun of introducing me to Frankie, she's cool about him, indifferent, as if he's played his part and now it's time for him to move offstage. This follows a precedent, a pattern that repeats itself with many people and places Brooke brings into my life. Museums, galleries, celebrities, writers, shows, friends—I often get more from them than she does. Just as I start to enjoy something, to learn from it, she casts it aside.

It makes me wonder if we're a good fit. I don't think so. And yet I can't step back, can't suggest we take a break, because I'm already distancing myself from tennis. With no Brooke and no tennis, I'll have nothing. I fear the void, the darkness. So I cling to Brooke, and she clings back, and though the clinging seems loving, it's more like the clinging in that painting in the Louvre. Holding on for dear life.

As Brooke and I approach our two-year anniversary, I decide that we should formalize our clinging. Two years is a meaningful benchmark in my love life. In every previous relationship two years has been the make-or-break moment—and I've always chosen break. Every two years I grow tired of the girl I'm dating, or she grows tired of me, as if a timer goes off in my heart. I was with Wendi two years, and then she declared our relationship open, which prefigured the end. Before Wendi I was with a girl in Memphis for exactly two years, and then I bolted. Why my love life runs in two-year cycles, I don't know. I wasn't even aware of the pattern until Perry pointed it out.

Whatever the reason, I'm determined to change. At twenty-six I believe this pattern needs to be broken, now, or I'll be thirty-six, looking back on a series of two-year relationships that went nowhere. If I'm going to have a family, if I'm going to be happy, I've got to break this cycle, which means pushing myself past the two-year mark, forcing myself to commit.

Of course, technically, it hasn't been two years with Brooke. With our hectic schedules, with my playing and her filming, we've actually spent only a few months together. We're still getting to know each other, still learning. Part of me knows I shouldn't force a decision. Part of me simply doesn't want to be married right now. But who cares what I want? When is what I want ever a good index of what I should do? How often do I enter a tournament, wanting to play, only to lose in the early rounds? How often do I enter reluctantly, feeling like hell, only to win? Maybe marriage—the ultimate match play, the ultimate single elimination tournament—is the same way.

Besides, everyone around me is getting married. Perry, Philly, J.P. In fact, Philly and J.P. met their wives together, on the same night. After the Summer of Revenge, it's the Winter of Marriage.

I ask Perry for advice. We talk for hours in Vegas and on the phone. He leans toward marriage. Brooke is the one, he says. How are you going to do better than a Princeton-educated supermodel? After all, didn't we fantasize about her years ago? Didn't he predict that she'd come along? And now here she is—destiny. What's the problem? He reminds me of *Shadowlands*. C. S. Lewis doesn't become fully alive, doesn't grow up, until he opens himself to love. Love is how we grow up, the movie says. And as Lewis reminds his students: *God wants us to grow up.*

Perry says he knows of an excellent jeweler in Los Angeles. The same jeweler Perry used when he got engaged. Set aside the question of whether or not to propose, he says, and just focus for a moment on the ring.

I know the kind of ring Brooke wants—round, Tiffany cut—because she's told me. Straight out. She's never shy about sharing her opinions on jewels, clothes, cars, shoes. In fact, the most animated talks we have are about *things*. We used to talk about our dreams, our childhoods, our feelings. Now we avidly discuss the best sofas, the best stereos, the best cheeseburgers, and while I find such talk interesting, an important aspect of the art of living, I fear Brooke and I put undue emphasis on it.

I gird myself, phone the jeweler and tell her I'm in the market for an engagement ring. The words come out croaky. I feel my heart pound. I ask myself, Shouldn't this be a joyous moment—one of the great moments of life? Before I can answer, the jeweler is peppering me with her own questions. Size? Carat? Color? Clarity? She keeps talking about clarity, asking me about clarity.

I think: *Lady, you're asking the wrong guy about clarity.*

I say: All I know is round, Tiffany cut.

When do you need it?

Soon?

Can do. I think I've got *just* the ring.

Days later, the ring arrives by courier. It's in a big box. I walk around with it in my pocket for two weeks. The box feels leaden, and dangerous, as do I.

Brooke is away, filming a movie. We talk every night on the phone, and sometimes I cradle the phone with one hand and fondle the ring with the other. She's in the Carolinas, where it's bitter cold, but the script calls for the weather to be balmy, so the director forces her and the other actors to suck ice cubes. It keeps their breath from fogging.

Better than licking hands.

She says a few of her lines for me, and we laugh because they sound fake. They sound like lines.

After we hang up I go for a drive, the heater turned up high, the lights of the Strip winking like diamonds. I replay our conversation, and I can't tell the difference between the lines in her script and the lines we've just spoken to each other. I pull the ring box from my coat pocket and open it. The ring catches and reflects the light. I set it on the dashboard.

Clarity.

AS BROOKE WRAPS HER FILM, I conclude a miserable stretch of tennis that has sportswriters openly, sometimes gleefully, saying I'm done. Three slams, they say. That's far more than we thought he'd win. Brooke says we need to get away. Far away. This time we choose Hawaii. I pack the ring.

My stomach rolls as our plane swoops toward the volcanoes. I gaze at the palm trees, the foaming coastline, the misty rain forests, and think: another island paradise. Why do we always feel compelled to run off to island paradises? It's as though we have Blue Lagoon Syndrome. I fantasize about the engine sputtering, the plane spiraling down into the mouth of a volcano. To my chagrin we land safely.

I've rented a bungalow at the Mauna Lani resort. Two bedrooms, a kitchen, a dining room, a pool, a full-time chef. Plus, a long stretch of white beach all to ourselves.

We spend the first few days hanging around the bungalow, relaxing by the pool. Brooke's engrossed in a book about how to be single and happy in your thirties. She holds the book over her face, licking her finger and loudly turning the pages. It doesn't cross my mind that this might be a pointed hint. Nothing crosses my mind except the proposal I'm about to deliver.

Andre, you seem distracted.

No. I'm here.

Everything all right?

Please leave me alone, I think, I'm trying to decide when and where to propose to you.

I'm like a murderer, plotting, thinking constantly of the time and the place. Except that a murderer has a motive.

On the third night, though we're planning to eat dinner in the bungalow, I suggest we dress up as if it's a special occasion. Great idea, Brooke says. She emerges from the bedroom an hour later in a flowing white dress that falls to her ankles. I wear a linen shirt and beige pants, the perfectly wrong outfit, because the pockets of the pants are shallow and the ring box doesn't fit. I keep my hand over the pocket to hide the bulge.

I stretch as though I'm about to play a match. I shake out my legs, then suggest a stroll. Yes, Brooke says, that sounds like a lovely idea. She takes a sip of wine, smiles casually, no idea what's coming. We walk for ten minutes until we reach a part of the beach where we can't see any sign of civilization. I crane my neck to make sure no one is coming. No tourists. No paparazzi. The coast is clear. I think of that line from *Top Gun*. I had the shot, there was no danger, so I took it.

I fall a few steps behind Brooke and drop to one knee on the sand. She turns, looks down, and all the color drains from her face as the colors of the sunset grow more vivid.

Brooke Christa Shields?

She's mentioned in conversation many times that any man who proposes to her had better use her full legal name, Brooke Christa Shields. I never knew why, and never thought to ask, but now it comes back to me.

I repeat, Brooke Christa Shields?

She puts a hand on her forehead. Wait, she says. What? Are you—? Wait. I'm not ready.

That makes two of us.

She's wiping away tears as I pull the ring box from my pocket and crack it open and remove the ring and slide it onto her finger.

Brooke Christa Shields? Will you—

She's pulling me to my feet. I'm kissing her and thinking, I really wish I'd thought this through. Is this the person that Andre Kirk Agassi is supposed to spend the next ninety years with?

Yes, she says. Yes, yes, yes.

Wait, I think. Wait, wait, wait.

SHE SAYS SHE WANTS a do-over.

One day later she tells me she was in such shock on the beach, she couldn't hear me. She wants me to repeat the proposal, word for word.

I need you to say it again, she insists, because I can't believe it really happened.

Me neither.

She's planning the wedding before we're off the island. And when we get back to Los Angeles, I resume the unplanned, unceremonious end of my tennis career. I moonwalk through one tournament after another. I'm losing in early rounds, and therefore I'm home a lot, which tickles Brooke. I'm placid, numb, and I have plenty of time to talk about wedding cakes and invitations.

We fly to England for the 1996 Wimbledon. Just before the start of the tournament Brooke insists we go for high tea at the Dorchester hotel. I beg off, but she insists. We're surrounded by older couples, all wearing tweed and bowties and ribbons. Half of them look asleep. We eat finger sandwiches with the crusts cut off, heaping plates of egg salad and scones with jam and butter—all things expressly engineered to clog the human artery, without the benefit of tasting good. The food is making me cranky, and the setting feels ridiculous, like a children's tea party in a nursing home. But just as I'm about to suggest that we ask for the check I notice that Brooke's ecstatic. She's having a grand time. She wants more jam.

In the first round I face Doug Flach, ranked number 281, a qualifier who's in over his head, though you'd never know it to watch him against me. He plays as if he's channeling Rod Laver, and I play like Ralph Nader. We're on Graveyard Court. By now you'd think I'd have my own plaque here. I lose as fast as I can, and Brooke and I hurry back to Los Angeles, to engage in more deep conversations about Battenburg lace and chiffon-lined tents.

As summer approaches, there is only one elaborate pageant that interests and inspires me. And it's not my wedding. It's the Atlanta Olympics. I don't know why. Maybe it feels like something new. Maybe it feels like something that has nothing to do with me. I'll be playing for my country, playing for a team with 300 million members. I'll be closing a circle. My father was an Olympian, now me.

I plan a regimen with Gil, an Olympian's regimen, and give all-out effort in our training sessions. I spend two hours with Gil each morning, then hit with Brad for two hours, then run up and down Gil Hill in the hottest part of the day. I want the heat. I want the pain.

As the Games begin, sportswriters kill me for skipping the opening ceremonies. Perry kills me for it too. But I'm not in Atlanta for opening ceremonies, I'm here for gold, and I need to hoard what little concentration and energy I can muster these days. The tennis is being played in Stone Mountain, an hour's drive from the opening ceremonies downtown. Stand around in the Georgia heat and humidity, wearing a coat and tie, waiting for hours to walk around the track, then drive to Stone Mountain and give my best? No. I can't. I'd love to experience the pageantry, to savor the spectacle of the Olympics, but not before my first match. This, I tell myself, is focus. This is what it means to put substance above image.

With a good night's sleep under my belt I win my first-rounder against Jonas Björkman, from Sweden. In the second round I cruise past Karol Kucera, from Slovakia. In the third round I face a stiffer test from Andrea Gaudenzi, from Italy. He has a muscle-bound game. He likes to trade body blows, and if you respect him too much he gets more macho. I don't show him any respect. But the ball doesn't respect me. I'm making all sorts of unforced errors. Before I know what's happening, I'm down a set and a break. I look to Brad. *What should I do?* He yells: Stop missing!

Oh. Right. Sage advice. I stop missing, stop trying to hit winners, put the pressure back on Gaudenzi. It's really that simple, and I scrape out an ugly, satisfying win.

In the quarters I'm on the verge of elimination against Ferreira. He's up 5–4 in the third, serving for the match. But he's never beaten me before, and I know exactly what's going on inside his body. Something my father used to say comes back to me: If you stick a piece of charcoal up his ass, you'll pull out a diamond. (Round, Tiffany cut.) I know Ferreira's sphincter is squeezing shut, and this makes me confident. I rally, break him, win the match.

In the semis I meet Leander Paes, from India. He's a flying jumping bean, a bundle of hyperkinetic energy, with the tour's quickest hands. Still, he's never learned to hit a tennis ball. He hits off-speed, hacks, chips, lobs—he's the Brad of Bombay. Then, behind all his junk, he flies to the net and covers so well that it all seems to work. After an hour you feel as if he hasn't hit one ball cleanly—and yet he's beating you soundly. Because I'm prepared, I stay patient, stay calm, and beat Paes 7–6, 6–3.

In the final I play Sergi Bruguera, from Spain. The match is delayed by thunderstorms, and the forecasters say it will be five hours before we can get on the court. So I wolf down a spicy chicken sandwich from Wendy's. Comfort food. On the day of a match, I don't worry about calories and nutrition. I worry about having energy and feeling full. Also, because of my nerves, it's rare that I'm hungry on match day, so any time I have an appetite I try to capitalize. I give my stomach whatever it asks for. Swallowing the last bite of spicy chicken, however, the clouds part, the storm blows away, and the heat comes. Now I have a spicy chicken sandwich sitting on my gut, it's ninety degrees, and the air is as thick as gravy. I can't move—and I have to play for a gold medal? So much for comfort food; I'm in extreme gastric discomfort.

But I don't care. Gil asks how I feel, and I tell him: A-OK. I'm going to hustle for every ball, I'm going to make this guy run, and if he thinks he's taking this medal back to Spain, he's got another think coming.

Gil grins from ear to ear. That's my boy.

It's one of the rare times, Gil says, that he sees no fear in my eyes as I walk onto the court.

From the opening serve, I'm pounding Bruguera, moving him from corner to corner, making him cover a parcel of real estate the size of Barcelona. Every point is a blow to his midsection. In the middle of the second set we have a titanic rally. He wins the point to get back to deuce. He takes so much time getting ready for the next point that I could argue with the umpire. By rights I should argue, and Bruguera should get a warning. Instead I use the moment to wander over to the ballboy, grab a towel, whisper to Gil, How's our friend looking over there?

Gil smiles. He nearly laughs, except that Gil never laughs during a fight.

Even though Bruguera has won the point, Gil sees, and I see, that winning the point will cost him the next six games.

Gil shouts: That's my boy!

As I mount the review stand, I think: What will this feel like? I've watched this on TV so many times, can it possibly live up to my expectations? Or, like so many things, will it fall short?

I look left and right. Paes, the bronze winner, is on one side. Bruguera, the silver winner, is on the other. My platform is a foot higher—one of the few times I'm taller than my opponents. But I'd feel ten feet tall on any surface. A man drapes the gold medal around my neck. The national anthem starts. I feel my heart swell, and it has nothing to do with tennis, or me, and thus it exceeds all my expectations.

I scan the crowd and spot Gil, Brooke, Brad. I look for my father, but he's hiding. He told me the night before that I've managed to reclaim something taken from him years ago, and yet he doesn't want to be visible, doesn't want to detract from the specialness of my moment. He doesn't understand that this moment is special precisely because it's not mine.

. . .

DAYS LATER, for reasons I can't begin to comprehend, the Olympic afterglow is gone. I'm on the court in Cincinnati, losing my mind. Playing for myself again, I'm smashing my racket in a fit of rage. I go on to win the tournament, however, which seems laughable, and only aggravates my sense that it's all a joke.

Then, in August, at the RCA Championships in Indianapolis, playing a first-round match against Daniel Nestor, a Serb from Canada, I'm well ahead. But I feel unduly piqued that he's just broken my serve. I can't let go of my sudden anger. I look up at the sky and fantasize about flying away. Since I can't fly away, at least this tennis ball can fly away. Be free, little ball. I whack it high above the stands and out of the stadium.

Automatic warning.

The umpire, Dana Laconto, says into the microphone, Code violation. Warning. Abuse of ball.

Fuck you, Dana.

He calls over the ref. He tells the ref that Agassi said, Fuck you, Dana.

The referee approaches and asks, Did you say that?

Yes.

This match is over.

Fine. Fuck you too. And fuck the umpire you rode in on.

The fans start a riot. They don't understand what's happening, because they can't hear me. They only know that they paid to see a match and now it's being canceled. They're booing, firing seat cushions and water bottles onto the court. The mascot of the RCA Championships is a Spuds MacKenzie dog, which now trots onto the court, dodging seat cushions and water bottles. He reaches the middle of the net, lifts his hind leg, and pees.

I couldn't agree more.

He makes a jaunty exit. I'm right behind him, ducking my head, dragging my tennis bag. The crowd is going berserk, like the crowd in a gladiator movie. They're showering the court with garbage.

In the locker room Brad says, What the—?

They defaulted me.

Why?

I tell him.

He shakes his head.

His seven-year-old son, Zach, is crying because the people are being mean to Uncle Andre. And because Spuds MacKenzie peed on the net. I send them both away, then sit in the locker room for an hour, head bowed. So here we are. A new low. Fine. I can handle this. I can actually get comfortable here. I can settle in. Rock bottom can be very cozy, because at least you're at rest. You know you're not going anywhere for a while.

But rock bottom is still a ways down. I go to the 1996 U.S. Open, and right away there's controversy. Something about seeding. A few of my fellow players complain that I've gotten special treatment, that I was bumped up in the draw because tournament officials and CBS want to see me and Pete in the final. Muster says I'm a prima donna. I take particular glee, therefore, in knocking his hair-mussing ass out of the quarters, continuing to keep my promise that I would never lose to him again.

I reach the semis against Chang. I can't wait to put a beating on him after losing to him months ago at Indian Wells. It should be no problem. He's on the back nine of his career, Brad says. So am I, people say. But I have a gold medal. I almost wish I could wear it during the match. Chang, however, doesn't give a damn about my gold medal. He fires sixteen aces, wriggles out of three break points, forces me into forty-five unforced errors. Seven years after winning his last slam, Chang is almighty, omnipotent. He is risen, and I am fallen.

The next morning, sportswriters trash me. I quit. I tanked. I didn't care. It almost seems as if they're angry with me. And I know why. As a result of my loss, they now have to deal with Chang for one more day.

I don't watch the final on TV when Pete beats Chang in straight sets. But I do read about it. Every article says matter-of-factly that Pete is the best player of his generation.

AS THE YEAR WINDS DOWN I go to Munich, where the boos are deafening. I lose to Mark Woodforde, whom I beat 6–0, 6–0, two short years ago. Brad is apoplectic. He begs me to tell him what's wrong.

I don't know.

Tell me, man. Tell me.

I would if I could.

We agree that I should rest, pull out of the Australian Open.

Go home, he says. Get some rest. Spend some time with your fiancée. That'll cure whatever ails you.

20

BROOKE AND I BUY A HOUSE in Pacific Palisades. It's not the house I wanted. I had my heart set on a big rambling farmhouse with a family room off the kitchen. But she loved this one, so here we are, living in a multilevel, French Country knockoff set against the side of a cliff. It has no flow, and it feels sterile, the ideal house for a childless couple who plan to spend lots of time in different rooms.

The real estate agent gushed about the breathtaking views of the skyline. In the foreground is Sunset Boulevard. At night I can see the Holiday Inn where I stayed after our first date. Many nights I stare at the hotel and wonder what would have happened if I'd kept driving, if I'd never phoned Brooke again. I decide that the view from our new house is better when fog or smog prevents me from seeing that Holiday Inn.

At the close of 1996 we throw a combination housewarming–New Year's Eve party, invite the gang from Vegas and Brooke's Hollywood friends. We confer with Gil about security. After a new batch of scary letters, we have to guard against intruders, so Gil spends most of the night standing at the foot of the driveway, screening people as they arrive. McEnroe shows up, and I kid him about getting past Gil. He sits on the deck, talking tennis, my least favorite topic these days, so I drift in and out. I spend the night mixing margaritas, watching J.P. slap his drums with a steel Buddy Rich–type brush, and sitting before the fireplace. I stoke it, feed it, stare deep into the flames. I tell myself that 1997 is going to be better than 1996. I vow that 1997 is going to be my year.

BROOKE AND I ARE AT THE GOLDEN GLOBE AWARDS when I get a call from Gil. His twelve-year-old daughter, Kacey, has been in an accident. She was snow sledding on a church trip at Mt. Charleston, an hour north of Vegas, and went straight into a frozen snowbank. She broke her neck. I leave Brooke and fly to Vegas, arriving at the hospital in my tuxedo. I find Gil and Gaye in the hallway, looking as if they're barely hanging on. We hug, and they tell me it's bad, very bad. Kacey's going to need surgery. Doctors say there's a chance she'll be paralyzed.

We spend days at the hospital, talking to doctors, trying to keep Kacey comfortable. Gil needs to go home, get some sleep. He's out on his feet, but he won't leave, he's going to stand guard over his daughter. I get an idea. I have a big pimped-out minivan, which I bought from Perry's father. It has a satellite dish and a foldout bed. I park it right outside the hospital, outside the front door, and I tell Gil: Now, when visiting hours are over, you don't have to go home, you can just go downstairs and catch a few hours' shut-eye in the back of your new van. And, since it's all metered parking in front of the hospital, I've filled the van's cup holders with quarters.

Gil gives me a strange look, and I realize it's the first time that he and I have ever switched roles. For a few days, it's me making *him* stronger.

WHEN THE HOSPITAL releases Kacey a week later the doctors say she's out of the woods. Her surgery was a success and she'll be up and around in no time. Still, I want to follow her home, stick around Vegas, see how she recovers.

Gil won't hear of it. He knows I'm due in San Jose.

I tell Gil I'm going to pull out of the tournament.

Absolutely not, he says. There's nothing to do now but wait and pray. I'll phone you with updates. Go. Play.

I've never had an argument with Gil, and I won't let this be the first. Reluctantly I go to San Jose and play my first match in three months. I face Mark Knowles, one of my old roommates at the Bollettieri Academy. After a solid doubles career he's trying to break into the singles bracket. He's a great athlete, but I shouldn't have any trouble with him. I know his game better than he knows it himself. And yet he takes me to a third set. Even though I win, it's not an easy win, so it sticks in my craw. I hack my way through the tournament, seemingly on a collision course with Pete, but I falter in the semis against Greg Rusedski, from Canada. My mind hurries back to Vegas, hours ahead of my body.

I'M AT THE BACHELOR PAD, watching TV with Slim, my assistant. I'm in a bad way. Kacey isn't doing well, and the doctors don't know why.

Gil is on the brink. Meanwhile, my wedding looms. I think all the time about postponing it, or calling it off altogether, but I don't know how.

Slim is stressed too. He was with his girlfriend recently, he says, and the condom broke. Now, she's late. During a commercial he stands up and announces that there's only one thing to do. Get high.

He says, You want to get high with me?

High?

Yeah.

On what?

Gack.

What the hell's gack?

Crystal meth.

Why do they call it gack?

Because that's the sound you make when you're high. Your mind is going so fast, all you can say is gack, gack, gack.

That's how I feel all the time. What's the point?

Make you feel like Superman, dude. I'm telling you.

As if they're coming out of someone else's mouth, someone standing directly behind me, I hear these words: You know what? Fuck it. Yeah. Let's get high.

Slim dumps a small pile of powder on the coffee table. He cuts it, snorts it. He cuts it again. I snort some. I ease back on the couch and consider the Rubicon I've just crossed. There is a moment of regret, followed by vast sadness. Then comes a tidal wave of euphoria that sweeps away every negative thought in my head, every negative thought I've ever had. It's a cortisone shot to the subcortex. I've never felt so alive, so hopeful— and above all, I've never felt such energy. I'm seized by an urge, a desperate desire to clean. I go tearing around my house, cleaning it from top to bottom. I dust the furniture. I scour the tub. I make the beds. I sweep the floors. When there's nothing left to clean, I do laundry. All the laundry. I fold every sweater and T-shirt and still I haven't made a dent in my energy. I don't want to sit down. If I had table silver I'd polish it. If I had leather shoes I'd shine them. If I had a giant jug of coins I'd roll them into paper wrappers. I look high and low for Slim—he's out in the garage, taking apart the engine of his car and putting it together again. I tell him I could do anything right now, anything, man, anything, anything, *anyfuckingthing.* I could get in the car and drive to Palm Springs and play eighteen holes, then drive home and make lunch and go for a swim.

I don't sleep for two days. When I finally do, it's the sleep of the dead and the innocent.

. . .

PLAYING WEEKS LATER, I struggle against Scott Draper. Left-handed, talented, he's a good player, but I've beaten him soundly in the past. I shouldn't have any trouble with him, and yet he's cleaning my clock. I'm so far from being able to beat Draper, in fact, I honestly wonder if it was me who beat him the last time. How could I have been that much better such a short time ago? He's outplaying me in every phase of the game.

Afterward, reporters ask if I'm OK. They don't sound accusatory or mean. They sound like Perry and Brad. They're actually concerned, trying to figure out what's wrong.

Brooke is remarkably unconcerned. I lose all the time now, and the only time I don't lose is when I pull out of a tournament, and her only comment is that she enjoys having me around more. Also, since I'm generally playing less often, she says I'm not as moody.

Her oblivion is partly due to the wedding planning, but also her rigorous premarital training regimen. She's working with Gil to get in shape for that white dress. She's running, lifting, stretching, counting every calorie. For added motivation, she tapes a photo on the refrigerator door, and around the photo she puts a magnetic heart frame. It's a photo of the perfect woman, she says. The perfect woman with the perfect legs—the legs Brooke wants.

Astonished, I stare at the photo. I reach out and touch the frame.

Is that—?

Yep, Brooke says. Steffi Graf.

I PLAY DAVIS CUP IN APRIL, looking for a spark. I practice hard, train hard. We're up against the Netherlands. My first match, in Newport Beach, is against Sjeng Schalken. He's six foot five but serves like a man five foot six. Still, he strikes the ball cleanly, and like me he's a punisher, a baseliner who stays back and tries to run an opponent into the ground. I know what I'm in for. The day is sunny, windy, and weird— Dutch fans wear wooden shoes and wave tulips. I beat Schalken in three wearying sets.

Two days later I play Jan Siemerink, aka the Garbage Man. He's a lefty, an excellent volleyer, who gets to the net quick and covers it well. But that's the only part of his game that isn't comically, fundamentally unsound. Every Siemerink forehand looks mishit, every backhand seems shanked. Even his serve has a wacky, slingy quality. Garbage. I start the match confident, then recall that his lack of form is a powerful weapon. His abysmal shotmaking keeps you always off balance. Your timing never feels right. After two hours, I'm wrong-footed, breathing hard, and have a splitting headache. I'm also down two sets to love. Still, somehow I win, making me 24–4 in Davis Cup play, one of the best records ever compiled by an American. Sportswriters praise this small part of my game, and ask why I can't translate it to the rest of my game. Even if their praise is tempered, I bask in it. It feels good. I give a small thanks for Davis Cup.

On the other hand, Davis Cup plays havoc with my manicure schedule. Brooke has made many requests of me for the wedding, but her non-negotiable demand is that my nails be perfect. I pick at my cuticles, a lifelong nervous habit, and when she puts a wedding band on my finger, she says, she wants my hands looking their best. Just before my match with the Garbage Man, and again after the match, I submit. I sit myself in the manicurist's chair, watch the woman work at my cuticles, and tell myself this feels as off balance and wrong-footed as my match against the Garbage Man.

I think: Now *this* is what I call garbage.

WITH FOUR HELICOPTERS full of paparazzi circling overhead, on April 19, 1997, Brooke and I get married. The ceremony takes place in Monterey, in a tiny church that's stiflingly, criminally hot. I'd give anything for a puff of fresh air, but the windows must remain shut to block out the noise of the helicopters.

The heat is one reason I break out in a sweat during the ceremony. The main reason, however, is that my body and nerves are shot. As the priest drones on, sweat drips from my brow, from my chin, from my ears. Everyone is looking. They're sweating too, but not like me. The jacket of my new Dunhill tuxedo is soaked. Even my shoes squish when I walk. They're also fitted with lifts, another non-negotiable demand from Brooke. She's nearly six feet tall and she doesn't want to tower over me in our photos, so she's wearing old-fashioned pumps with minimal heels, and I'm wearing what feel like stilts.

Before we leave the church, a decoy bride, a stand-in for Brooke, leaves first. To throw the paparazzi off the scent. The first time I heard about this plan, I tuned it out, refused to pay attention. Now, as I see the

Brooke look-alike leaving, I have a thought no man should have on his wedding day: I wish I were leaving too. I wish I had a decoy groom to take my place.

A horse-drawn carriage is standing by to whisk Brooke and me to the reception, at a ranch called Stonepine. But first we have a short car ride to the carriage. I sit in the car beside Brooke, staring into my lap. I feel mortified about my attack of hysterical sweats. Brooke tells me it's OK. She's very sweet, but it's not OK. Nothing is OK.

Into the reception we go, into a solid wall of noise. I see a whirling carousel of faces—Philly, Gil, J.P., Brad, Slim, my parents. There are famous people I don't know, have never met, but vaguely recognize. Friends of Brooke? Friends of friends? Some of the Friends from *Friends*? I catch sight of Perry, my best man and the self-anointed wedding producer. He wears a Madonna headset so he can be in constant communication with the photographers and florists and caterers. He's so jacked up, so high-strung, he's making me more nervous, which I didn't think was possible.

At the end of the night, Brooke and I stagger up to our bridal suite, which I've arranged to have filled with hundreds of candles. Too many candles—the room is an oven. It's hotter than the church. Again I start to sweat. We start to blow out the candles, and the smoke detectors go off. We disable the smoke detectors and open the windows. While the room cools we go downstairs, back to the reception, to spend our wedding night eating chocolate mousse with the wedding party.

The following afternoon, at a barbecue for friends and family, Brooke and I make a grand entrance. As per Brooke's plan, we wear cowboy hats and denim shirts and arrive on horses. Mine is named Sugar. Her sad glassy eyes remind me of Peaches. People surround me, talk at me, congratulate me, slap me on the back, and I need to run away. I spend a good portion of the barbecue with my nephew, Skyler, son of Rita and Pancho. We get hold of a bow and arrow and take target practice with a distant oak.

While drawing back the bow, I feel a sudden twinge in my wrist.

I PULL OUT OF THE 1997 FRENCH OPEN. Of all the surfaces, clay is the worst on a tender wrist. There is no way I can last five sets against the dirt rats, who've been practicing and drilling on clay while I've been getting manicures and riding Sugar.

But I will go to Wimbledon. I want to go. Brooke has landed an acting job in England, which means she can accompany me. This will be good, I think. A change of venue. A trip, our first as husband and wife, to somewhere other than an island.

Though, come to think of it, England is an island.

In London we spend several happy nights. Dinner with friends. An experimental play. A walk along the Thames. The stars are lined up for a good Wimbledon. And then I decide that I'd rather jump in the Thames. Out of nowhere I can't bring myself to practice.

I tell Brad and Gil I'm pulling out of the tournament. I'm in vapor lock.

Brad says, What the hell does vapor lock mean?

I've played this game for a lot of reasons, I say, and it just seems like none of them has ever been my own.

The words come tumbling out, with no forethought, just as they did that night with Slim. But they sound remarkably true. So much, in fact, that I write them down. I repeat them to reporters. And to mirrors.

After pulling out of the tournament I stay on in London, waiting for Brooke to finish filming. We go out one night with a group of actors to a world-famous restaurant Brooke is eager to try. The Ivy. Brooke and the actors talk over each other while I silently hunker down at one end of the table, eating. Grazing, actually. I order five courses, and for dessert I shovel three sticky toffee puddings into my mouth.

Slowly, an actress notices how much food is disappearing at my end of the table. She looks at me, alarmed.

Do you always, she asks, eat like this?

I'M PLAYING IN D.C. and my opponent is Flach. Brad tells me to go out and avenge last year's Wimbledon loss, but I can't imagine anything mattering less. Revenge? Again? Haven't we been down that road before? It makes me sad, and weary, that Brad can be so blinded by his Bradness, that he can be so oblivious to what I'm feeling. Who does he think he is—Brooke?

I lose to Flach, of course, then tell Brad I'm shutting down for the summer.

Brad says, The whole summer?

See you in the fall.

Brooke is in Los Angeles, but I spend most of my time in Vegas. Slim is there, and we get high a lot. It's a welcome change to have energy, to feel happy, to clear away the vapor lock. I like feeling inspired again, even if the inspiration is chemically induced. I stay awake all night, several nights in a row, relishing the silence. No one phoning, no one faxing, no one bothering me. Nothing to do but dance around the house and fold laundry and think.

I want to get clear of the void, I tell Slim.

Yeah, he says. Yeah. The void.

Apart from the buzz of getting high, I get an undeniable satisfaction from harming myself and shortening my career. After decades of merely dabbling in masochism, I'm making it my mission.

But the physical aftermath is hideous. After two days of being high, of not sleeping, I'm an alien. I have the audacity to wonder why I feel so rotten. I'm an athlete, my body should be able to handle this. Slim gets high all the time, and he seems fine.

Then all at once Slim is not fine. He becomes unrecognizable, and drugs aren't fully to blame. He was already frantic about the prospect of becoming a father; now he phones me one night from the hospital and says, It happened.

What.

She had the baby. Months ahead of time. A boy. Andre, it only weighs one pound, six ounces. The doctors don't know if he's going to make it.

I speed down to Sunrise Hospital, the hospital where Slim and I were born twenty-four hours apart. I stare through the glass at what they tell me is a baby, though it's only the size of my open palm. The doctors tell Slim and me that the baby is very sick. They have to give him an IV of antibiotics.

The next morning the doctors tell us that the IV popped out. It dripped on the baby's leg, and now the leg is burned. Also, the baby's not breathing on his own. They need to put him on a ventilator. It's risky. The doctors worry that the baby's lungs aren't developed enough for the ventilator, but without the ventilator he'll die.

Slim says nothing. Do whatever you think best, I tell the doctors.

As feared, hours later one of the baby's lungs collapses. Then the other. Now the doctors say the lungs *really* can't handle the ventilator, but without the ventilator the baby will die. They simply don't know what to do.

There's one final hope. A machine that might do the work of a ventilator without harming the lungs. A machine that takes the blood from the baby, oxygenates it, then flows it back into the baby. But the nearest such machine is in Phoenix.

I arrange a medical airplane. A team of doctors and nurses unhooks the baby from the ventilator and carries him like an egg to the tarmac.

Then Slim, his girlfriend, and I board a separate plane. A nurse gives us a number to call when we land, to find out if the baby has survived the flight.

As the wheels touch down in Phoenix, I take a breath and dial.

Is he—?

He made it. But now we need to get him onto the machine.

At the hospital we sit and sit. The clock doesn't move. Slim chain-smokes. His girlfriend weeps quietly over a magazine. I step away for a moment to phone Gil. Kacey isn't doing well, he says. She's in constant pain. He doesn't sound like Gil. He sounds like Slim.

I return to the waiting room. A doctor appears, pulling down his mask. I don't know if I can handle more bad news.

We managed to get him hooked to the machine, the doctor says. So far, so good. The next six months will tell.

I rent a house near the hospital for Slim and his girlfriend. Then I fly back to Los Angeles. I should sleep on the flight, but instead I stare at the back of the seat in front of me and think how fragile it all is. *The next six months will tell.* To which of us does that dire statement not apply?

At home, sitting in our kitchen, I tell Brooke the entire sad, awful, miraculous story. She's fascinated—but mystified.

She asks, How could you get so involved?

How could I not?

WEEKS LATER, Brad talks me into coming back, briefly, to play at the ATP Championships in Cincinnati. I face Gustavo Kuerten, a Brazilian. It takes him forty-six minutes to beat me. My third first-round loss in a row. Gullickson announces that he's dropping me from the Davis Cup team. I'm one of the best American players ever, but I don't blame him. Who could blame him?

At the 1997 U.S. Open I'm unseeded for the first time in three years. I'm wearing a peach shirt, and they can't keep them in stock at the concession stand. Astonishing. People still want to dress like me. People want to look like me. Have they taken a good look at me lately?

I reach the round of sixteen and play Rafter, who's having his break-out year. He reached the semis of the French Open, and he's my personal favorite to win this tournament. He's a great serve-and-volleyer, reminiscent of Pete, but I always thought Rafter and I made a better rivalry, aesthetically, because Rafter is more consistent. Pete can play a lousy thirty-eight minutes, then one lights-out minute and win the set,

250

whereas Rafter plays well all the time. He's six foot two, with a low center of gravity, and he can change direction like a sports car. He's one of the hardest guys on the tour to pass, and even harder to dislike. He's all class, win or lose, and today he wins. He gives me a gentlemanly handshake and a smile in which there is an unmistakable trace of pity.

I'M PLAYING STUTTGART IN TEN DAYS. I should lie low, rest, practice, but instead I need to go to North Carolina, a little town called Mount Pleasant, because of Brooke. She's tight with David Strickland, an actor on her new TV show, *Suddenly Susan,* and David's traveling to North Carolina to spend his birthday with family. Brooke wants us to tag along. She thinks it would do us good, hanging out in the country, breathing fresh air, and I can't think of a good reason to say no.

Mount Pleasant is a quaint Southern town, but I don't see any mount and it's not all that pleasant. The Strickland house is comfortable, with old wood floors and soft beds and a warm, enveloping smell of cinnamon and pie crust. But somewhat incongruously it sits on a golf course, its back porch only twenty yards from one of the greens, so there's always someone in my peripheral vision, lining up a putt. The lady of the house, Granny Strickland, is ample-bosomed, apple-cheeked, straight out of Mayberry, and she's forever standing at her stove, baking something or whipping up another batch of paella. Not exactly training food, but to be polite I clean my plate and ask for seconds.

Brooke seems to be in heaven, and part of me understands. The house is surrounded by rolling hills and ancient trees, the leaves have turned nine different kinds of orange, and she loves David. They have a special bond, a secret language of inside jokes and comic banter. Now and then they slip into their characters from the show, doing a scene, then laughing themselves hoarse. Then they quickly explain what they've just done and said, trying to bring me up to speed, so I don't feel left out. But it's always too little, too late. I'm the third wheel, and I know it.

At night the temperature drops. The cool air has a piney, earthy scent that makes me sad. I stand on the back porch, looking at the stars, wondering what's wrong with me, why this setting has no power to charm me. I think about that moment, so many years ago, when Philly and I decided I was going to quit. When that call came for me to play here, in North Carolina. The rest is history. Over and over, I ask myself—what if?

I decide that I need to work. Work, as always, is the answer. After all, Stuttgart is only days off. It would be nice to win. I phone Brad, and he locates a tennis court an hour or so away. He also scrounges up a sparring partner, a young amateur who'd love nothing more than to hit with me each morning. I drive through the morning mist, toward the Blue Ridge Mountains, and meet the amateur. I thank him for taking the time, but he says the pleasure is all his. It will be my honor, Mr. Agassi. I feel virtuous—I'm getting my work done, even here in this remote outpost— and then we start hitting. At the higher altitude, the ball flies every which way, defying gravity. It's like playing in outer space. Hardly worth the effort.

Then the young pro blows out his shoulder.

I spend the next two days of our Southern sojourn scarfing paella and brooding. When I grow so bored that I think I might bang my head against a pine tree, I walk out to the golf course and try to birdie the hole off the porch.

At last it's time for me to leave. I kiss Brooke goodbye, kiss Granny Strickland goodbye, and notice that both kisses have the same amount of passion. I fly to Miami to connect with a direct flight to Stuttgart. Walking up to the gate, who should I see but Pete. As always, Pete. He looks as if he's done nothing for the last month but practice, and when he wasn't practicing, he was lying on a cot in a bare cell, thinking about beating me. He's rested, focused, wholly undistracted. I've always thought the differences between Pete and me were overblown by sportswriters. It seemed too convenient, too important for fans, and Nike, and the game, that Pete and I be polar opposites, the Yankees and Red Sox of tennis. The game's best server versus its best returner. The diffident Californian versus the brash Las Vegan. It all seemed like horseshit. Or, to use Pete's favorite word, nonsense. But at this moment, making small talk at the gate, the gap between us appears genuinely, frighteningly wide, like the gap between good and bad. I've often told Brad that tennis plays too big a part in Pete's life, and not a big enough part in mine, but Pete seems to have the proportions about right. Tennis is his job, and he does it with brio and dedication, while all my talk of maintaining a life outside tennis seems like just that—talk. Just a pretty way of rationalizing all my distractions. For the first time since I've known him—including the times he's beaten my brains out—I envy Pete's dullness. I wish I could emulate his spectacular lack of inspiration, and his peculiar lack of *need* for inspiration.

I LOSE TO MARTIN in the first round of Stuttgart. Driving away from the stadium, Brad is in a mood I've never seen. He looks at me with astonishment, and sadness, and a Rafter-like pity. As we pull up to the hotel, he asks me up to his room.

He rummages in the minibar and extracts two bottles of beer. He doesn't glance at the labels. He doesn't care that they're German. When Brad drinks German beer without noticing or complaining, something is up.

He's wearing jeans and a black turtleneck. He looks somber, severe— and older. I've aged him.

Andre, we've got a big decision to make, and we're going to make it before we leave this room tonight.

What's up, Brad?

We ain't continuing like this. You're better than this. At least, you used to be better. You either need to quit—or start over. But you can't go on embarrassing yourself like this.

What—?

Let me finish. You have game left. At least I think you do. You can still win. Good things can still happen. But you need a full overhaul. You need to go back to the beginning. You need to pull out of everything and regroup. I'm talking square one.

When Brad talks about pulling out of tournaments, I know it's serious.

Here's what you'd need to do, he says. You'd need to train like you haven't trained in years. Hard core. You'd need to get your body right, get your mind right, then start at the bottom. I'm talking challengers, against guys who never dreamed they'd get a chance to meet you, let alone play you.

He stops. He takes a long sip of beer. I say nothing. We've come to the crossroads, this is it, and it feels as if we've been headed here for months. Years. I stare out the window at the Stuttgart traffic. I hate tennis more than ever—but I hate myself more. I tell myself, So what if you hate tennis? Who cares? All those people out there, all those millions who hate what they do for a living, they do it anyway. Maybe doing what you hate, doing it well and cheerfully, is the point. So you hate tennis. Hate it all you want. You still need to respect it—and yourself.

I say, OK, Brad, I'm not ready for it to be over. I'm all in. Tell me what to do, and I'll do it.

21

CHANGE.

Time to change, Andre. You can't go on like this. Change, change, change—I say this word to myself several times a day, every day, while buttering my morning toast, while brushing my teeth, less as a warning than as a soothing chant. Far from depressing me, or shaming me, the idea that I must change completely, from top to bottom, brings me back to center. For once I don't hear that nagging self-doubt that follows every personal resolution. I won't fail this time, I can't, because it's change now or change never. The idea of stagnating, of remaining *this Andre* for the rest of my life, that's what I find truly depressing and shameful.

And yet. Our best intentions are often thwarted by external forces— forces that we ourselves set in motion long ago. Decisions, especially bad ones, create their own kind of momentum, and momentum can be a bitch to stop, as every athlete knows. Even when we vow to change, even when we sorrow and atone for our mistakes, the momentum of our past keeps carrying us down the wrong road. Momentum rules the world. Momentum says: Hold on, not so fast, I'm still running things here. As a friend likes to say, quoting an old Greek poem: The minds of the ever-lasting gods are not changed suddenly.

Weeks after Stuttgart, walking through LaGuardia Airport, I get a phone call. It's a man with a gruff voice, a voice of judgment and con-demnation. A voice of Authority. He says he's a doctor working with the ATP. (I think what those letters stand for: Association of Tennis Profes-sionals.) There is doom in his voice, as if he's going to tell me I'm dying. And then that's exactly what he tells me.

It was his job to test my urine sample from a recent tournament. It's my duty, he says, to inform you that you've failed the standard ATP drug test. The urine sample you submitted has been found to contain trace amounts of crystal methylene.

I fall onto a chair in the baggage claim area. I'm carrying a backpack, which I slip off my shoulder and drop to the ground.

Mr. Agassi?

Yes. I'm here. So. What now?

Well, there is a process. You'll need to write a letter to the ATP, admitting your guilt or declaring your innocence.

Uh huh.

Did you know there was a likelihood that this drug was in your system?

Yes. Yes, I knew.

In that case, you'll need to explain in your letter how the drug got there.

And then?

Your letter will be reviewed by a panel.

And then?

If you knowingly ingested the drug—if you, as it were, plead guilty—you'll be disciplined, of course.

How?

He reminds me that tennis has three classes of drug violation. Performance-enhancing drugs, of course, would constitute a Class 1, he says, which would carry suspension for two years. However, he adds, crystal methylene is a clear case of Class 2. Recreational drugs.

I think: Recreation. *Re-creation.*

I say: Meaning?

Three months' suspension.

What do I do once I've written this letter?

I have an address for you. Have you got something to write on?

I fish in my backpack for my notebook. He gives me the street, city, zip code, and I scribble it all down, in a daze, with no intention of actually writing the letter.

The doctor says a few more things, which I don't hear, and then I thank him and hang up. I stumble out of the airport and hail a cab. Driving into Manhattan, staring out the smudged window, I tell the back of the cabdriver's head: So much for change.

I go straight to Brooke's brownstone. Luckily, she's in Los Angeles. I'd never be able to hide my emotions from her. I'd have to tell her everything, and I couldn't handle that right now. I fall onto the bed and immediately pass out. When I wake an hour later, I realize it was just a nightmare. What a relief.

It takes several minutes to accept that, no, the phone call was real. The doctor was real. The meth, all too real.

My name, my career, everything is now on the line, at a craps table where no one wins. Whatever I've achieved, whatever I've worked for, might soon mean nothing. Part of my discomfort with tennis has always been a nagging sense that it's meaningless. Now I'm about to learn the true meaning of meaninglessness.

Serves me right.

I lie awake until dawn, wondering what to do, whom to tell. I try to imagine how it will feel to be publicly shamed, not for my clothes or game, not for some marketing slogan someone hung on me, but for my utter stupidity, mine alone. I'll be an outcast. I'll be a cautionary tale.

Still, though I'm in pain, during the next few days I don't panic. Not yet, not quite. I can't, because other more harrowing problems crowd in from all sides. People around me, people I love, are hurting.

Doctors need to operate a second time on little Kacey's neck. The first operation was clearly botched. I arrange for her to fly to Los Angeles, to have the best care, but during her post-surgery recuperation period she's immobilized again, lying on her back in a hospital bed, and she's suffering terribly. Unable to move her head, she says her scalp and skin burn. Also, her room is unspeakably hot, and she's like her father: she can't take heat. I kiss her cheek and tell her, Don't worry. We'll fix it.

I look at Gil. He's shrinking before my eyes.

I run to the nearest appliance store and buy the biggest, baddest air-conditioning unit they have. Gil and I install it in Kacey's window. When I turn the knob up to Max Cool and press Power, Gil and I clap hands and Kacey smiles as the cold air pushes the bangs from her pretty round face.

Next I run to a toy store, the swimming section, and buy one of those tiny inner tubes for toddlers. I slide the inner tube under Kacey, positioning her head in the center, then blow it up until it gently and gradually lifts her head without altering the angle of her neck. A look of pure relief, and gratitude, and joy, washes over her face, and in this look, in this courageous little girl, I find the thing I've been seeking, the philosopher's stone that unites all the experiences, good and bad, of the last few years. Her suffering, her resilient smile in the face of that suffering, my part in easing her suffering—this, *this* is the reason for everything. How many times must I be shown? This is why we're here. To fight through the pain and, when possible, to relieve the pain of others. So simple. So hard to see.

I turn to Gil and he sees it all, and his cheeks are glistening with tears.

Later, while Kacey sleeps, while Gil pretends not to sleep in a corner, I sit in a hard-backed chair at her bedside, a legal pad in my lap, and write a letter to the ATP. It's a letter filled with lies interwoven with bits of truth.

I acknowledge that the drugs were in my system—but I assert that I never knowingly took them. I say Slim, whom I've since fired, is a known drug user, and that he often spikes his sodas with meth—which is true. Then I come to the central lie of the letter. I say that I recently drank accidentally from one of Slim's spiked sodas, unwittingly ingesting his drugs. I say that I felt poisoned, but thought the drugs would leave my system quickly. Apparently they did not.

I ask for understanding, and leniency, and hastily sign it: Sincerely.

I sit with the letter on my lap, watching Kacey's face. I feel ashamed, of course. I've always been a truthful person. When I lie, it's almost always unknowingly, or to myself. But imagining the look on Kacey's face as she learns that Uncle Andre is a drug user, banned three months from tennis, and then multiplying that look by a few million faces, I don't know what else to do but lie.

I promise myself that at least this lie is the end of it. I'll send the letter, but I won't do anything more. I'll let my lawyers handle the rest. I won't go before any panel and lie to anyone's face. I'll never lie about this publicly. From here on, I'll leave it in the hands of fate and men in suits. If they can settle it privately, quietly, fine. If not, I'll live with what comes.

Gil wakes. I fold the letter and step with him into the hallway.

Under the fluorescent lights, he looks drawn, pale. He looks—I can't believe it—*weak*. I'd forgotten: it's in hospital hallways that we know what life is about. I put my arms around him and tell him I love him and that we'll get through this.

He nods, thanks me, mumbles something incoherent. We stand in silence for the longest time. In his eyes I can see his thoughts circling the abyss. Then he tries to distract himself. He needs to talk about something, anything, other than the fear and worry. He asks how it's going with me.

I tell him that I've decided to recommit myself to tennis, start at the minor leagues and work my way back. I tell him that Kacey has inspired me, shown me the way.

Gil says he wants to help.

No, you've got your hands full.

Hey. Stand on my shoulders, remember? Reach?

I can't believe he still has faith; I've given him so many reasons to doubt. I'm twenty-seven, the age when tennis players start to fade, and I'm talking about a second chance, and yet Gil doesn't frown, doesn't arch an eyebrow.

Let's throw down, he says. It's on.

WE START FROM THE BEGINNING, as if I'm a teenager, as if I've never worked out, because that's how I look. I'm slow, fat, frail as a kitten. I haven't picked up a dumbbell in a year. The heaviest thing I've lifted is Kacey's air conditioner. I need to rediscover my body, add gingerly and gradually to its strength.

But first: We're in Gil's gym. I'm sitting on the free bench, he's leaning against the leg extension. I tell him what I've done to my body. The drugs. I tell him about the pending suspension. I can't ask him to lead me out of the depths unless he knows how deep I've fallen. He looks as crushed as he looked in his daughter's hospital room. To me, Gil has always resembled that statue of Atlas, but now he looks as if he literally shoulders the weight of the world, as if he's bench-pressing the problems of six billion. His voice chokes.

I've never been so disgusted with myself.

I tell him I'm done with drugs, I'll never touch them again, but it goes without saying. He knows this as well as I do. He clears his throat, thanks me for being honest, then pushes it all aside. Where you've been, he says, doesn't matter. From now on, we're all about where you're going.

Where we're going, I say.

Right.

He draws up a plan. He outlines a proper diet. And no more Mr. Nice Guy, he says. No more lapses, no more fast food, no more shortcuts.

You'll even have to cut back on the booze, he says.

Above all, he's going to keep me on a strict schedule. Eat, exercise, lift, hit, at precise times of day.

As part of my new ascetic lifestyle, I'll be seeing less of my wife. I wonder if she'll notice.

I PUT IN A FIERCE, rugged month with Gil, every bit as rugged as our mini boot camp in early 1995, and then I go to a challenger, the bottom of

258

the pro tennis ladder. The winner's check is $3,500. The crowd is smaller than the crowd at a typical high school football game.

The venue is UNLV. Familiar territory for such an unfamiliar moment. As Gil and I pull into the parking lot, I think of how far I've come, and how far I haven't. These are the same courts I played on when I was seven. This is where I came the day Gil quit his job to work with me. I stood right over there, outside his office, hopping on one foot because I was so excited about the road that lay before us. Now, just a three wood from that spot, I'm playing hackers and has-beens.

In other words, my peers.

A challenger is the definition of small-time, and nowhere is this more evident than in the players' lounge. The pre-match meal is airplane food: rubber chicken, limp veggies, flat soda. Once upon a time, at slams, I would walk up and down the endless buffet line, chatting with white-hatted chefs while they made me feathery omelets and homemade pasta. All gone.

The indignities don't stop there. At a challenger, there are fewer ball boys. It makes sense, since there are practically no balls. You get only three per match. On either side of your court are rows of courts with other matches taking place simultaneously. As you toss a ball to serve, you see the players to your left and right. You hear them arguing. They don't care if they're interrupting your concentration. Fuck you and your concentration. Now and then a ball comes dribbling past your feet from another court, and you hear, A little help! You need to stop whatever you're doing and throw the ball back. Now *you're* the ball boy. Again.

You also operate your own scoreboard. Manually. During the changeover, I flip the little plastic numbers, which feel like part of a children's game. Fans laugh and yell things. How the mighty have fallen! *Image Is Everything,* eh, buddy? A high-ranking official says publicly that Andre Agassi playing a challenger is like Bruce Springsteen playing a corner bar.

So what's wrong with Springsteen playing a corner bar? I think it would be cool if Springsteen played a corner bar now and then.

I'm ranked number 141 in the world, the lowest I've been ranked in my adult life, the lowest I've dreamed of being ranked. Sportswriters say I'm humbled. They love saying this. They couldn't be more wrong. I was humbled in the hotel room with Brad. I was humbled smoking meth with Slim. Now I'm just glad to be out here.

Brad feels the same way. He doesn't find anything demeaning about the challenger. He's reenergized, rededicated, and I love him for it. He's excited for this challenger, coaching me as if we're at Wimbledon. He doesn't doubt that this is step one on the road all the way back to number one. Inevitably, I put his faith to the test right away. I'm a shadow of my former self. My legs and arms might be on the mend, but my mind is still grossly out of shape. I reach the final, and then my mind gives out. Shaking from the pressure, the strangeness, the ridicule from the stands, I lose.

Brad is undiscouraged. Some technique will need relearning, he says. Shot selection, for instance. You need to retrain that muscle with which a tennis player decides in the heat of battle that this shot is the right one and that shot is the wrong one. You need to remember that it doesn't matter if you hit the best shot in the world—remember? If it's the wrong moment, it's the wrong shot.

Every shot is an educated guess, and I'm no longer educated. I'm as green as I was in juniors. It took me twenty-two years to discover my talent, to win my first slam—and only two years to lose it.

ONE WEEK AFTER VEGAS I play a challenger in Burbank. The venue is a public park. Center court has a large tree on one side that casts a twenty-foot shadow. I've played on thousands of courts in my career, and this is the sorriest one of all. In the distance I hear kids playing kickball and dodgeball, cars backfiring, boom boxes blaring.

The tournament runs through Thanksgiving weekend, and I reach the third round, which falls on Thanksgiving Day. Rather than eating turkey at home, I'm scuffling in a Burbank public park, ranked 120 spots lower than I was two Thanksgivings ago. Meanwhile, in Göteborg, Davis Cup is under way. Chang and Sampras versus Sweden. It's sad, but appropriate, that I'm not there. I don't belong there. I belong here, under the ridiculous courtside tree. Unless I can accept that I'm where I'm supposed to be, I'll never belong *there* again.

Warming up before my match, I realize that I'm only four minutes from the studio where Brooke shoots *Suddenly Susan,* on which Perry is now a producer. The show has become a smash hit, and Brooke's busy, working twelve hours a day. Still, it seems odd that she doesn't pop over, watch a few points. Even when I get home she doesn't ask about the match.

Then again, I don't ask about *Suddenly Susan* either.

We talk about things. We talk about nothing.

. . .

THE ONLY TIME I BREAK TRAINING is to meet with Perry and lay the groundwork for my charitable foundation. This is what we talked about fifteen years ago, two idealistic teenagers with their mouths full of Chipwiches. We wanted to reach a plateau from which we could give back, and we've finally arrived. I've negotiated a long-term deal with Nike, which will pay me tens of millions over the next decade. I've bought my parents a house. I've taken care of everyone on my team. Now I'm financially able to think larger, to widen my lens, and in 1997, though I've hit rock bottom, or because I've hit rock bottom, I'm ready.

My primary concern is children at risk. Adults can always ask for help, but children are voiceless, powerless. So the first project my foundation undertakes is a shelter for abused and neglected children who've been placed in the protective custody of the courts. The shelter includes a cottage for medically fragile children, and a makeshift school. Next we launch a program to clothe three thousand inner-city children each year. Then a series of scholarships to UNLV. Then a Boys and Girls Club. My foundation takes a 2,200-square-foot building that's falling apart and turns it into a 25,000-square-foot showplace, with a computer lab, a cafeteria, a library, and tennis courts. Colin Powell speaks at the dedication.

I spend many carefree hours at the new Boys and Girls Club, meeting children, listening to their stories. I take them onto the tennis court, teach them the proper grip, watch their eyes sparkle because they've never held a racket before. I sit with them in the computer room, where the demand for online time is so great that they stand in long lines, patiently waiting their turn. It shocks me, pains me, to see how resolved they are to learn. Other times I simply station myself in the rec center of the Boys and Girls Club, playing ping-pong with the children. I never walk into that rec center without thinking of the rec center at the Bollettieri Academy, where I was so scared that first night, my back against the wall. The memory makes me want to adopt every scared child I see.

One day in the rec center I sit with Stan, the man who runs the Boys and Girls Club. I ask him, What more can we do? How can we make a bigger difference in their lives?

Stan says, You have to figure out a way to occupy more of their day. Otherwise it's one step forward, two steps back. You really want to make a difference? You want to have a lasting impact? You need more of their day. In fact, you need *all* of their day.

So in 1997 I huddle again with Perry, and we hit on the idea of adding education to our work. Then we decide to *make* education our work. But how? We briefly consider opening a private school, but the bureaucratic and financial obstacles are too much. By chance I catch a story on *60 Minutes* about charter schools, and it's the eureka moment. Charter schools are partly state funded, partly privately funded. The challenge is raising money, but the benefit is retaining full control. With a charter school we could do things the way we want. We'd be free to build something unique. Special. And if it works, it can spread like wildfire. It can be a model for charter schools around the nation. It can change education as we know it.

I can't believe the irony. A *60 Minutes* piece caused my father to send me away, to break my heart, and now a *60 Minutes* piece lights the way home, gives me the map to find my life's meaning, my mission. Perry and I resolve to build the best charter school in America. We resolve to hire the best teachers, pay them well, and hold them accountable for grades and test scores. We resolve to show the world what can be done when you set standards outrageously high and open the purse strings. We shake on it.

I'll give millions of my own money to launch the school, but we'll need to raise many more millions. We'll issue a $40 million bond, then pay it off by parlaying and trading on my fame. At last my fame will have a purpose. All those famous people I've met at parties and through Brooke—I'll ask them to give their time and talent to my school, to visit the children, and to perform at an annual fund-raiser, which we're calling the Grand Slam for Children.

WHILE PERRY AND I are scouting locations for our school, I get a call from Gary Muller, a South African who used to play and coach on the tour. He's organizing a tennis event in Cape Town to raise money for the Nelson Mandela Foundation. He asks if I'd like to take part.

We don't know if Mandela's going to be there, he says.

If there's even a remote chance, I'm in.

Gary calls right back. Good news, he says. You're going to get to meet The Man.

You're kidding.

He's confirmed. He's coming to the event.

I grip the phone tighter. I've admired Mandela for years. I've followed his struggles, his imprisonment, his miraculous release and stunning political career, with awe. The idea of actually meeting him, speaking to him, makes me dizzy.

I tell Brooke. It's the happiest she's seen me in a long time, which makes her happy. She wants to come. The event happens to be a short flight from where she stayed while filming her Africa movie, back in 1993, when we first started faxing.

She immediately goes shopping for matching safari outfits.

J.P. shares my reverence for Mandela, so I invite him to join us on the trip, and bring his wife, Joni, whom Brooke and I both love. The four of us fly to South America, then catch another plane to Johannesburg. Then we hop a rickety prop plane into the heart of Africa.

A storm forces us to make an unscheduled landing. We batten down in a straw-roofed hut in the middle of nowhere, and over the sound of the thunder we can hear hundreds of animals run for cover. Looking out of the hut, over the vast savannah, watching storm clouds whirl along the horizon, J.P. and I agree this is one of those moments. We're both reading Mandela's memoir, *Long Walk to Freedom*, but feeling like heroes in a Hemingway novel. I think about something Mandela said once in an interview: No matter where you are in life, there is always more journey ahead. And I think of one of Mandela's favorite quotes, from the poem Invictus, which sustained him during those moments when he thought his journey had been cut short: *I am the master of my fate: I am the captain of my soul.*

After the storm passes we pile back into the prop plane and fly to a game reserve. We spend three days on safari. Every morning, before dawn, we climb into a Jeep. We drive and drive, then abruptly stop. We sit for twenty minutes in pitch dark, the engine running. As the dawn slowly breaks we find that we're on the banks of a vast fog-covered marsh, surrounded by dozens of different kinds of animals. We see hundreds of impala. We see at least seventy-five zebras. We see scores of giraffes as tall as two-story buildings, dancing around us and gliding among the trees, nibbling from the highest branches, a sound like celery being crunched. We feel the landscape speaking to us: All these animals, beginning their day in a dangerous world, exude tremendous calm and acceptance—why can't you?

With us are a driver and a shooter. The shooter is named Johnson. We love Johnson. He's our African Gil. He stands guard. He knows we love him, and he smiles with the pride of a crack shot. He also knows the landscape better than the impalas do. At one point he waves his hand at

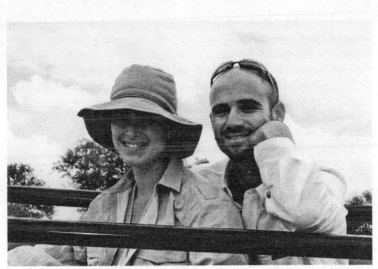

In South Africa, on safari with Brooke, late 1997,
days before meeting Mandela

the trees and a thousand small monkeys, as if on cue, fall to the ground, like autumn leaves.

We're driving deep into the bush one morning when the Jeep shudders, swerves, and we go spinning off to the right.

What happened?

We nearly ran over a lion sleeping in the middle of the road.

The lion sits up and stares with an expression that says, *You woke me.* His head is enormous. His eyes are the color of lemon-lime Gatorade. The smell of him is a musk so primal that it makes us lightheaded.

He has hair like I used to have.

Do not make a sound, the driver whispers.

Whatever you do, Johnson whispers, do not stand up.

Why?

The lion looks at us as one big predator. Right now he's afraid of us. If you stand, he'll see that we're several smaller people.

Fair enough.

After a few minutes, the lion backs away, into the bush. We drive on.

Later, returning to our campsite, I lean into J.P. and whisper: I need to tell you something.

Fire away.

I'm going through—well, a tough time right now. I'm trying to put some bad stuff behind me.

What's the problem?

I can't go into it. But I wanted to apologize if I seem—different.

Well, now that you mention it, you do. You have. But what's going on?

I'll tell you when I know you better.

He laughs.

Then he sees that I'm not kidding. He asks, Are you OK?

I don't know. I honestly don't know.

I want to tell him about the depression, the confusion, the time with Slim, the pending suspension from the ATP. But I can't. Not now. Not until it's all farther behind me. At the moment it feels like the lion, still inches away and glowering. I don't want to give voice to my problems, for fear of rousing them, making them pounce. I just want to alert J.P. to their presence.

I also tell him that I'm doubling down on tennis, and if I can pull through this tough time, if I can come back, everything is going to be different. I'm going to be different. But even if I can't, even if I'm finished, even if I lose everything, I'm still going to be different.

He says, Finished?

I just wanted you to know.

It's like a confession, a testimony. J.P. looks at me with sadness. He squeezes my arm and tells me, in so many words, that I am the captain of my fate.

WE TRAVEL TO CAPE TOWN, where I play tennis with obvious impatience, like a child doing chores on Saturday morning. Then, at last, it's time. We helicopter to a compound, and Mandela himself greets us at the helipad. He's surrounded by photographers, dignitaries, reporters, aides—and he towers above them all. He looks not only taller than I expected, but stronger, healthier. He looks like a former athlete, which surprises me, given his years of hard labor and torture. But of course he is a former athlete, a boxer in his youth—and in prison, he says in his memoir, he kept fit by running in place in his cell and playing tennis occasionally on a crude, makeshift court. For all his strength, however, his smile is sweet, almost angelic.

I tell J.P. he seems saintly to me. Gandhi-like, void of all bitterness. His eyes, though damaged by years of working in the harsh glare of the prison's lime quarry, are filled with wisdom. His eyes say that he's figured something out, something essential.

I babble as he fixes me with those eyes and shakes my hand and tells me he admires my game.

We follow him into a great hall, where a formal dinner is served. Brooke and I are seated at Mandela's table. Brooke sits on my right, Mandela on her right. Throughout the meal he tells stories. I have many questions, but I don't dare interrupt him. He talks about Robben Island, where he was held for eighteen of his twenty-seven years in prison. He talks about winning over a few of the guards. As a special treat, they would sometimes let him walk to the edge of a small lake with a fishing pole, to catch his own dinner. He smiles at the memory, almost nostalgic.

After dinner Mandela stands and gives a stirring talk. His theme: we must all care for one another—this is our task in life. But also we must care for ourselves, which means we must be *careful* in our decisions, *careful* in our relationships, *careful* in our statements. We must manage our lives carefully, in order to avoid becoming victims. I feel as if he's speaking directly to me, as if he's aware that I've been careless with my talent and my health.

He talks about racism, not just in South Africa but around the world. It's nothing but ignorance, he says, and education is the only remedy. In prison, Mandela spent his few free hours educating himself. He created a kind of university, and he and his fellow prisoners were professors to each other. He survived the loneliness of constant confinement by reading; he especially loved Tolstoy. One of the harshest punishments his guards devised was taking away his right to study for four years. Again his words seem to shimmer with personal relevance. I think of the work Perry and I have undertaken in Vegas, our charter school, and I feel invigorated. Also embarrassed. For the first time in many years I'm acutely aware of my lack of education. I feel the weight of this lack, the misfortune of it. I see it as a crime in which I've been complicit. I think of how many thousands in my hometown are victims of this crime right now, deprived of an education, unaware how much they're losing.

Finally, Mandela talks about the road he's traveled. He talks about the difficulty of all human journeys—and yet, he says, there is clarity and nobility in just being a journeyer. When he stops speaking and takes his chair I know that my journey, compared with his, is nothing, and yet that's not his point. Mandela is saying that every journey is important, and that no journey is impossible.

Bidding Mandela goodbye, I'm magnetized. I'm pointed in the right direction. A friend later shows me a passage in the Pulitzer Prize–winning novel *A Death in the Family,* in which a woman deep in mourning thinks:

> Now I am more nearly a grown member of the human race . . .
> she thought that she had never before had a chance to realize the
> strength human beings have, to endure; she loved and revered all
> those who had ever suffered, even those who had failed to endure.

This is close to what I feel as I leave Mandela. This is what I think when the helicopter lifts away from his compound. I love and revere those who suffer, who have ever suffered. I am now more nearly a grown member of the human race.

God wants us to grow up.

NEW YEAR'S EVE, the last hours of this dreadful year, 1997. Brooke and I throw another New Year's party, and the next morning I wake early. I pull the covers over my head, then remember that I scheduled a practice with a kid on the tour, Vince Spadea. I decide to cancel. No. I yell at myself. You cannot cancel. You're not that person anymore. You're not going to start 1998 by oversleeping and canceling a practice.

I force myself out of bed and meet Spadea. Even though it's only practice, we both want it. He turns it into a battle, which I appreciate, especially when I win. Walking off the court, I feel winded but strong. The old kind of strong.

This is going to be my year, I tell Spadea—1998 is my year.

Brooke comes with me to the 1998 Australian Open and watches me dispatch my first three opponents, and unfortunately watches as I face Alberto Berasategui, from Spain. I go up two sets to love, then unaccountably, impossibly, for no reason, I lose. Berasategui is a nasty opponent, but still, I had him. It's an unthinkable loss, one of the few times I've ever lost a match when ahead two sets to none. Is this a detour in the comeback or a dead end?

I go to San Jose and play well. I meet Pete in the final. He seems glad to have me back, glad to see me again on the other side, as if he's missed me. I have to admit, I've missed him too. I win, 6–2, 6–4, and toward the end, part of him seems to be pulling for me. He knows what I'm attempting, how far I have to go.

I tease him in the locker room about how easy it was to beat him.

How does it feel to lose to someone outside the top hundred?

I'm not too worried about it, he says. It's not going to happen again.

Then I tease him about recent reports of his personal life. He's broken up with the law student and he's said to be dating an actress.

Bad move, I tell him.

The words catch us both off guard.

In the media room, reporters ask me about Pete and Marcelo Ríos, who are dueling for the number one rank: Which of them do you think will ultimately be number one?

Neither.

Nervous laughter.

I think I'm going to be number one.

Raucous laughter.

No. Really. I mean it.

They stare, then dutifully write my insane prediction in their notebooks.

In March I go to Scottsdale and win my second straight tournament. I beat Jason Stoltenberg, from Australia. A classic Aussie, he's solid, steady, with an enviable all-around game that forces opponents to execute. He's a good gut check for me, a good test of my nerves, and I pass. Anyone who crosses me right now is going to have to deal with something they don't want to deal with.

I go to Indian Wells and beat Rafter, but lose to a young phenom named Jan-Michael Gambill. They say he's the best of the young bucks coming up. I look at him and wonder if he knows what lies ahead, if he's ready—if anyone can possibly be ready.

I go to Key Biscayne. I want to win, I'm crazy to win. It's not like me to want a win this badly. What I normally feel is a desire not to lose. But warming up before my first-rounder, I tell myself I want this, and I realize precisely why. It's not about my comeback. It's about my team. My *new* team, my real team. I'm playing to raise money and visibility for my school. After all these years I've got what I've always wanted, something to play for that's larger than myself and yet still closely connected to me. Something that bears my name but isn't about me. The Andre Agassi College Preparatory Academy.

At first I didn't want my name on the school. But friends persuaded me that my name can bring cachet and credibility. My name might make raising money easier. Perry chooses the word *Academy*, and it's not until later that I appreciate the way this forever links my school to

my past, to Bradenton Academy and the Bollettieri Academy, my childhood prisons.

I DON'T HAVE MANY FRIENDS IN LOS ANGELES, and Brooke has
countless friends, so most nights find her out being sociable and me at
home, alone.

Thank God for J.P. He lives in Orange County, so it's easy enough for
him to drive north now and then, sit with me by the fire, smoke a cigar,
and talk about life. His pastoring days seem like ancient history, but during our fireside talks it feels as if he's speaking to me from an invisible
pulpit. Not that I mind. I like being his solitary congregation, his flock of
one. In early 1998 he covers all the big topics. Motivation, inspiration,
legacy, destiny, rebirth. He helps me sustain the sense of mission I felt in
Mandela's presence.

One night I tell J.P. that I feel a remarkable confidence in my game,
and a new purpose for being on the court—so how come I still feel all
this fear? Doesn't the fear ever go away?

I hope not, he says. Fear is your fire, Andre. I wouldn't want to see you
if it ever completely went out.

Then J.P. looks around the house, takes a pull on his cigar, and says he
can't help but notice my wife is never around. Whenever he comes over,
no matter the day or time, Brooke seems to be out with friends.

He asks if it bothers me.

Hadn't noticed.

I GO TO MONTE CARLO in April 1998 and lose to Pete. He pumps his
fist. No more pulling for me—the rivalry is back on.

I go to Rome. I'm lying on my hotel bed, resting after a match.

Back-to-back phone calls.

First, Philly. He's sniffling, on the verge of all-out tears. He tells me his
wife, Marti, just gave birth to a baby girl. They're calling her Carter
Bailey. My brother sounds different. Happy, of course, and busting with
pride, but also: Philly sounds as though he feels blessed. Philly sounds as
though he feels supremely *lucky*.

I tell him how overjoyed I am for him and Marti, and I promise to get
home as soon as I can. Brooke and I will come straight over and see my
brand-new niece, I say, my voice catching in my throat.

The phone rings again. Is it an hour later? Three? In my memory it will always feel like part of the same foggy moment, though the two calls might be days apart. It's my lawyers, they're on speaker phone. Andre? Can you hear us? Andre?

Yes, I hear you. Go ahead.

Well, the ATP has read and carefully reviewed your heartfelt assertion of innocence. I'm pleased to say that your explanation has been accepted. Your failed test is thrown out. Henceforth the matter will be considered closed.

I'm not suspended?

No.

I'm free to go on with my career? My life?

Yes.

I ask several more times. You're sure? You mean, this is really over?

As far as the ATP is concerned, yes. They believe and accept your explanation. Gladly. I think everyone is eager to move on and put this behind them.

I hang up and stare into space, thinking again and again: New life.

I GO TO the 1998 French Open, and against Marat Safin, from Russia, I hurt my shoulder. I always forget how weighty the ball can be on this particular clay. It's like hitting a shotput. The shoulder is agony, but I'm grateful for the hurt. I will never again take for granted the privilege of hurting on a tennis court.

The doctor says I have an impingement. Pressure on the nerve. I shut myself down for two weeks. No practice, no sparring, nothing. I miss the game. What's more, I let myself miss it. I enjoy and celebrate missing it.

At Wimbledon I face Tommy Haas, from Germany. In the third set, during a fierce tiebreak, the linesman makes an atrocious blunder. Haas hits a ball clearly long and wide, but the linesman calls it in, giving Haas a commanding 6–3 lead. It's the worst call of my career. I know the ball was out, know it without question, but all my arguing is for nothing. The other linesman and the umpire uphold the call. I go on to lose the tiebreak. Now I'm down two sets to one, a steep hole.

Officials pause the match, postpone the end because of darkness. Back at my hotel, on the news, I see that the ball was several inches out. I can only laugh.

The next day, taking the court, I'm still laughing. I still don't care about the call. I'm just happy to be here. Maybe I don't know yet how to be happy and play well at the same time: Haas wins the fourth set. Afterward, he tells reporters he grew up idolizing me. I used to look up to Agassi, he says—it's a very special win for me because he won Wimbledon in 1992 and I can say I beat Andre Agassi, a former number one who's won a couple of Grand Slams.

It sounds like a eulogy. Does the guy think he beat me or buried me?

And did anyone in the press room bother to tell him I've actually won *three* slams?

BROOKE LANDS A ROLE in an indie film called *Black and White*. She's elated, because the director is a genius and the theme is race relations and she'll get to ad-lib her lines and wear her hair in dreadlocks. She's also living in the woods for a month, bunking with her fellow actors, and when we talk on the phone she says they all stay in character, 24–7. Doesn't that sound cool?

Cool, I say, rolling my eyes.

On her first morning home, eating breakfast in the kitchen, she's full of stories about Robert Downey Jr. and Mike Tyson and Marla Maples and other stars of the movie. I try to be interested. She asks about my tennis, and she tries to be interested. We're tentative, like strangers. We're not like spouses sharing a kitchen; more like teens sharing a hostel. We're courteous, polite, even kind, but the vibe feels brittle, as if everything could shatter any minute.

I put another log in the kitchen fireplace.

So I have something to tell you, Brooke says. While I was away, I got a tattoo.

I spin around. You're kidding.

We go to the bathroom where there's more light, and she pulls down the waistline of her jeans and shows me. On her hip. A dog.

Did it cross your mind to run that by me?

The exact wrong thing to say. Controlling, she calls it. Since when does she need my permission to decorate *her* body? I go back to the kitchen, pour myself a second cup of coffee, and stare harder into the fire. Stare *harder*.

BECAUSE OF SCHEDULING CONFLICTS, Brooke and I couldn't take our honeymoon right after the wedding. But now, with her done filming and me just *done*, it seems like the perfect time. We decide to go to Necker

Island, in the British Virgin Islands, southeast of Indigo Island. It's owned by billionaire Richard Branson, and he tells us we'll love it.

He says, It's an island paradise!

From the moment we land, we're out of sync. We can't get comfortable. We can't agree how to spend our time. I want to relax. Brooke wants to go scuba diving. And she wants me to go with her. Which means taking a class. I tell her that of all the things I want to do on my honeymoon, taking a class is right up there with having a colonoscopy.

While watching *Friends*.

She insists.

We spend hours at the pool, an instructor teaching us about wet suits and tanks and masks. Water keeps leaking into my mask because I have a five-o'clock shadow and my bristles prevent the mask from lying flush against my skin. I go up to the room and shave.

When I come back down the instructor says the final phase of training is an underwater card game. If you can sit calmly playing cards at the bottom of the pool, and if you can play a full game without needing to surface, then you're a scuba diver. So here I am, in full scuba gear, in the middle of the Caribbean, sitting at the bottom of a pool and playing Go Fish. I don't feel like a scuba diver. I feel like Dustin Hoffman in *The Graduate*. I climb out of the pool and tell Brooke, I can't do this.

You never want to try anything new.

Enjoy. Go out to the middle of the ocean if you want. Say hi to the Little Mermaid. I'll be in the room.

I walk into the kitchen and order a large plate of French fries. Then I go up to the room, kick off my shoes, stretch out on the couch, and watch TV for the rest of the day.

We leave the island paradise three days early. Honeymoon over.

I'M IN D.C. FOR THE 1998 LEGG MASON. Another July heat wave, another withering D.C. tournament. Other players are carping about the heat, and ordinarily I'd be carping too, but I feel only a cool gratitude and a steely resolve, which I maintain in part by waking early every morning, writing out my goals. After putting them on paper, saying them aloud, I also say aloud: No shortcuts.

Just before the tournament starts, during a final practice with Brad, I give a halfhearted effort. Perry drives me back to the hotel. I stare out the window, silent.

Pull over, I say.

Why?

Just pull over.

He steers onto the shoulder.

Drive two miles ahead and wait for me.

What are you talking about? Are you crazy?

I'm not done. I didn't give my best today.

I run two miles through Rock Creek Park, the same park where I gave my rackets away in 1987. With every step I'm close to passing out, but I don't care. This run, even if it brings on heatstroke, will give me peace of mind tonight in that all-important ten minutes before I fall asleep. I now live for that ten minutes. I'm all about that ten minutes. I've been cheered by thousands, booed by thousands, but nothing feels as bad as the booing inside your own head during those ten minutes before you fall asleep.

When I get to the car, my face is bright purple. I slide into the passenger seat, turn up the air-conditioning, and smile at Perry.

That's how we *do* it, he says, handing me a towel as he pulls away.

I reach the final. I face Draper again. I remember wondering not too long ago how I ever beat him. I remember shaking my head in disbelief that I'd ever gotten past him. One of the low points of my life. Now I take him out in fifty minutes, 6–2, 6–0. I win the tournament for the fourth time.

At the Mercedes-Benz Cup I reach the semis without losing a set and ultimately win the whole thing. At the du Maurier Open in Toronto I face Pete again. He plays great in the first set but wears down in the second. I beat him, which costs him the number one ranking and moves me up to number nine.

I meet Krajicek in the semis. He's still feeling good about winning the 1996 Wimbledon, the only Dutchman ever to do it. In the process he beat Pete in the quarters, handing Pete his first Wimbledon loss in years. But I'm not Pete, and I'm not me. Krajicek is down a set, serving at 3–4 in the second set, love–40. Triple break point. I rope the best return of my adult life. The ball seems to clear the net by a centimeter and leaves a smoking skid mark. It's a true old-fashioned rug-burner. Krajicek shuts his eyes, shoves out his racket, hits a wild volley. It could go anywhere, he has no idea where it might go, but it's a winner. If his racket had been open another half degree, the ball would have hit somebody in the front row and I would have broken serve and taken control of the match. Instead he wins the point, holds serve, beats me in three sets, ends my streak of consecutive matches at fifteen. In the old days I'd have had trouble getting over it. Now I tell Brad: That's tennis, right, BG?

ENTERING THE 1998 U.S. OPEN, I'm number eight in the world. The crowd is fully behind me, which always lifts my spirits, makes me lighter on my feet. In the round of sixteen I meet Kucera, who seems to be trying to irk me with his serve. He tosses the ball, then stops, catches it, and tosses it again. I'm down two sets to love, sorely annoyed by this guy. Then I remember: the better you play Kucera, the better he plays. Hit shit to him, he hits shit back. That's it—I'm playing too well! I'm also serving too well. When it's my serve, I imitate Kucera. The crowd laughs. Then I hit big goofy moonballs. I irk Kucera, irritate my way back into the match.

Rain falls. The match is held over until tomorrow.

Brooke and I go out for a late dinner with her friends. Actors. It's always actors. The sky has cleared, so we eat outside at a downtown restaurant with tables on the roof. Afterward, we're standing in the street, saying goodnight.

Good luck tomorrow! the actors shout as they jump into cabs, off to do some more drinking.

Brooke watches them, turns to me. Her bottom lip is out. She's torn. She looks like a child caught between what she should do and what she wants to do.

I take a swig from my liter bottle of Gil Water. Go, I say.

Really? You won't mind?

No, I lie. Have fun.

I take a cab to Brooke's apartment. She sold the brownstone and bought this place on the Upper East Side. I miss the brownstone. I miss the front stoop where Gil stood guard. I even miss the eyeless, hairless African masks, if only because they were there when Brooke and I didn't wear masks with each other. I finish my Gil Water, slide into bed. I drift off but snap awake when Brooke comes home hours later.

Go back to sleep, she whispers.

I try. I can't. I get up and take a sleeping pill.

The next day I have a titanic battle with Kucera. I manage to tie the match. But he has more verve, more stamina. He outduels me in a tough fifth set.

. . .

I'M SITTING IN A CORNER of our bathroom in Los Angeles, watching Brooke get ready to go out. I'm staying home—again. We talk about why this is always so.

She accuses me of refusing to participate in her world. She says I'm not open to new experiences, new people. I'm not interested in meeting her friends. I could be rubbing elbows every night with geniuses—writers, artists, actors, musicians, directors. I could be attending art gallery openings, world premieres, new plays, private screenings. But all I want to do is stay home, watch TV, and maybe, just maybe, if I'm feeling social, have J.P. and Joni over for dinner.

I can't lie. That does sound like a perfect night.

Andre, she says, they're all bad for you. Perry, J.P., Philly, Brad—they coddle you, humor you, enable you. Not one of them has your best interests at heart.

You think all my friends are bad for me?

All but Gil.

All?

All. Especially Perry.

I know she's been feuding with Perry, that he gave up his producer role on *Suddenly Susan*. I know she's irked that I haven't automatically taken her side in the feud. But I had no idea she was ready to write off everyone else on my team.

Standing, turning from the mirror, she says: Andre, I consider you a rose among thorns.

A rose among—?

An innocent, surrounded by people who are bleeding you dry.

I'm not so innocent. And those thorns have helped me since I was a boy. Those thorns have saved my life.

They're holding you back. They're keeping you from growing. From evolving. You're unevolved, Andre.

PERRY AND I CHOOSE to set the academy in the worst neighborhood of West Las Vegas, where it can serve as a beacon. After months of scouting locations, trying to find a lot that's for sale and affordable and capable of accommodating an evolving campus, we find an eight-acre parcel that meets all our requirements. It's in the center of an urban wasteland, surrounded by pawnshops and homes on the verge of being torn down. It's on the site of the original Las Vegas, the long-forgotten outpost where settlers first arrived, which was later abandoned. I like that our school will be placed on a site that has a history of abandonment. Where better to initiate the kind of change we envision in the lives of children?

At the groundbreaking ceremony, dozens of politicians and dignitaries and neighborhood leaders are on hand. Reporters, TV cameras, speeches. We push the golden shovel into the litter-strewn dirt. I look around, and I can actually hear the sound of children in the future, laughing and playing and asking questions. I can feel the procession of lives that will cross this spot, and go forward from this spot. I become lightheaded, thinking of the dreams that will be formed here, the lives that will be shaped and saved. I'm so overcome by the thought of what will happen here, in a few years, and many decades after I'm gone, that I don't hear the speeches. The future drowns out the present.

Then someone jolts me from my reverie, tells me to stand over here for a group picture. A flash goes off, a happy occasion, but daunting. We have so far to go. The fight to get the school opened, accredited, funded, will be rough. If not for my progress these last few months, fighting to reconstitute my tennis career, to recapture my health and balance, I don't know that I'd have the stomach.

People ask me where Brooke is, why she isn't here for the groundbreaking. I tell them the truth. I don't know.

NEW YEAR'S EVE, the close of 1998. Brooke and I throw our traditional New Year's Eve party. No matter how disconnected we may be, she insists that during holidays we give no sign of trouble to our friends and family. It feels as if we're actors and our guests are an audience. And yet, even when the audience isn't here, she playacts, and I follow along. Hours before our guests arrive, we pretend to be happy—a dress rehearsal of sorts. Hours after they're gone, we continue pretending. A kind of cast party.

Tonight there seem to be more of Brooke's friends and family than mine in the audience. Included in this group is Brooke's new dog, an albino pit bull named Sam. It growls at my friends. It growls as if it's been briefed on what Brooke thinks of all of them.

J.P. and I sit in a corner of the living room, eyeballing the dog, which is lying at Brooke's feet, eyeballing us.

That dog would be cool, J.P. says, if it were sitting *here.* He points to the ground beside my feet.

I laugh.

No. Really. That's not a cool dog. That's not *your* dog. This is not *your* house. This is not *your* life.

Hm.

Andre, there are red flowers on this chair.

I look at the chair where he's sitting and see it as if for the first time.

Andre, he says. Red flowers. *Red flowers.*

AS I PACK FOR THE 1999 AUSTRALIAN OPEN, Brooke frowns and stomps around the house. She's irritated by my attempted comeback. It can't be that she resents my hitting the road, given all the tension between us. So I can only assume she thinks I'm wasting my time. She's certainly not alone.

I kiss her goodbye. She wishes me luck.

I reach the round of sixteen. The night before my match I phone her.

This is hard, she says.

What is?

Us. This.

Yes. It is.

There's so much distance between us, she says.

Australia is far.

No. Even when we're in the same room—distance.

I think: You said all my friends suck. How could there not be distance?

I say: I know.

When you get home, she says, we should talk. We need to talk.

What about?

She repeats, When you get home. She sounds overwhelmed. Is she crying? She tries to change the subject. Who do you play?

I tell her. She never recognizes the names or understands what they mean.

She asks, Is it on TV?

I don't know. Probably.

I'll watch.

OK.

OK.

Goodnight.

Hours later I play Spadea, my practice partner from New Year's Day one year ago. He isn't half the player I am. There have been days in my prime when I could have beaten him with a spatula. But I've been on the road for thirty-two of the last fifty-two weeks, not to mention the training with Gil, the struggles with the school, and the maneuvering with Brooke. My mind is still on the phone with Brooke. Spadea edges me in four sets.

The newspapers are cruel. They point out that I've been ousted early from my last six slams. Fair enough. But they say I'm embarrassing myself. Too long at the fair, they say. Agassi doesn't seem to know when to hang it up. He's won three slams. He's nearly twenty-nine years old. How much more does he really hope to accomplish?

Every other article contains the threadbare phrase: At an age when most of his peers are thinking about retiring—

I walk in the door and call out Brooke's name. Nothing. It's midmorning, she must be at the studio. I spend the day waiting for her to come home. I try to rest, but it's hard with an albino pit bull eyeing you.

When Brooke gets home, it's dark and the weather has turned bad. A rainy, wintry night. She suggests we go out for dinner.

Sushi?

Lovely.

We drive to one of our favorite places, Matsuhisa, sit at the bar. She orders sake. I'm starved. I ask for all my favorites. The blue fin sashimi, the crab toro cucumber avocado hand roll. Brooke sighs.

You always order the same thing.

I'm too hungry and tired to bother about her disapproval.

She sighs again.

What's wrong?

I can't even look you in the eye right now.

Her eyes are wet.

Brooke?

No, really, I can't look at you.

Easy does it. Take a deep breath. Please, please, try not to cry. Let's get the check and go. Let's just talk about this at home.

I don't know why, but after all that's been written about me in the last few days, it's important that tomorrow's newspapers don't report that I was seen fighting with my wife.

In the car Brooke is still crying. I'm not happy, she says. We're not happy. We haven't been happy for so very long. And I don't know if we can ever be happy again if we stay together.

So. There it is. That's that.

I walk into the house, a zombie. I pull a suitcase out of the closet, which I notice is so organized, so neat, it's unsettling. I realize how difficult it must be for Brooke, living with my losses, my silences, my peaks and valleys. But I also notice how little space in this closet is allotted to me. Symbolic. I think of J.P. *This is not your house.*

I grab the few hangers holding my clothes and carry them downstairs.

Brooke is in the kitchen, sobbing. Not crying as she did at the restaurant and in the car, but sobbing. She's sitting on a stool at the butcher block island. Always an island. One way or another, we spend all our time together on islands. We *are* islands. Two islands. And I can't recall when it was different.

She asks, What are you doing? What's going on?

What do you mean? I'm leaving.

It's raining. Wait until morning.

Why wait? No time like the present.

I make a pile of essentials: clothes, blender, Jamaican coffee beans, French press—and a gift Brooke recently gave me. The scary painting Philly and I saw years ago at the Louvre. She commissioned an artist to make an exact replica. I look at the man hanging from the cliff. How has he not fallen off that cliff by now? I throw everything in the backseat of my car, a mint-condition convertible Eldorado Cadillac, 1976, the last year they made them. The car is a pure lustrous white, lily white, so I named it Lily. I turn Lily's key, and the dashboard lights come on like an old TV set. The odometer reads 23,000 miles. It strikes me that Lily is the exact opposite of me. Old, with low mileage.

I peel out of the driveway.

A mile from the house I start crying. Through my tears, and the gathering fog, I can barely see the chrome wreath of the hood ornament. But I keep going, and going, until I reach San Bernardino. The fog is now snow. The pass through the mountains is closed. I phone Perry and ask him if there's another way to Vegas.

What's wrong?

I tell him. Trial separation, I say. We don't know each other anymore.

I think about the day Wendi and I broke up, when I pulled over and phoned Perry. I think of all that's happened since—and yet here I am, pulled over again, phoning Perry with a broken heart.

He says there's no other way to get to Vegas, so I need to make a U-turn, head back toward the coast, and stop at the first motel that has a room. I drive slowly, picking my way through the snow, the car spinning and skidding on the slick highway. I stop at every motel. No vacancy.

Finally I get the last available bed at a fleabag in Nowhere, California. I lie on the smelly bedspread, interrogating myself. How the hell did you get here? How did it come to this? Why are you reacting like this? Your marriage is far from perfect, you're not even sure why you got married in the first place, or if you ever wanted to *get* married—so why are you such an emotional wreck thinking it might be over?

Because you hate losing. And divorce is one tough loss.

But you've suffered tough losses before—why does this one feel different?

Because you don't see any way that, as a result of this loss, you can improve.

I PHONE BROOKE TWO DAYS LATER. I'm contrite, she's hardened.

We both need time to think, she says. We shouldn't talk for a while. We need to go inside ourselves, not interfere with each other.

Inside ourselves? What does that even mean—for how long?

Three weeks.

Three? Where do you come up with that number?

She doesn't answer.

She suggests I use the time to see a therapist.

SHE'S A SMALL DARK WOMAN in a small dark office in Vegas. I sit on a love seat—how exquisitely ironic. She sits in a chair three feet away. She listens without interrupting. I'd rather she interrupted. I want answers. The more I talk, the more acutely aware I become of talking to myself. As always. This isn't the way to save a marriage. Marriages don't get saved or solved by one person talking.

I wake later that night on the floor. My back is stiff. I go out to the living room and sit on the couch with a pad and pen. I write pages and pages to Brooke. Another pleading handwritten letter, but this one is all true. In the morning I fax the pages to Brooke's house. I watch the pages go through the fax machine and I think of how it all started, five years ago, sliding the pages into Philly's fax machine, holding my breath, waiting for the witty, flirty reply from a hut somewhere in Africa.

This time there is no reply.

I fax her again. Then again.

She's much farther away than Africa.

I phone.

I know you said three weeks, but I need to talk to you. I think we should meet, I think we need to be working through these things together.

Oh Andre, she says.

I wait.

Oh Andre, she says again. You don't understand. You just don't get it. This isn't about us—this is about you individually and me individually.

I tell her she's right, I don't understand. I tell her I don't see how we got here. I tell her how unhappy I've been for so long. I tell her I'm sorry that we've grown distant, that I've grown cold. I tell her about the whirl, the constant whirl, the centrifugal force of this fucked-up tennis life. I tell her that I haven't known who I am for the longest time, maybe ever. I tell her about the search for a self, the endless monologue in my head, the depression. I tell her everything in my heart, and it all comes out halting, clumsy, inarticulate. It's embarrassing, but necessary, because I don't want to lose her, I've had enough losing, and I know if I'm honest she'll give me a second chance.

She says that she's sorry I'm suffering, but she can't solve it. She can't fix me. I need to fix myself. By myself.

Listening to the dial tone, I feel resigned, calm. The phone call now seems like the brief, curt handshake at the net between two mismatched opponents.

I eat something, watch TV, go to bed early. In the morning I phone Perry and tell him I want the fastest divorce in the history of divorce.

I give my platinum wedding band to a friend and point him to the nearest pawnshop. Take their first offer, I tell him. When he brings me the cash I make a donation to my new school in the name of Brooke Christa Shields. For better or for worse, in sickness and in health, she will forever be one of the original benefactors.

22

THE FIRST TOURNAMENT of my new, Brooke-less life is San Jose. J.P. drives up from Orange County for a few days of emergency counseling. He encourages, advises, cajoles, promises that better days are ahead. He understands that I have good moments and bad. One moment I say, To hell with her, and the next moment I miss her. He says it's all par for the course. He tells me that for the last few years my mind has been a swamp—stagnant, fetid, seeping in every direction. Now it's time for my mind to be a river—raging, channeled, and therefore pure. I like it. I tell him I'll try to keep this image in mind. He talks and talks, and as long as he's talking, I'm OK. I'm in control. His advice feels like an oxygen cup on my mouth.

Then he leaves, drives back to Orange County, and I'm a mess again. I'm standing on the court, in the middle of a match, thinking about everything but my opponent. I'm asking myself, If you took a vow, before God and your family, if you said I do, and now you don't, what does that make you?

A failure.

I walk in circles, cursing myself. The linesman hears me call myself an obscene name and walks past me, across the court, to the umpire's chair. He reports me to the umpire for using foul language.

The umpire gives me a warning.

Now here comes the linesman, walking back across the court, past me, to resume his position. I glare. The mealy-mouthed fink. The pathetic tattletale. I know I shouldn't, I know there will be hell to pay, but I can't hold it in.

You're a *cocksucker*.

He stops, turns, marches straight back to the umpire, reports me again.

This time I'm docked a point.

The linesman comes back again, past me, to resume his position.

I say, You're *still* a cocksucker.

He stops, turns, walks back to the umpire, who heaves a sigh and pitches forward in his chair. The umpire calls over the supervisor, who also sighs, then beckons me.

Andre. Did you call the linesman a cocksucker?

Do you want me to lie or tell you the truth?

I need to know if you said it.

I said it. And you want to know something? He *is* a cocksucker.

They kick me out of the tournament.

I HEAD BACK TO VEGAS. Brad phones. Indian Wells is coming up, he says. I tell Brad that I'm going through some stuff right now, but I can't tell him what. And Indian Wells is out of the question.

I have to get well, get right, which means spending lots of time with Gil. Every night we buy a sack of hamburgers and drive around the city. I'm breaking training, big time, but Gil sees again that I need comfort food. He also sees that he might lose a finger if he tries to take the hamburger away from me.

We drive into the mountains, up and down the Strip, listening to Gil's special CD. He calls it *Belly Cramps*. Gil's philosophy in all things is to seek the pain, woo the pain, recognize that pain is life. If you're heartbroken, Gil says, don't hide from it. Wallow in it. We hurt, he says, so let's hurt. *Belly Cramps* is his medley of the most painful love songs ever written. We listen to them over and over until we know the lyrics by heart. After a song has played Gil will speak the lyrics. For my money, his speaking is better than anyone's singing. He puts all recording artists to shame. I'd rather hear Gil talk a song than Sinatra croon it.

With each passing year Gil's voice grows deeper, richer, and softer, and when he speaks the chorus of a torch song he sounds as if he's channeling Moses and Elvis. He deserves a Grammy for his rendition of Barry Manilow's Please Don't Be Scared:

> *Cause feeling pain's a hard way*
> *To know you're still alive.*

But his take on Roy Clark's version of We Can't Build a Fire in the Rain knocks me out every time. One line in particular resonates with us both:

Just going through the motions and pretending
we have something left to gain.

When I'm not with Gil, I'm locked in my new house, the one I bought with Brooke for those infrequent occasions when we came home to Vegas. Now I think of it as Bachelor Pad II. I like the house, it's more my style than the French Country place where she and I lived in Pacific Palisades, but it doesn't have a fireplace. I can't think without a fireplace. I must have fire. So I hire a guy to build one.

While it's under construction the house is a disaster area. Huge plastic sheets hang from the walls. Tarps cover the furniture. A thick coat of dust lies everywhere. One morning, staring into the unfinished fireplace, I think about Mandela. I think about the promises I've made to myself and others. I reach for the phone and dial Brad.

Come to Vegas. I'm ready to play.

He says he's on his way.

Unbelievable. He could dump me—no one would blame him—but instead he drops everything the moment I call. I love the guy. Now, while he's on his way, I worry that he won't be comfortable, because of all the construction. Then I smile. I have two leather club chairs set in front of a large-screen TV, and a wet bar stocked with Bud Ice. All Brad's basic needs will be met.

Five hours later he comes through the door, flops into one of the club chairs, opens a beer, and instantly looks as if he's nestled in his mother's arms. I join him in a beer. Six o'clock rolls around. We switch to frozen margaritas. At eight o'clock we're still in the club chairs, Brad flipping channels, looking for sports highlights.

I say, Listen, Brad, I need to tell you something. It's something I should have told you a while ago.

He's staring at the TV. I'm staring into the unfinished fireplace, imagining flames.

You see that game the other night? he asks. No one is beating Duke this year.

Brad, this is important. Something you need to know. Brooke and I—we're done. We're not going to make it.

He turns. He looks me dead in the eye. Then he puts his elbows on his knees and hangs his head. I had no idea he'd take it this hard. He stays this way for three full seconds. Finally he looks up and gives me a big, toothy smile.

He says, It's going to be a great year.

What?

We're going to have a *great* year.

But—

This is the best thing that's ever happened to your tennis.

I'm miserable. What are you talking about?

Miserable? Then you're looking at this all wrong. You don't have kids. You're free as a bird. If you had kids, OK, there would be real problems. But this way, you get off scot free.

I guess.

You've got the world by the balls. You're *solo*, rid of all that drama!

He looks deranged. He looks delirious. He tells me we have Key Biscayne coming up, then clay season, then—good things. About to happen.

This burden is off you now, he says. Instead of lying around Vegas, feeling *your* pain, let's go put some pain on your opponents.

You know what? You're right. That calls for another batch of margaritas!

At nine o'clock I say, We should think about food.

But Brad is peacefully, contentedly licking salt from the rim of his glass, and he's found tennis on the TV, a night match in Indian Wells. Steffi Graf versus Serena Williams.

He wheels and gives me the toothy smile again.

That's your play right there!

He points to the TV.

He says, Steffi Graf! *That's* who you should be with.

Yeah. Right. She wants no part of me.

I've told Brad the stories. The 1991 French Open. The 1992 Wimbledon Ball. I've tried and tried. No dice. Steffi Graf is like the French Open. I just can't get across that particular finish line.

That's all in the past, Brad says. Besides, your approach back then was so un-Andre. Asking once and backing off? Strictly amateur. Since when do you let other people run your game? Since when do you take no for an answer?

I nod. Maybe.

You just need a look, Brad says. A crack of light. A window. An opening.

The next tournament where Steffi and I are both scheduled to play is Key Biscayne. Brad tells me to relax, he'll get me close. He knows Steffi's coach, Heinz Gunthardt. He'll talk to Heinz about setting up a practice session.

· · ·

THE MOMENT WE ARRIVE IN KEY BISCAYNE, Brad phones Heinz, who's surprised by the proposition. He says no. He says Steffi would never agree to break her regular preparation schedule for a practice session with a stranger. She's too regimented. Also, she's shy. She'd be highly uncomfortable. But Brad is persistent, and Heinz must have some trace of romantic in him. He suggests Brad and I book the court for right after Steffi's practice session, then arrive early. Heinz will then casually suggest that Steffi hit a few balls with me.

It's all set, Brad says. High noon. You. Me. Steffi. Heinz. Let's get this party started.

FIRST THINGS FIRST. I phone J.P. and tell him to get his ass to Florida, pronto. I need advice. I need a sounding board. I need a wingman. Then I hit the court and practice for my practice session.

On the appointed day, Brad and I get to the court forty minutes early. I've never been so breathless. I've played seven times in the final of a Grand Slam and I never felt like this. We find Heinz and Steffi deeply absorbed in their practice session. We stand off to the side, watching. After a few minutes Heinz calls Steffi to the net and says something to her. He points to us.

She looks.

I smile.

She doesn't.

She says a few words to Heinz, and Heinz says a few words, and then she shakes her head. But when she jogs back to the baseline, Heinz waves me onto the court.

I tie my shoes quickly. I pull a racket out of the bag and walk onto the court—then impulsively whip off my shirt. It's shameless, I realize, but I'm desperate. Steffi looks and does a barely detectable double take. Thank you, Gil.

We start to hit. She's flawless, of course, and I'm struggling to get the ball over the net. *The net is your biggest enemy.* Relax, I tell myself. Stop thinking. Come on, Andre, it's only a practice session.

But I can't help myself. I've never seen a woman so beautiful. Standing still, she's a goddess; in motion, she's poetry. I'm a suitor, but also a fan. I've wondered for so long what Steffi Graf's forehand feels like. I've watched her on TV and at tournaments and I've wondered how that ball feels when it comes flying off her racket. A ball feels different off every player's racket—there are minute but concrete subtleties of force and spin. Now, hitting with her, I feel her subtleties. It's like touching her, though we're forty feet apart. Every forehand is foreplay.

She hits a series of backhands, carving up the court with her famous slice. I need to impress her with my ability to take that slice and do whatever I want with it. But it's harder than I thought. I miss one. I yell to her: You're not going to get away with that again!

She says nothing. She hits another slice. I sit down on my backhand and hit the ball as hard as I can.

She nets the return.

I yell: That shot pays a lot of bills for me!

Again, nothing. She merely hits the next one deeper and slicier.

Generally, during my practice sessions, Brad likes to keep busy. He chases balls, offers pointers, runs his mouth. Not this time. He's sitting in the umpire chair, his eyes peeled, a lifeguard on a shark-infested beach.

Whenever I look in his direction he mutters one word. *Beautiful.*

Around the edges of the court, people are beginning to gather, to gawk. A few photographers snap photos. I wonder why. Is it the rarity of a male and female player practicing? Or is it that I'm catatonic and missing every third ball? From a distance, it looks as if Steffi is giving a lesson to a shirtless, grinning mute.

After we hit for one hour and ten minutes, she waves and comes to the net.

Thank you very much, she says.

I trot to the net and say, The pleasure was all mine.

I manage to act nonchalant, until she starts to use the net post to stretch out her legs. All the blood rushes to my head. I need to do something physical or I might lose consciousness. I've never stretched before, but now seems like a good time to start. I put a leg on the net post and pretend my back is flexible. We stretch, talk about the tour, complain about the travel, compare notes on different cities we've enjoyed.

I ask, What's your favorite city? When tennis is over, where do you imagine living?

Oh. It's a tie, I think. Between New York and San Francisco.

I think: Have you ever thought of living in Las Vegas?

I say: My two favorites also.

She smiles. Well, she says. Thanks again.

Any time.

We do the European double-cheek kiss.

Brad and I take the ferry back to Fisher Island, where J.P. is waiting. The three of us spend the rest of the night talking about Steffi as if she's an opponent, which she is. Brad treats her like Rafter or Pete. She has strengths, she has weaknesses. He breaks down her game, coaches me up. Now and then J.P. phones Joni, puts her on speaker, and we try to get the female point of view.

The conversation continues over the next two days. At dinner, in the steam room, at the hotel bar, the three of us talk about nothing but Steffi. We're plotting, using military jargon, like *recon* and *intel*. I feel as if we're planning a land and sea invasion of Germany.

I say, She seemed kind of cool to me.

Brad says, She has no idea you split from your missus. It hasn't been in the papers yet. Nobody knows. You need to let her know your status, and tell her how you feel about her.

I'll send her flowers.

Yes, J.P. says. Flowers are good. But you can't send them under your name. It might get leaked to the press. We'll have Joni send them, with your name on the card.

Good thinking.

Joni goes to a shop in South Beach and, under my directive, buys every rose in the place. She essentially orders a rose garden transplanted to Steffi's room. On the card I thank Steffi for the practice session and invite her to dinner. Then I sit back and wait for the call.

There is no call. All day.

Or the next day.

No matter how much I stare at it, and shout at it, the phone refuses to ring. I pace, pick my cuticles until they bleed. Brad comes to my room and worries that he might need to give me a sedative.

I shout, This is bullshit! OK, she's not interested, I get it, but how about a thank you? If she doesn't call by tonight, I swear, I'm calling her.

We move to the patio. Brad looks off and says, Uh-oh.

What?

J.P. says, I think I see your flowers.

They point to the patio of a room across the way. Steffi's room, obviously, because there on the patio table are my giant bouquets of long-stemmed red roses.

Not sure that's a good sign, J.P. says.

No, Brad says. NG. Not good.

.   .   .

WE DECIDE THAT I'LL wait for Steffi to win her first match—a fore-gone conclusion—and when she does, I'll phone. J.P. preps me for the call. He plays the role of Steffi. We rehearse every scenario. He throws me every line she might possibly utter.

Steffi beats her hapless first-round opponent in forty-two minutes. I've tipped the ferry captains to phone me the moment they see her step on the ferry. Fifty minutes after the match I get a call: She's aboard.

I give her fifteen minutes to reach the island, ten minutes to go from the dock to the hotel, and then I phone the operator and ask for her room. I know her room number because I can still see my damn flowers sitting dejectedly on the patio table.

She picks up the phone on the second ring.

Hi. It's Andre.

Oh.

I just wanted to call and make sure you got my flowers.

I did.

Oh.

Silence.

She says, I don't want any misunderstandings between us. My boyfriend is here.

I see. Well, OK, I understand.

Silence.

Good luck with the tournament.

Thank you. You too.

Yawning canyon of silence.

Well, goodbye.

Bye.

I fall on the couch and stare at the floor.

I have one question for you, J.P. says. What could she possibly have said that would put that look on your face? What scenario did we not rehearse?

Her boyfriend is here.

Oh.

Then I smile. I take a page from Brad's positive-thinking playbook: maybe she's sending me a message. *Obviously* her boyfriend was sitting right there.

So?

So she couldn't talk, and rather than say, I have a boyfriend, case closed, leave me alone, she said, My boyfriend is *here*.

So?

I think she's saying there's a chance.

J.P. says he'll fix me a drink.

THE TOURNAMENT PROVIDES a small measure of distraction. Sadly, the distraction lasts only a few hours. In the first round, against Dominik Hrbaty, from Slovakia, I can think only of Steffi and her boyfriend enjoying or awkwardly ignoring my roses. Hrbaty whoops me in three sets.

I'm out of the tournament. I should leave Fisher Island. But I stick around, sitting on the beach, plotting with J.P. and Brad.

Steffi's boyfriend probably showed up unexpectedly, Brad says. Plus, she still doesn't know you're divorced. She still thinks you're married to Brooke. Give it time. Let the news come out. Then make your move.

You're right, you're right.

Brad mentions Hong Kong. In light of my performance against Hrbaty, clearly I need another tournament before we head into clay season. Let's go to Hong Kong, he says. Let's not sit around anymore thinking and talking about Steffi.

Next thing I know I'm settling into a seat on an airplane bound for China. I look at the screen at the head of the cabin. *Estimated flight time: 15 hrs, 37 mins.*

I look at Brad. Fifteen hours and thirty-seven minutes? To obsess about Steffi? I don't think so.

I unbuckle my seat belt and stand.

Where are you going?

I'm getting off this plane.

Don't be ridiculous. Sit down. Relax. We're here. We're all packed. Let's go play.

I ease back into my seat, order two Belvederes, swallow a sleeping pill, and after what feels like a month I'm on the other side of the earth. I'm in a car being whisked along a Hong Kong highway, looking up at the soaring International Finance Centre.

I phone Perry. When is the news of my divorce going to break?

The lawyers are hashing out the details, he says. Meantime, you and Brooke need to work on the statement.

We fax drafts back and forth. Her team, my team. Lawyers and publicists have a go at it. Brooke adds a word, I delete a word. Faxes and more faxes. What began with faxes ends with faxes.

The statement is about to be released, Perry says. It should be in the papers any day now.

Brad and I run down to the lobby every morning, buy up all the newspapers, then sit over breakfast and scan every page, looking for the headline. For the first time in my memory I can't wait for newspapers to report about my private life. Each day I say a prayer: Let this be the day that Steffi learns I'm free.

Day after day, it's not there. It's like waiting for Steffi's call. If only I had hair, so I could pull it out. Finally, the cover of *People* carries a photo of Brooke and me. The headline reads: *Suddenly Split.* It's April 26, 1999, three days before my twenty-ninth birthday, almost exactly two years after our wedding.

Reborn, renewed, I win Hong Kong—but on the flight home I can't lift my arm. I rush from the airport to Gil's house. He examines the shoulder, grimaces. He doesn't like the look of it.

We might need to shut everything down and skip the entire clay season.

No, no, no, Brad says. We have to be in Rome for the Italian Open.

Please. I never win that thing. Let's forget it.

No, Brad says. Let's go to Rome, see how the shoulder does. You didn't want to go to Hong Kong, right? But you won, right? I see a trend developing.

I let him drag me onto a plane, and in Rome I lose in the third round to Rafter, whom I just beat at Indian Wells. Now I really want to shut it down. But Brad talks me into going to play the World Team Cup in Germany. I don't have the strength to argue with him.

The weather in Germany is cold, dreary, meaning the ball plays heavy. I look at Brad with murder in my eye. I can't believe he's dragged me to Düsseldorf with a sore shoulder. In the middle of the first set, down 3–4, I can't take another swing. I quit. That's it. We're going home, I tell Brad. I have to get my shoulder right. And I have to figure out this thing with Steffi.

As we board the flight from Frankfurt to San Francisco, I'm not speaking to Brad. I'm mad as hell. We have twelve hours ahead of us, side by side, and I tell him: Here's how it's going to be, Brad. I haven't slept all night, because of this shoulder. I'm going to swallow two sleeping pills right now and I'm not going to listen to you for the next twelve hours and it's going to be heaven. You hear me? And when we land, the *first thing* I want you to do is pull me out of the French Open.

He leans into me and badgers me for two hours. You're *not* going back to Vegas. You're *not* pulling out. You're coming with me to my house in

San Francisco. I've got the guest cottage set up with plenty of firewood, the way you like it, and then you and I are flying back to Paris and you're going to play. It's the only slam you don't have, and you've always wanted it, and you can't win it if you don't play.

French Open? Please. You must be kidding. That ship has sailed.

How do you know? Who's to say this isn't your year?

Trust me. In no sense is 1999 my year.

Look, you were just starting to show glimpses of the player you used to be. I saw something in you I hadn't seen in years. We have to stay after that.

I see right through him. It's not that he thinks the French Open is remotely winnable. But if I pull out of the French Open, it will be easier to pull out of Wimbledon, and there goes the whole year. Goodbye come-back. Hello retirement.

Landing in San Francisco, I'm once again too tired to argue. I slide into Brad's car, and he drives me to his place and puts me in the cottage. I sleep for twelve hours. When I wake a chiropractor is there, ready to treat me.

It's not going to work, I say.

It's going to work, Brad says.

I get treatments twice a day. The rest of the time I watch the fog and stoke the fire. By Friday I do feel better. Brad smiles. We hit balls on his backyard court, twenty minutes, then I hit a few serves.

Call Gilly, I say. Let's go to Paris.

IN OUR PARIS HOTEL Brad is looking over the draw.

I ask, How is it?

He says nothing.

Brad?

Couldn't be worse.

Seriously?

Nightmare. Your first-rounder is Franco Squillari, lefty, from Argentina, probably the roughest guy in the draw who's not seeded. An absolute beast on clay.

I can't believe you talked me into this.

We practice Saturday and Sunday. Monday we start. I'm in the locker room, getting my feet taped, and I realize I forgot to pack underwear in my tennis bag. The match is in five minutes. Can I play without underwear? I don't even know if it's physically possible.

Brad jokes that I can borrow his.

I will never want to win that badly.

Then I think: This is perfect. I didn't want to be here anyway, I shouldn't be here, I'm playing the quintessential dirt rat in the first round on center court. Why shouldn't I go commando?

There are sixteen thousand people in the stands, screaming like peasants overrunning Versailles. Before I've broken a sweat I'm down a set and a break. I look to my box, stare at Gil and Brad. *Help me.* Brad stares back, stone-faced: Help yourself.

I hitch up my shorts, take the deepest breath possible and let it out slowly. I tell myself that it can't get any worse. I tell myself: Just win one set. Winning one set off this guy would be an accomplishment. One set—try for that. Scaling down the task makes it seem manageable and makes me looser. I start ripping my backhand, hitting my spots. The crowd stirs. They haven't seen me play well here in a long time. Something inside me stirs too.

The second set turns into a street fight and a wrestling match and pistols at fifty paces. Squillari doesn't give an inch and I have to bludgeon the set from him, 7–5. Then a shocking thing happens. I win the third set. Now I start to feel hope, actual hope, rising from my toes. My body is tingling. I glance at Squillari—he's hopeless. His face is expressionless. One of the fittest guys on the tour, he's unable to take a step. He's done. In the fourth set I roll him, and all at once I'm walking off the court with one of the most improbable wins of my career.

Back at the hotel, covered with clay, I tell Gil: Did you see him? Did you see that dirt rat cramp? We made him cramp, Gil!

I saw.

The elevator is tiny. There's room for five normal-sized humans, or else me and Gil. Brad tells us to go ahead, he'll catch the next one. I hit the button, and on the way up Gil leans against one corner of the elevator, I lean against the other. I feel him staring.

What?

Nothing.

He keeps staring.

What is it, Gil?

Nothing. He smiles and says again: Nothing.

In the second round, I stick with no underwear. (I will never don underwear again. Something works, you don't change.) I play Arnaud Clément, from France. I win the first set 6–2. I'm up in the second, playing the best I've ever played on clay. I'm rocking him to sleep. Then Clément wakes up. He wins the second set—and the third. How did that just happen? I'm serving at 4–5, love–30, in the fourth set. I'm two points from being bounced out of this tournament.

I think: Two points. *Two points.*

He hits a forehand inside-out winner. I walk over and check the mark. It's out. I circle the mark with the racket. The linesman runs out to confirm. He examines it, like Hercule Poirot. He puts up his hand. Out!

If that thing had caught the line I'd be down triple match point. Instead I'm at 15–30. What a difference. What if—?

But I plead with myself to stop thinking about what if. Don't think, Andre. Turn off your mind. I play two minutes of the best tennis I'm capable of playing. I hold. We're at 5–all.

Clément is serving. If I were a different player, he would have the edge. But I'm my father's son. I'm a returner. I let nothing past me. Then I run him from side to side. Back and forth. His tongue starts to hang from his mouth. Just when he and the crowd think I can't run him any more, I run him a little more. He's a metronome. Then he's a goner. He pitches forward as if shot in the head. His cramps have cramps. He calls for medical treatment.

I break him. Then I hold easily to win the fourth set.

I win the fifth set 6–0.

In the locker room, Brad is talking to himself, to me, to anyone who will listen.

His back tire blew out! Did you see? Holy shit! His back tire—*boom.*

Reporters ask if I feel lucky that Clément cramped.

Lucky? I worked hard for those cramps.

At the hotel, riding the tiny elevator with Gil, my face is covered with clay. My eyes and ears and mouth are filled with clay. My clothes are spotted with clay. I look down. I never noticed before how Roland Garros clay, when it dries, looks like blood. I'm trying to brush it off when I feel Gil staring again.

What is it?

Nothing, he says, smiling.

IN THE THIRD ROUND I'm playing Chris Woodruff. I've played him once before, here, in 1996 and lost. A disastrous loss. I secretly liked my chances that year. This time I know from the start that I'm going to win. I have no doubt that I'll have my revenge, served ice cold. I beat him 6–3, 6–4, 6–4, on the same court where he beat me. Brad requested it, because he wanted me to remember, to make it personal.

I'm in the round of sixteen at the French Open for the first time since 1995. My reward is Carlos Moyá, the defending champion.

Not to worry, Brad says. Even though Moyá's the champ, and real good on the dirt, you can take away his time. You can bull-rush him, stand inside the baseline, hit the ball early and apply pressure. Go after his backhand, but if you have to bring it to his forehand, do it with purpose, with heat. Don't just go there—drive it hard up Main Street. Make him feel you.

In the first set, it's me feeling Moyá. I lose the set fast. In the second set I fall down two breaks. I'm not playing my game. I'm not doing anything Brad said to do. I look up at my box and Brad screams: *Come on! Let's go!*

Back to basics. I make Moyá run. And run. I establish a sadistic rhythm, chanting to myself: Run, Moyá, run. I make him run laps. I make him run the Boston Marathon. I win the second set, and the crowd is cheering. In the third set I run Moyá more than I've run the last three opponents combined, and suddenly, all at once, he's cooked. He wants no part of this. He didn't sign on for anything like this.

As the fourth set opens, I'm oozing confidence. I hop up and down. I want Moyá to see how much energy I've got left. He sees, and he sighs. I put him away and sprint to the locker room. Brad gives me a fist bump that almost breaks my fist.

In the hotel elevator, I feel Gil staring again.

Gil, what is it?

I have a feeling.

What feeling?

I feel like you're on a collision course.

With what?

Destiny.

I'm not sure I believe in destiny.

We'll see. We can't build a fire in the rain . . .

WE HAVE TWO DAYS OFF. Two days to relax and think about something besides tennis. Brad discovers that Springsteen is in our hotel. He's playing a concert in Paris. Brad suggests we attend. He scores us three seats, down front.

At first I'm not sure. I don't know if it's such a good idea to go out and paint Paris red. But the TV has mostly news about the tournament, which isn't good for my mood either. I remember the tennis official who mocked my playing a challenger, comparing it to Springsteen playing a corner bar. Yes, I say. Let's take the night off. Let's go see the Boss.

Brad, Gil, and I enter the arena a few seconds before Springsteen comes onstage. As we run down the aisle, several people spot me and point. A man yells my name. Andre! *Allez, Andre!* A few more men take up the cry. We slip into our seats. A spotlight scans the crowd—and suddenly lands on us. Our faces appear on the giant video screen above the stage. The crowd roars. They begin to chant: *Allez, Agassi! Allez, Agassi!* Some sixteen thousand people—about the same number as the crowd at Roland Garros—are chanting, cheering, stomping their feet. *Allez, Agassi!* It has a lilt the way they chant it, a bouncing rhythm like a children's nursery rhyme. *Deet-deet, da da da.* It's contagious. Brad chants too. I stand, wave. I'm honored. Inspired. I wish I could play the next match right now. Here. *Allez, Agassi!*

I stand once more, my heart in my throat. Then, at last, the Boss comes on.

IN THE QUARTERS I face Marcelo Filippini, from Uruguay. The first set is easy. The second set is easy. I run him, he crumbles. *Tramps like us, baby, we were born to run.* I enjoy this as much as winning—cutting the legs out from under my opponents, seeing the many years with Gil pay dividends in one concentrated two-week span. I win the third set without any resistance from Filippini, 6–0.

You're maiming guys! Brad shouts. Oh my God, Andre, you're freaking maiming them.

I'm in the semis. My opponent is Hrbaty, who just whooped me in Key Biscayne, when I was in a stupor over Steffi. I win the first set, 6–4. I win the next set, 7–6. Clouds roll in. A light drizzle starts to fall. The ball is getting heavier, which keeps me from playing offense. Hrbaty takes advantage and wins the third set, 6–3. In the fourth he goes up 2–1, and a match that I had won is slipping, slipping away. He's down a set, but clearly he's seized the momentum. I feel as if I'm just hanging on.

I look to Brad. He points to the skies. Stop the match.

I signal the supervisor and umpire. I point to the clay, which is mud. I tell them I'm not playing under these conditions. It's dangerous. They examine the mud like miners panning for gold. They confer. They halt play.

At dinner with Gil and Brad, I'm in a foul mood because I know the match was turning against me. Only the rain saved me. Otherwise we'd be at the airport right now. And now I can't believe I have all night to stew over the match, to worry about tomorrow.

I stare at my food, silent.

Brad and Gil discuss me as if I'm not at the table.

He's OK physically, Gil says. He's in fine condition. So give him a good speech, Brad. Coach him up.

What do you want me to say?

Think of something.

Brad takes a swig of beer and turns to me. OK, Andre. Look. Here's the deal. I need twenty-eight minutes from you tomorrow.

What?

Twenty-eight minutes. It's a sprint through the tape. You can do it. You've got five games to win, that's all, and that shouldn't take any more than twenty-eight minutes.

The weather. The ball.

The weather is going to be fine.

They're saying rain.

No, it's going to be fine. Just give us twenty-eight great minutes.

Brad knows my mind, the way it works. He knows that order, specificity, a clear and precise goal, are like candy to me. But does he also know the weather? For the first time it crosses my mind that Brad isn't a coach but a prophet.

Back at the hotel, Gil and I squeeze into the elevator.

It's going to be OK, Gil says.

Yeah.

Before bed, he forces me to drink my Gil Water.

I don't want to.

Drink it.

When I'm so hydrated that I'm pissing pure cottony white, he lets me go to sleep.

The next day I come out tight. Down 1–2 in the fourth, serving, I fall behind two break points. No, no, no. I fight back to deuce. I hold. The set is now tied. Having averted disaster, I'm suddenly loose, happy. It's so typical in sports. You hang by a thread above a bottomless pit. You stare death in the face. Then your opponent, or life, spares you, and you feel so blessed that you play with abandon. I win the fourth set and the match. I'm in the final.

My first look is to Brad, who's excitedly pointing to his watch and the digital play clock on the court.

Twenty-eight minutes. On the dot.

. . .

My opponent in the final is Andrei Medvedev, from Ukraine, which is not possible. It's simply not possible. Just months ago, in Monte Carlo, Brad and I bumped into Medvedev in a nightclub. He'd suffered a heartbreaking loss that day and was drinking to numb the pain. We invited him to join us. He threw himself into a chair at our table and announced that he was quitting tennis.

I can't play this fucking game anymore, he said. I'm old. The game has passed me by.

I talked him out of it.

How dare you, I said. Here I am, twenty-nine, injured, divorced, and *you're* bitching about being washed up at twenty-four? Your future is bright.

My game is shit.

So? Fix it.

He asked me for tips, pointers. He asked me to analyze his game, just as I'd once asked Brad to analyze mine. And I was Brad-esque. I was brutally honest. I told Medvedev he had a huge serve, a big return, and a world-class backhand. His forehand was not his best shot, of course, that was no secret, but he could hide it, because he was big enough to push opponents around.

You're a good mover! I shouted. Get back to the basics. Keep moving, slam your first serve, and rip the backhand up the line.

Ever since that night he's followed my advice to the letter and he's been on fire. He's been winning consistently on the tour and dominating guys in this tournament. Each time we've bumped into each other in the locker room, or around Roland Garros, we've exchanged sly winks and waves.

I never once dreamed we were on a collision course.

So Gil was wrong. I haven't been on a collision course with destiny, but with a fire-breathing dragon that I helped to build.

Everywhere I go, Parisians rush up and wish me luck. The tournament is the talk of the city. In restaurants and cafés, on the street, they yell my name, kiss my cheek, urge me onward. The story of my reception at the Springsteen concert has made the newspapers. The people, the press, are fascinated by my improbable run. Everyone can identify with it. They see something of themselves in my comeback, in my return from the dead.

It's the night before the final and I'm sitting in my hotel room, watching TV. I shut it off. I go to the window. I feel sick. I think about this last year, these last eighteen months, these last eighteen years. Millions of balls, millions of decisions. I know this is my final chance to win the French Open, my final chance to win all four slams and complete the set, which means my final shot at redemption. The idea of losing scares me, and the thought of winning scares me nearly as much. Would I be grateful? Would I be worthy? Would I build on it—or squander it?

Also, Medvedev is never far from my thoughts. He has my game. I gave it to him. He even has my first name. Andrei. It's going to be Andre versus Andrei. Me versus my doppelgänger.

Brad and Gil knock at the door.

Ready for dinner?

I hold the door open and tell them to come in for one second.

They stand just inside the door and watch me open the minibar. I pour myself a huge vodka. Brad's mouth falls open as I down the drink in one gulp.

What the hell do you think—?

I'm sick nervous, Brad. I haven't been able to eat a bite all day. I need to eat, and the only way I can eat is if I take the edge off.

Don't worry, Gil says to Brad. He's fine.

At least drink a big glass of water too, Brad says.

After dinner, when I get back to my room, I take a sleeping pill and slide into bed. I phone J.P. He says it's early afternoon where he is.

What time is it there?

It's late. It's so very late.

How are you feeling?

Please, *please,* talk to me for a few minutes about anything but tennis.

Are you OK?

Anything but tennis.

OK. Well. Let's see. How about I read you a poem? I've been reading a lot of poetry lately.

Yeah. Good. Whatever.

He goes to his bookshelf, takes down a book. He reads softly.

> *Though much is taken, much abides; and though*
> *We are not now that strength which in old days*
> *Moved earth and heaven, that which we are, we are;*
> *One equal temper of heroic hearts,*

> Made weak by time and fate, but strong in will
> To strive, to seek, to find, and not to yield.

I fall asleep without hanging up the phone.

GIL KNOCKS AT MY DOOR, dressed as if he's meeting de Gaulle. He's got the nice black sport coat, the creased black slacks—the black hat. And he's wearing the necklace I gave him. I'm wearing the matching earring. Father, Son, Holy Ghost.

In the elevator he says: It's going to be OK.

Yeah.

But it's not OK. I know it during warm-ups. I'm soaked in sweat. I'm sweating as if I'm about to get married. I'm so overcome with nerves that my teeth are clicking. The sun is bright, which should make me happy, because the ball will be drier and lighter. But the warmth of the day is also making me sweat that much more.

As the match begins, I'm a sweat-soaked wreck. I'm making stupid mistakes, rookie mistakes, every kind of error and fuck-up you can make on a tennis court. It takes just nineteen minutes to lose the first set, 6–1. Medvedev, meanwhile, couldn't look calmer. And why not? He's doing everything he's supposed to do, everything I told him to do in Monte Carlo. He's directing the pace, moving nimbly, ripping the backhand up the line whenever he chooses. His game is cool, precise, pitiless. If I move in, if I try to take over a point by creeping forward, he hits a crushing backhand past me.

He's wearing plaid shorts, as if we're at the beach, and in fact he looks as if he's frolicking on the Riviera. He's fresh, vigorous, having a holiday. He could be out here for days and days and not get tired of this.

As the second set starts, dark clouds appear. Suddenly a light rain falls. Hundreds of umbrellas appear in the stands. Play is halted. Medvedev runs into the locker room, and I follow.

No one is in there. I walk up and down. Water drips from a faucet. The sound pings off the metal lockers. I sit on a bench, sweating, staring into an open locker.

In come Brad and Gil. Brad, wearing a white jacket and white hat, a stark contrast against Gil's all-black ensemble, slams the door as hard as he can and yells, What's going on?

He's too good, Brad. He's just too good. I can't beat him. This fucker is six-five, serving bombs, never missing. He's hurting me with his serve, he's hurting me with his backhand, I can't get back in the point on his serve. I don't have this.

Brad says nothing. I think of Nick, standing in about the same spot, saying nothing to me during the rain delay when I lost to Courier eight years ago. Some things never change. Same elusive tournament, same queasy feeling, same callous reaction from my coach.

I yell at Brad: Are you kidding me? You're going to pick this moment, of all moments, to decide not to talk? Of all times, *this* is the moment you're finally going to shut the hell up?

He stares. Then starts screaming. Brad, who never raises his voice to *anybody,* comes apart.

What do you want me to say, Andre? What is it that you want me to *say?* You tell me he's too good. How the fuck would you know? You can't judge how he's playing! You're so confused out there, so blind with panic, I'm surprised you can even see him. Too good? You're *making* him look good.

But—

Just start letting go. If you're going to lose, at least lose on your own terms. Hit the fucking ball.

But—

And if you're not sure where to hit it, here's an idea. Just hit it to the same place he hits it. If he hits a backhand crosscourt, you hit a backhand crosscourt. Just hit yours a little better. You don't have to be better than the whole fucking world, remember? You just have to be better than one guy. There isn't one shot he has that you don't have. Fuck his serve. His serve will break down when you start making your shots. Just hit. Just fucking hit. If we're going to lose today, fine, I can live with it, but let's lose on our terms. The last thirteen days, I've seen you lay it on the line. I've seen you rip it, under pressure, maim guys. So please stop feeling sorry for yourself, and stop telling me he's too good, and for the love of God stop trying to be perfect! Just see the ball, hit the ball. Do you hear me, Andre? See the ball. Hit the ball. Make this guy deal with you. Make him *feel* you out there. You're not moving. You're not hitting. You may think you are, but trust me, you're just standing there. If you're going down, OK, go down, but go down with guns blazing. Always, always, always, go down with both guns *blaaazing.*

He opens a locker and slams it shut. The door flaps and clangs.

The referee appears.

We're back on court, gentlemen.

Brad and Gil walk out of the locker room. I notice that as they slip through the door Gil gives Brad's back a furtive pat.

I walk slowly onto the court. We have a brief warm-up, then resume play. I've forgotten the score. I have to look at the scoreboard to remind myself. Oh yes. I lead, 1–0, in the second set. But Medvedev is serving. I think again of the final against Courier in 1991, the rain delay that disrupted my rhythm. Maybe this will be payback. Tennis karma. Maybe, as that rain delay befuddled me, this rain delay will help me right myself.

But Medvedev is counting on his own Ukrainian karma. He picks up right where he left off, keeps the pressure on, forces me continually to retreat and play defense, which is not my game. The day is now heavily overcast, and damp, which seems to further strengthen Medvedev. He likes the pace slow. He's an angry elephant, taking his sweet time, crushing me underfoot. In the first game after the delay, he serves the ball 120 miles an hour. Within seconds the score is even at 1–1.

Then he breaks me. Then he holds, then breaks me again, going on to win the second set with remarkable ease, 6–2.

In the third set, we hold serve through five games. Suddenly, inexplicably, for the first time in the match, I break him. I'm ahead, 4–2. I hear gasps and murmurs in the crowd.

But Medvedev breaks me right back. He holds and knots the set at 4–all.

The sun reappears. It's shining brightly, and the clay begins to dry. The pace of play picks up considerably. I'm serving, and at 15–all we play a frantic point, which I win with a beautiful backhand volley. Now, at 30–15, I hear Brad telling me to see the ball, hit the ball. I let it fly. I cut loose my first serve with an extra loud grunt. Out. I hurry the second serve. Out again. Double fault. 30–30.

So. There you have it. I'm still going to lose—Medvedev is now just six points from the championship—but I'm going to lose on Brad's terms instead of mine.

I serve again. Out. I stubbornly refuse to take anything off the second serve. Out again. Two double faults in a row.

Now it's 30–40. Break point. I walk in circles, squeezing my eyes, on the verge of tears. I need to pull myself together. I toe the line, toss the ball into the air, and miss yet another serve. I've now missed five straight serves. I'm falling apart. I'm one missed serve away from Medvedev serving for the French Open.

He leans in, ready to obliterate this second serve. As a returner you're always guessing about your opponent's psyche, and Medvedev knows my psyche is in tatters after missing five serves in a row. He's guessing, there-fore, with a high degree of certainty, that I won't have the stomach to be aggressive. He expects a nice soft kick serve. He thinks I have no other choice. He steps up, well inside the baseline, sending me a message that he anticipates a softie, and when he gets hold of it he's going to ram it down my throat. He wears a look on his face that unmistakably says: Go ahead, bitch. Be aggressive. I dare you.

This moment is the crucial test for both of us. This is the turning point in the match, perhaps in both of our lives. It's a test of wills, of heart, of manhood. I toss the ball in the air and refuse to back down. Con-trary to Medvedev's expectations, I serve hard and aggressive to his back-hand. The ball takes a wicked skidding bounce. Medvedev stretches out and shovels the ball to the center of the court. I hit a forehand behind him. He gets there, hits a backhand at my feet. I bend, play an awkward forehand volley that lands on the line, he shovels it over the net, and then I tap it ever so lightly back over, where it dies, a huge winner for such a soft shot.

I go on to hold serve.

I have a bounce in my step as I walk to my chair. The crowd is going crazy. The momentum hasn't shifted, but it's twitched. That was Medvedev's moment, and he missed it, and I think I can see on his face that he knows it.

Allez, Agassi! Allez!

One good game, I think. Play one good game, and you'll have won a set, and then at least you can walk out of here holding your head up.

The clouds have blown away. The sun has dried the clay hard and the pace is now lightning fast. I catch Medvedev sneaking a worried look at the sky as we retake the court. He wants those rain clouds to return. He wants no part of this blazing sun. He's starting to sweat. His nostrils are flaring. He looks like a horse—like a dragon. *You can beat the dragon.* He falls behind love–40. I break him and win the third set.

Now we play on my terms. I move Medvedev side to side, hit the ball big, do everything Brad said to do. Medvedev is a step slower, notably dis-tracted. He's had too long to think about winning. He was five points away, five points, and it's haunting him. He's going over and over it in his mind. He's telling himself, *I was so close. I was there. The finish line!* He's living in the past, and I'm in the present. He's thinking, I'm feeling. Don't think, Andre. Hit *harder*.

In the fourth set, I break him again. Then we settle into a dogfight. We play good solid tennis, each of us sprinting and grunting and digging deep. The set could go either way. But I have one distinct advantage, a secret weapon I can pull out any time I need a point—my net play. Everything I do at the net is working, and it's clearly troubling Medvedev, messing with his head. He becomes skittish, almost paranoid. If I merely pretend to rush the net, he flinches. I jump, he lunges.

I win the fourth set.

I break him early in the fifth set and go up 3–2. It's happening. It's turning. The thing that should have been mine in 1990 and 1991 and 1995 is coming around again. I'm up 5–3. He's serving, 40–15. I have two match points. I need to win this thing right now, or I'm going to have to serve out the match, and I don't want that. If I don't win this thing right now, maybe I don't win at all. If I don't win this thing right now, I'll be in Medvedev's shoes, haunted by how close I was. If I don't win this thing right now, I'll have to think about the French Open in my old age, in my rocking chair, mumbling about Medvedev with a plaid blanket over my legs. I've already obsessed about this tournament for the last ten years. I can't bear the idea of obsessing about it for another eighty. After all this work and sweat, after this improbable comeback and this miraculous tournament, if I don't win this thing right now, I'll never be happy, truly happy, again. And Brad will have to be institutionalized. The finish line is close enough to kiss. *I feel it pulling me.*

Medvedev wins both match points. He staves off death. We're back to deuce. I win the next point, however. Match point, again.

I yell at myself: Now. *Now.* Win this now.

But he wins the next point, then wins the game.

The changeover takes an eternity. I mop my face with a towel. I look at Brad, expecting him to be disconsolate, as I am. But his face is determined. He holds up four fingers. *Four more points.* Four points equals all four slams. *Come on! Let's go!*

If I'm going to lose this match, if I'm doomed to live with withering regret, it won't be because I didn't do what Brad said. I hear his voice in my ear: Go back to the well.

Medvedev's forehand is the well.

We walk onto the court. I'm going to hit everything to Medvedev's forehand, and he knows I'm going to. On the first point he's tight, tentative on a passing shot up the line. He puts the ball into the net.

He wins the next point, however, when I net my running forehand.

Suddenly I rediscover my serve. Out of nowhere I uncork a big first serve that he can't handle. He hits a tired forehand that flies long. I hit my next first serve, even bigger, and he nets a forehand.

Championship point. Half the crowd is yelling my name, the other half is yelling, *Ssssh*. I hit another sizzling first serve, and when Medvedev steps to the side and takes a chicken-wing swing, I'm the second person to know that I've won the French Open. Brad is the first. Medvedev is third. The ball lands well beyond the baseline. Watching it fall is one of the great joys of my life.

I raise my arms and my racket falls on the clay. I'm sobbing. I'm rubbing my head. I'm terrified by how good this feels. Winning isn't supposed to feel this good. Winning is never supposed to matter this much. But it does, it does, I can't help it. I'm overjoyed, grateful to Brad, to Gil, to Paris—even to Brooke and Nick. Without Nick I wouldn't be here. Without all the ups and downs with Brooke, even the misery of our final days, this wouldn't be possible. I even reserve some gratitude for myself, for all the good and bad choices that led here.

I walk off the court, blowing kisses in all four directions, the most heartfelt gesture I can think of to express the gratitude pulsing through me, the emotion that feels like the source of all other emotions. I vow that I will do this from now on, win or lose, whenever I walk off a tennis court. I will blow kisses to the four corners of the earth, thanking everyone.

WE HAVE A SMALL PARTY at an Italian restaurant, Stressa, in downtown Paris, close to the Seine, close to the spot where I gave Brooke the tennis bracelet. I'm drinking champagne out of my trophy. Gil is drinking a Coke and he's physically incapable of not smiling. Every now and then he puts his hand on mine—it's as heavy as a dictionary—and says, You did it.

We did it, Gilly.

McEnroe is there. He hands me a phone and says: Someone wants to say hello.

Andre? Andre! Congratulations. I got such joy watching you tonight. I envy you.

Borg.

Envy? Why?

Doing something so few of us have done.

The sun is coming up when Brad and I walk back to the hotel. He puts his arm around me and says, The journey ended the right way.

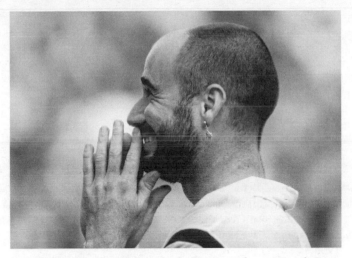

Seconds after beating Andrei Medvedev to capture the 1999 French Open

How so?

He says, Usually in life the journey ends the wrong fucking way. But this one time it ended the right way.

I throw an arm around Brad. It's one of the few things the prophet has gotten wrong all month. The journey is just beginning.

23

ON THE CONCORDE BACK TO NEW YORK, Brad tells me it's destiny—*destiny*. He's had a couple of beers.

You won the 1999 French Open on the men's side, he says. And who should happen to have won it on the women's side? Who? Tell me.

I smile.

That's right. Steffi Graf. It's destiny you end up together. Only two people in the history of the world have won all four slams and a gold medal—you and Steffi Graf. The Golden Slam. It's destiny that you two should be married.

In fact, he says, here's my prediction. He takes the Concorde promotional literature from the seat pocket and scribbles on the upper right-hand corner: *2001—Steffi Agassi.*

What the hell does that mean?

You guys will be married by 2001. And you'll have your first kids together in 2002.

Brad, she has a boyfriend. Have you forgotten?

After the two weeks you've just had, you're going to tell me anything is impossible?

Well, I'll say this. Now that I've won the French Open, I do feel slightly more—I don't know. Worthy?

There. Now you're talking.

I don't believe people are destined to win tennis tournaments. Destined to come together, maybe, but not destined to hit more winners and aces than their opponent. Still, I'm reluctant to question anything Brad says. So, just in case, and because I like the way it looks, I tear off the corner of the Concorde program on which he's written his latest prophecy and I put it in my pocket.

We spend the next five days on Fisher Island, recuperating and celebrating. Mostly the latter. The party keeps growing. Brad's wife, Kimmie, flies in. J.P. and Joni fly in. Late at night we crank the stereo, listening over and over to Sinatra singing That's Life, Kimmie and Joni dancing like go-go girls atop the table and bed.

Then I take to the grass courts at the hotel. I hit with Brad for several days, and we board a plane for London. Halfway across the Atlantic, I realize that we're going to land on Steffi's birthday. What are the chances? What if we bump into her? It would be nice to have something for her.

I look at Brad, sleeping. I know he'll want to go straight from the airport to the practice courts at Wimbledon, so there won't be time to stop at a stationery store. I should make some kind of birthday card now. But with what?

I notice that the airplane's first-class menu is kind of cool. On the cover is a photo of a country church under a sliver of moon. I combine two covers into one card and along the inside I write: *Dear Steffi, I wanted to take this opportunity to wish you a happy birthday. How proud you must feel. Congratulations on what I know is only a sliver of what is out there for you.*

I punch holes in the two menus. Now I just need something to hold them together. I ask the flight attendant if she has any string or ribbon. Maybe some tinsel? She gives me a bit of raffia coiled around the neck of a champagne bottle. I carefully weave the raffia through the holes. It feels as though I'm stringing a tennis racket.

When the card is finished I wake Brad and show him my handiwork.

Old World craftsmanship, I say.

He twirls a knuckle in his eye, nods approvingly. All you need is a look, he says. An opening. I tuck the card in my tennis bag and wait.

THERE ARE THREE LEVELS of practice courts at the Wimbledon practice site, Aorangi Park. It's a tiered mountain, an Aztec temple of tennis courts. Brad and I hit on the middle tier for half an hour. When we're done I pack my tennis bag, taking my time, as always. It's hard to get reorganized after a transatlantic flight. I'm carefully arranging, rearranging, slipping my wet shirt into a plastic bag, when Brad begins punching my shoulder.

She's coming, dude, she's coming.

I look up like an Irish setter. If I had a tail it would be wagging. She's thirty yards off, wearing tight-fitting blue warm-up pants. I notice for the first time that she walks slightly pigeon-toed, like me. Her blond hair is pulled back in a ponytail and gleaming in the sun. It looks, yet again, like a halo.

I stand. She gives me the European double-cheek kiss.

Congratulations on the French, she says. I was so happy for you. I had tears in my eyes.

Me too.

She smiles.

Congratulations to you as well, I say. You paved the way. You warmed up the court for me.

Thank you.

Silence.

Luckily, no fans or photographers are around, so she seems relaxed, in no hurry. I'm oddly relaxed as well. Brad, however, is making small squeaking noises, like air being slowly let out of a balloon.

Oh, I say. Hey. I just remembered. I have a gift for you. I knew it was your birthday, so I made you a card. Happy Birthday.

She takes the card, looks at it for several seconds, then looks up, touched.

How did you know it was my birthday?

I just—know.

Thank you, she says. Really.

She walks away quickly.

THE NEXT DAY she's coming off the practice courts just as Brad and I arrive. This time there are mobs of fans and reporters all around and she seems painfully self-conscious. She slows, gives us a half wave, and in a stage whisper says: How can I reach you?

I'll give my number to Heinz.

OK.

Goodbye.

Bye.

After practice Perry and Brad and I sit around the house we've rented, debating when she's going to call.

Soon, Brad says.

Very soon, Perry says.

The day passes without a call.

Another day passes.

I'm in agony. Wimbledon starts Monday, and I can't sleep, can't think. Sleeping pills are powerless against this kind of anxiety.

She had better call, Brad says, or you're going to lose in the first round.

Saturday night, just after dinner, the phone rings.

Hello?

Hi. It's Stefanie.

Stefanie?

Stefanie.

Stefanie—*Graf?*

Yes.

Oh. You go by Stefanie?

She explains that her mother called her Steffi years ago, and the press picked it up and it stuck. But she thinks of herself as Stefanie.

Stefanie it is, I say.

While talking to her I go skiing around the living room in my sweat socks. I schuss across the wood floors. Brad pleads with me to stop, to sit in a chair. He's sure I'm going to break a leg or tweak a knee. I settle into an easy cross-country motion around the perimeter of the room. He smiles and tells Perry, We're going to have a good tournament. It's going to be a *good* Wimbledon.

Sssh, I tell him.

Then I lock myself in a back room.

Listen, I tell Stefanie, back in Key Biscayne you said you didn't want any misunderstandings with me. Well, I don't want any misunderstandings with you either. So I need to tell you, I just need to say before we go any further, that I think you are *beautiful.* I respect you, I admire you, and I would absolutely love to get to know you better. That's my goal. That's my only agenda. That's where I am. Tell me this is possible. Tell me we can go to dinner.

No.

Please.

It's not possible—not here.

Not here. OK. Can we go somewhere else?

No. I have a boyfriend.

I think: the boyfriend. Still. I've read about him. Race-car driver. The same boyfriend she's had for six years. I try to come up with something clever to say, some way of telling her to open herself to the *possibility* of being with me. With the silence stretching to an uncomfortable length, the moment sliding away, all I can come up with is this:

310

Six years is a long time.

Yes, she says. Yes it is.

If you're not moving forward, you're moving backward. I've lived that.

She doesn't say anything. But it's the way she doesn't say anything. I've struck a chord.

I continue. It can't be exactly what you're looking for. I mean, I don't want to make any assumptions—but.

I hold my breath. She doesn't contradict me.

I say, I don't want to be disrespectful, or take liberties, but just, can you just, please, could you, maybe, I don't know, just get to *know* me?

No.

Coffee?

I can't be in public with you. It wouldn't be right.

What about letters? Can I write you?

She laughs.

Can I send you stuff? Can I *let* you know me before you decide if you want to *get* to know me?

No.

Not even letters?

There is someone who reads my mail.

I see.

I knock my fist against my forehead. Think, Andre, *think*.

I say, OK, look, how about this. You're playing your next tournament in San Francisco. I'll be there practicing with Brad. You said you love San Francisco. Let's meet in San Francisco.

This is—possible.

This is—*possible*?

I wait for her to elaborate. She doesn't.

So can I call you, or do you just want to call me?

Call me after this tournament, she says. Let's both play, and call me when you finish the tournament.

She gives me her cell phone number. I write it on a paper napkin, kiss it, and put it in my tennis bag.

I REACH THE SEMIS AND PLAY RAFTER. I beat him in straight sets. I don't have to wonder who's waiting for me in the final. It's Pete. As always, Pete. I stagger back to the house, thinking shower, food, sleep. The phone rings—I'm sure it's Stefanie, wishing me luck against Pete, confirming our San Francisco date.

But it's Brooke. She's in London and asks to come by and see me.

As I hang up the phone and turn, Perry is there, inches from my face.

Andre, please tell me you said no. Please tell me you're not letting that woman come here.

She's coming. In the morning.

Before you play the final at Wimbledon?

It'll be fine.

SHE ARRIVES AT TEN, wearing an enormous British hat with a wide, floppy brim and plastic flowers. I give her a quick tour of the house. We compare it to the houses she and I used to rent, back in the day. I ask if she'd like something to drink.

Do you have any tea?

Sure.

I hear Brad cough in the next room. I know what the cough means. It's the morning of the final. An athlete should never change his routine on the morning of a final. I've had coffee every morning of the tournament. I should be having coffee now.

But I want to be a good host. I make a pot of tea, and we drink it at a table under the kitchen window. We talk without saying anything. I ask if she has anything special she wanted to tell me. She misses me, she says. She wanted to tell me that.

She sees a stack of magazines on the corner of the table, copies of a recent *Sports Illustrated*. I'm on the cover. The headline is *Suddenly Andre.* (I'm suddenly starting to hate that word, *suddenly.*) Tournament officials sent them over, I tell her. They want me to autograph copies for fans and Wimbledon officials and staffers.

Brooke picks up one of the magazines, stares at my photo. I watch her stare. I think of that day thirteen years ago, sitting with Perry in his bedroom, beneath hundreds of *Sports Illustrated* covers, dreaming about Brooke. Now here she is, I'm on the cover of *Sports Illustrated,* Perry is a former producer of her TV show, and we're all barely speaking.

She reads the headline aloud. Suddenly Andre. She reads it again. Suddenly Andre?

She looks up. Oh, Andre.

What?

Oh, Andre. I'm so *so* sorry.

Why?

Here it is, your big moment, and they make it all about me.

. . .

STEFANIE IS IN THE FINAL TOO. She loses to Lindsay Davenport. She had been playing mixed doubles as well, with McEnroe, and they had reached the semis, but she pulled out because of a bad hamstring. I'm in the locker room, getting dressed for my match with Pete, and McEnroe is telling a group of players that Stefanie left him in the lurch.

Can you believe this *bitch*? She asks to play mixed doubles with me and I fucking do it and then we're in the semis and she backs out?

Brad puts a hand on my shoulder. Steady, champ.

I start strong against Pete. My mind is going in several directions at once—how dare Mac say those things about Stefanie? what was the deal with that hat Brooke was wearing?—but somehow I'm playing solid, crisp tennis. It's 3–all in the first set, Pete serving at love–40. Triple break point. I see Brad smiling, punching Perry, shouting, *Come on! Let's go!* I let myself think about Borg, the last person to win the French and Wimbledon back to back, a feat now within my grasp.

I imagine Borg phoning me again to congratulate me. Andre? Andre, it's me. Björn. I envy you.

Pete wakes me from my fantasy. Unreturnable serve. Unreturnable serve. Blur. Ace. Game, Sampras.

I stare at Pete in shock. No one, living or dead, has ever served like that. No one in the history of the game could have returned those serves.

He takes me out in straight sets, finishing me off with two aces, two fiery exclamation points at the end of a seamless performance. It's the first match I've lost in a slam in the last fourteen matches, a streak of dominance almost without precedence in my career. But history will record that it's Pete's sixth Wimbledon, and his twelfth slam overall, tying him for most all-time among men—as history should. Later, Pete tells me he never saw me hit the ball as hard and clean as I did those first six games, and it made him raise his game, amp up his second serve by twenty miles an hour.

In the locker room I need to take the standard drug test. I so badly want to piss and run back to the house and call Stefanie, but I can't, because I have a bladder like a whale. It takes forever. Finally my bladder cooperates with my heart.

I drop my bag in the front hall and lunge for the phone as if it's a drop shot. Fingers trembling, I dial. Straight to voice mail. I leave a message. Hi. It's Andre. Tournament's over. I lost to Pete. Sorry about your loss to Lindsay. Call me when you can.

I sit. I wait. A day passes. No call. Another day. No call.

I hold the phone in front of my face and tell it: Ring.

I dial her again, leave another message. Nothing.

I fly back to the West Coast. As I step off the plane, I check my messages. Nothing.

I fly to New York for a charity event. I check my voice mail every fifteen minutes. Nothing.

J.P. meets me in New York City. We hit the town. P. J. Clarke's and Campagnola. A big ovation when we walk in. I see my friend Bo Dietl, the cop-turned-TV personality. He's sitting at a long table with his crew: Mike the Russian, Shelly the Tailor, Al Tomatoes, Joey Pots and Pans. They insist we join them.

J.P. asks Joey Pots and Pans how he got his nickname.

I love to cook!

Later we all break up laughing when Joey's cell phone rings. He flips it open and yells, *Pots!*

Bo says he's having a party in the Hamptons this weekend. He insists that J.P. and I come. Pots is cooking, he says. Tell him your favorite food, whatever it is, he'll cook it. It makes me think of those long-ago Thursday nights at Gil's house.

I tell Bo we wouldn't miss it.

THE CROWD AT BO'S HOUSE is like the cast of *GoodFellas* meets *Forrest Gump*. We sit around the pool, smoking cigars, drinking tequila. Every now and then I pull Stefanie's number out of my pocket and study it. At one point I go into Bo's house and call her from his landline, in case she's screening my calls. Straight to voice mail.

Frustrated, restless, I drink three or four too many margaritas, then put my wallet and cell phone on a chair and do a cannonball into the pool, still dressed. Everyone follows. An hour later, I check my voicemail again. You have one new message.

For some reason my cell phone didn't ring.

Hi, she says. I'm sorry I haven't called you back. I got very sick. My body broke down after Wimbledon. I had to pull out of San Francisco and come home to Germany. But I'm feeling better now. Call me back when you can.

She doesn't leave her number, of course, because she already gave me her number.

I pat my pockets. Where did I put that number?

My heart stops. I remember writing it on a paper napkin, which was in my pocket when I jumped in the pool. Gingerly I reach into my pocket and pull out the napkin. It looks like Tammy Faye Bakker's makeup.

I remember that I phoned Stefanie once from Bo's landline. I grab him by the arm and tell him that whatever it takes, whatever favors he has to call in, whoever he needs to grease or bully or kill, he must get the phone records for his house, with all the outgoing phone calls from today. And he must do it right now.

Done, Bo says.

He reaches out to a guy who knows a guy who has a friend who has a cousin who works for the phone company. An hour later we have the records. The list of calls made from the house looks like the Pittsburgh white pages. Bo yells at his crew: I'm going to start keeping an eye on you mutts! No wonder my frigging phone bill is so high!

But there's the number. I write it down in six different places, including my hand. I dial Stefanie, and she answers on the third ring. I tell her what I've been through tracking her down. She laughs.

We're both playing near Los Angeles soon. Can we meet there? Maybe?

After your tournament, she says. Yes.

I FLY TO LOS ANGELES AND PLAY WELL. I meet Pete in the final. I lose 7–6, 7–6, and don't care. Running off the court, I'm the happiest guy in the world.

I shower, shave, dress. I grab my tennis bag and head for the door—and there's Brooke.

She heard I was in town and decided to come down and see me play. She gives me a head-to-toe.

Wow, she says. You're all dressed up. Got a big date?

Actually, yes.

Oh. With who?

I don't answer.

Gil, she says, who does he have a date with?

Brooke, I think you should probably ask Andre that.

She stares at me. I sigh.

I'm going out with Stefanie Graf.

Stefanie?

Steffi.

I know we're both thinking of the photo on the refrigerator door. I say, Please don't tell anybody, Brooke. She's a private person, and she doesn't like any attention.

I won't tell a soul.

Thank you.

You look nice.

Really?

Uh-huh.

Thanks.

I hoist my tennis bag. She walks me into the tunnel under the stadium, where players park their cars.

Hello, Lily, she says, putting a hand on the gleaming white hood of the Cadillac. The top is already down. I throw my bag on the backseat.

Have a nice time, Brooke says. She kisses me on the cheek.

I pull away slowly, glancing at Brooke in the rearview mirror. Once more I drive away from her in Lily. But I know this time will be the last, and that we'll never speak again.

ON THE WAY TO SAN DIEGO, where Stefanie is playing, I phone J.P., who gives me a pep talk. Don't try too hard, he says. Don't try to be perfect. Be yourself.

I think I know how to follow that advice on a tennis court, but on a date, I'm at a loss.

Andre, he says, some people are thermometers, some are thermostats. You're a thermostat. You don't register the temperature in a room, you change it. So be confident, be yourself, take charge. Show her your essential self.

I think I can do that. Should I pick her up with the top up or down?

Up. Girls worry about their hair.

Don't we all. But isn't it cooler with the top down?

Her hair, Andre, her hair.

I keep the top down. I'd rather be cool than chivalrous.

STEFANIE IS RENTING A CONDO at a large resort. I find the resort but can't find the condo, so I phone her for directions.

What kind of car are you driving?

A Cadillac as big as a Carnival cruise ship.

Ahh. Yes. I see you.

I look up. She's standing on a tall grassy hill, waving.

She shouts: Wait there!

She comes running down the hill and makes as if to jump in my car.

Wait, I say. I have something I want to give you. Can I come up a minute?

Oh. Um.

Just a minute.

Reluctantly, she walks back up the hill. I drive around and park outside the front door of her condo.

I present her with a gift, a box of fancy candles I bought for her in Los Angeles. She seems to like them.

OK, she says. Ready?

I was hoping we could have a drink first.

A drink? Like what?

I don't know. Wine?

She says she doesn't have any wine.

We could order room service.

She sighs. She hands me a wine list and asks me to pick out a bottle.

When the room-service guy knocks at the door, she asks me to wait in the kitchen. She says she doesn't want to be seen together. She feels uncomfortable about our date. Guilty. She can imagine the room-service guy going back to tell his fellow room-service guys. She has a boyfriend, she reminds me.

But we're just—

There's no time to explain, she says. She pushes me into the kitchen.

I can hear the poor room-service guy, slightly enamored of Stefanie, who's just as nervous, for very different reasons. She's trying to rush him, he's fumbling with the bottle, and of course he drops it. A 1989 Château Beychevelle.

When the guy leaves I help Stefanie pick up the pieces of broken glass.

I say, I think we're off to a fine start, don't you?

I'VE RESERVED A TABLE by the window at Georges on the Cove, overlooking the ocean. We both order chicken and vegetables on a bed of mashed potatoes. Stefanie eats faster than I and doesn't touch her wine. I realize she's not a foodie, not a three-course-meal-and-linger-over-coffee kind of girl. She's also fidgeting, because someone she knows is sitting behind us.

We talk about my foundation. She's fascinated to hear about the charter school I'm building; she has her own foundation, which gives psycho-logical counseling to children scarred by war and violence in places like South Africa and Kosovo.

The subject of Brad, naturally, comes up. I tell her about his tremen-dous coaching skills, his odd people skills. We laugh about his efforts to make tonight happen. I don't tell her about his prediction. I don't ask about her boyfriend. I ask what she likes to do in her free time. She says she loves the ocean.

Would you like to go to the beach tomorrow?

I thought you were supposed to go to Canada.

I could take a red-eye tomorrow night.

She thinks.

OK.

After dinner I drop her at the resort. She gives me the double-cheek kiss, which is starting to feel like a karate self-defense move. She runs inside.

Driving away, I phone Brad. He's already in Canada, and it's hours later there. I woke him. But he rouses himself when I tell him the date went well.

Come on, he says groggily, stifling a yawn. Let's go!

SHE SPREADS A TOWEL ON THE SAND and pulls off her jeans. Underneath she's wearing a white one-piece bathing suit. She walks out into the water, up to her knees. She stands with one hand on her hip, the other shielding her eyes from the sun, scanning the horizon.

She asks, You coming in?

I don't know.

I'm wearing white tennis shorts. I didn't think to bring a bathing suit, because I'm a desert kid. I don't do well in the water. But I'll swim to China right now if that's what it takes. In just my tennis shorts I walk out to where Stefanie's standing. She laughs at my swimwear, and pretends to be shocked that I'm going commando. I tell her I've been like this since the French Open, and I'm never going back.

We talk for the first time about tennis. When I tell her that I hate it, she turns to me with a look that says, Of course. Doesn't everybody?

I talk about Gil. I ask about her conditioning. She mentions that she used to train with Germany's Olympic track team.

What's your best race?

Eight hundred meters.

Whoa. That's a gut check. How fast can you run it?

She smiles shyly.

You don't want to tell me?

No answer.

Come on. How fast are you?

She points down the beach, at a red balloon in the distance.

See that red dot down there?

Yeah.

You'd never beat me to that.

Really.

Really.

She smiles. Off she goes. I go tearing after her. It feels as if I've been chasing her all my life, and now I'm literally *chasing* her. At first it's all I can do to keep pace, but near the finish line I close the gap. She reaches the red balloon two lengths ahead of me. She turns, and peals of her laughter carry back to me like streamers on the wind.

I've never been so happy to lose.

24

I'M IN CANADA, she's in New York. I'm in Vegas, she's in Los Angeles. We stay connected by phone. One night she asks for a rundown of my favorites. Song. Book. Food. Movie.

You've probably never heard of my favorite movie.

Tell me, she says.

It came out several years ago. It's called *Shadowlands*. It's about C. S. Lewis, the writer.

I hear a sound like the phone dropping.

That's impossible, she says. That's simply not *possible*. That's *my* favorite movie.

It's about committing, opening yourself to love.

Yes, she says. Yes, it is, I know.

We are like blocks of stone . . . blows of His chisel which hurt us so much are what make us perfect.

Yes. Yes. Perfect.

PLAYING IN MONTREAL, in the semis against Kafelnikov, I can't win a single point. He's number two in the world and he puts a beating on me that causes people in the stands to cover their eyes. I tell myself: I have no say in the outcome of this match. I have no vote about what's happening to me today. I'm not just being defeated, I'm being *disenfranchised*. But I'm OK. In the locker room I see Kafelnikov's coach, Larry, leaning against the wall, smiling.

Larry, that was the sickest display of tennis I've ever seen. I'm going to make you a promise. Tell your boy he has a couple of beatings coming from me.

Later in the day I get a call from Stefanie. She's at LAX.

I ask, How'd you do in your tournament?

I hurt myself.

Agh. I'm sorry.

Yes. That's it. I'm done.

Where are you headed?

Back to Germany. I have some—some unfinished business.

I know what this means. She's going to talk to her boyfriend, tell him about me, break things off. I feel a goofy smile spread across my face.

When she returns from Germany, she says, she'll meet me in New York. We can spend time together before the 1999 U.S. Open. She mentions that she'll need to call a news conference.

A news conference? For what?

My retirement.

Your—*you're retiring?*

That's what I just said. I'm done.

When you said *done,* I thought you meant done for the tournament! I didn't know you meant—done.

I feel bereft, thinking of tennis without Stefanie Graf, the greatest women's player of all time. I ask how it feels knowing she'll never swing a racket in competition again. It's the kind of question reporters ask me every day, but I can't help myself. I want to know. I ask with a mixture of curiosity and envy.

She says it feels fine. She's at peace, more than ready to be done.

I wonder if I'm ready. I meditate on my own tennis mortality. But a week later, I'm in Washington, D.C., playing Kafelnikov in the final. I beat him 7–6, 6–1, and afterward I give his coach, Larry, a look. A promise is a promise.

I realize I'm not done. I have promises yet to keep.

I'M ON THE VERGE of being number one again. This time it's not my father's goal, or Perry's, or Brad's, and I remind myself that it's not mine either. It would be nice, that's all. It would cap off the comeback. It would be a memorable milestone on the journey. I sprint up one side of Gil Hill, down the other. I'm training for the number one ranking, I tell Gil. And for the U.S. Open. And, in a funny way, for Stefanie.

I can't wait for you to meet her, I say.

She arrives in New York and I whisk her upstate to a friend's nineteenth-century farmhouse. It has fifteen hundred acres and several large stone fireplaces. In every room we can sit and stare into the flames and talk. I tell her I'm a firebug. Me too, she says. The leaves are just starting to turn, and each window frames a postcard view of red-gold woods and mountains. There is no one around for miles.

We spend our time walking, hiking, driving into nearby towns, puttering in antique shops. At night we lie on the couch and watch the original *Pink Panther*. After half an hour we're both laughing so hard at Peter Sellers that we have to stop the tape and catch our breath.

She leaves after three days. She has to go on holiday with her family. I beg her to come back for the final weekend of the U.S. Open. To be there for me. In my box. I wonder if I'm jinxing myself, presuming that I'll be playing on the final weekend, but I don't care.

She says she'll try.

I reach the semis. I'm scheduled to play Kafelnikov. Stefanie phones and says she'll come. But she won't sit in my box. She's not ready for that.

Well then, let me arrange a seat for you.

I'll find my own seat, she says. Don't worry about me. I know my way around that place.

I laugh. I guess so.

She watches from the upper deck, wearing a baseball cap pulled low over her eyes. Of course the CBS cameras pick her out of the crowd, and McEnroe, doing commentary, says U.S. Open officials should be ashamed, not getting Steffi Graf a better seat. I beat Kafelnikov again. Tell Larry I said hello.

In the final I face Martin. I thought it would be Pete. I said publicly that I wanted Pete, but he pulled out of the tournament with a bad back. So it's Martin, who's been there, across the net, at so many critical junctures. At Wimbledon, in 1994, when I was still struggling to absorb Brad's teachings, I lost to Martin in a nip-and-tuck five-setter. At the U.S. Open that same year, Lupica predicted that Martin would upend me in the semis, and I believed him, but still managed to beat Martin and win the tournament. In Stuttgart, in 1997, it was my appalling first-round loss to Martin that finally pushed Brad to the breaking point. Now it's Martin who will be a test of my newfound maturity, who will show if the changes in me are fleeting or meaningful.

I break him in the very first game. The crowd is solidly behind me. Martin doesn't hang his head, however, doesn't lose any poise. He makes me work for the first set, then comes out stronger in the second, taking it in a tight tiebreak. He then wins the third set—an even tighter tiebreak. He leads two sets to one, a commanding lead at this tournament. No one ever comes back from such a deficit in the final here. It hasn't happened in twenty-six years. I see in Martin's eyes that he's feeling it, and waiting for me to show the old cracks in my mental armor. He's waiting for me to crumble, to revert to that jittery, emotional Andre he's played so often in years past. But I neither fold nor yield. I win the fourth set, 6–3, and in the fifth set, with Martin looking spent, I'm on the balls of my feet. I win the set, 6–2, and walk away knowing I'm healed, I'm back, exulting that Stefanie was here to see it. I've made only five unforced errors in the final two sets. Not once all day have I lost my serve, the first five-setter of my career in which I haven't lost my serve, and it comes as I capture my fifth slam. When I get back to Vegas I want to put five hundred on number five at a roulette table.

In the press room, one reporter asks why I think the New York crowd was pulling for me, cheering so loudly.

I wish I knew. But I take a guess: They've watched me grow up.

Of course fans everywhere have watched me grow up, but in New York their expectations were higher, which helped accelerate and validate my growth.

It's the first time I've felt, or dared to say aloud, that I'm a grown-up.

STEFANIE FLIES WITH ME TO VEGAS. We do all the typical Vegasy things. We gamble, see a show, take in a boxing match with Brad and Kimmie. Oscar De La Hoya vs. Félix Trinidad—our first official public date. Our coming-out party. The next day a photo of us holding hands, kissing at ringside, appears in newspapers.

No turning back now, I tell her.

She stares, then slowly, thankfully, smiles.

She spends the weekend at my house. The weekend turns into a week. Then a month. J.P. phones one day and asks how things are going.

I've never been better.

When are you going to see Stefanie again?

She's still here.

What do you mean?

I cup my hand over my mouth and whisper: It's still Date Three. She hasn't left.

Well—what?

I assume she'll leave eventually, go back to Germany, get her stuff, but we don't talk about it, and I don't want to bring it up. I don't want to do anything to disrupt things.

The way you're not supposed to wake a sleepwalker.

But soon it's time for *me* to go back to Germany. To play Stuttgart. She wants to come along—she even agrees to sit in my box—and I'm delighted to have her there with me. After all, Stuttgart is an important city for us both. It's where she turned pro, and where I re-turned pro. And yet we don't talk about tennis on the flight. We talk kids. I tell her I want them—with her. A bold thing to say, but I can't help myself. She takes my hand, tears in her eyes, then looks out the window.

On our last morning in Stuttgart, Stefanie needs to get up early, she has an early flight. She kisses my forehead goodbye. I pull the pillow over my head and go back to sleep. When I wake an hour later and stumble to the bathroom, I see, lying in my open shaving kit, Stefanie's birth control pills. As if to say: I won't be needing these anymore.

I NOT ONLY REACH NUMBER ONE, I finish 1999 number one, the first time I've ever ended a year in the top slot. I snap Pete's streak of six year-end finishes at number one. I then win the Paris Open and become the first man ever to win the Paris Open and the French Open in the same year. But at the ATP World Tour Championship I lose to Pete. Our twenty-eighth meeting. He leads 17–11. In slam finals he leads 3–1. Not much of a rivalry, sportswriters say, since Pete usually wins. I can't argue, and I can't be upset about Pete anymore.

I do the only thing I can do. I go to Gil's house and burn muscles. I run up and down Gil Hill until I see visions. I run in the morning, I run in the evening. I run on Christmas Eve, Gil timing me with a stopwatch. He says I'm breathing so loudly when I reach the top of the hill that he can hear me from the bottom. I run until I lean over the sticker bushes and vomit. Finally he meets me at the summit and tells me to stop. We stand and look at all the Christmas lights in the distance, and then we watch for shooting stars.

I'm proud of you, he says. Being out here. Tonight. Christmas Eve. It says something.

I thank him for being out here *with* me. For giving up his Christmas Eve.

Must be so many other places that you'd rather be.

No place I'd rather be, he says.

As the 2000 Australian Open begins I beat Mariano Puerta in straight sets and he publicly praises my concentration. I feel it, I'm on a collision course with Pete again, and sure enough we face off in the semis. I've lost four of the last five times we've played, and he's as good this day as ever. He hits me with thirty-seven aces, more than he's ever notched against me. But I've got Christmas Eve with Gil. Two points from losing the match I mount a furious comeback. I win the match and become the first man since Laver to reach the final in four straight slams.

In the final I face Kafelnikov again. It takes time to warm up. I'm still rubbery after my tussle with Pete. I lose the first set, but find my stride, my touch, and take him in four. My sixth slam. At the post-match news conference I thank Brad and Gil for teaching me that my best is good enough. A fan shouts out Stefanie's name, asks what's the story there.

Mind your business, I say, joking. I'd actually like to tell the world about it. And I will. Soon.

Gil tells the *New York Times:* I really believe we will never see Andre stop fighting ever again.

Brad tells the *Washington Post:* He's got a 27–1 match record over the last four Grand Slams. Only Rod Laver, Don Budge, and Steffi Graf have ever done better.

Even Brad doesn't fully realize how floored I am to be mentioned in that company.

25

STEFANIE TELLS ME her father is coming to Vegas for a visit. (Her parents are long divorced, and her mother, Heidi, already lives fifteen minutes from us.) Thus, the unavoidable moment has arrived. Our fathers are going to meet. The prospect unnerves us both.

Peter Graf is suave, sophisticated, well read. He likes to make jokes, lots of jokes, none of which I get, because his English is spotty. I want to like him, and I see that he wants me to like him, but I'm uneasy in his presence, because I know the history. He's the German Mike Agassi. A former soccer player, a tennis fanatic, he started Stefanie playing before she was out of diapers. Unlike my father, however, Peter never stopped managing her career and her finances, and he spent two years in jail for tax evasion. The subject never comes up, but feels at times like the German *Elefant* in the room.

I should have expected it: the first thing Peter wants to see when he arrives in Nevada isn't Hoover Dam or the Strip but my father's ball machine. He's heard all about it, and now he wants to study it up close. I drive him to my father's house, and along the way he chatters amiably. But I don't understand much. Is it German? No, it's a hybrid of German and English and tennis. He's asking questions about my father's game. How often does my father play? How well does he play? He's trying to size up my father before we get there.

My father doesn't do well with people who don't speak perfect English, and he doesn't do well with strangers, so I know we have two strikes on us as we walk through my parents' front door. I'm relieved, however, to see that sport is a universal language, that these two men, both aficionados, both former athletes, know how to use their bodies to communicate, through swings and gestures and grunts. I tell my father that Peter would like to see the famous ball machine. My father is flattered. He takes us outside to his backyard court and wheels out the dragon. He revs the motor, raises the pedestal high. He's talking nonstop, giving Peter a lecture, shouting to be heard above the dragon—blissfully unaware that Peter doesn't understand a word.

Go stand there, my father tells me.

He hands me a racket, points me to the other side of the court, aims the machine at my head.

Demonstrate, he says.

I'm having shuddering, violent flashbacks, and only the thought of the tequila waiting for me back home keeps me functioning.

Peter positions himself behind me and watches while I hit.

Ahh, he says. *Ja.* Good.

My father cranks up the machine. He clicks the dial until the balls are coming almost in twos. My father must have added a gear to the dragon. I don't remember balls ever coming this fast. I don't have time to bring back my racket and hit the second ball. Peter scolds me for missing. He takes the racket from me, pushes me aside. *This,* he says, is the shot you should have had. You never had this shot. He shows me the famous Stefanie Slice, which he claims to have taught Stefanie. You need a quieter racket, he says. Like this.

My father is livid. In the first place, Peter isn't listening to my father's lecture. In the second place, Peter is interfering with my father's star pupil. My father comes around the net, shouting: That slice is bullshit! If Stefanie had *this* shot, she would have been better off. He then demonstrates the two-handed backhand he taught me.

With this shot, my father says, Stefanie would have won thirty-two slams!

The two men can't understand each other, and yet they're managing a heated argument. I turn my back, concentrate on hitting balls. I train all my attention on the dragon. Occasionally I hear Peter mention my rivals, Pete and Rafter, and then my father responds with Stefanie's nemeses, Monica Seles and Lindsay Davenport. My father then mentions boxing. He uses a boxing analogy, and Peter howls in protest.

I was a boxer too, Peter says—and I would have knocked you out.

You can say a lot of things to my father. But not that. Never that. I cringe, knowing what's coming. I wheel just in time to see Stefanie's sixty-three-year-old father take off his shirt and tell my sixty-nine-year-old father: Look at me. *Look* at the *shape* I'm in. I'm taller than you. I can keep you at bay with my jab.

My father says, You think so? Come on! You and me.

Peter is trash-talking in German, my father is trash-talking in Assyrian, and they're both putting up their fists. They're circling, feinting, bobbing and weaving, and just before one of them throws hands, I step in, push them apart.

My father shouts, This fucker is talking shit!

That may be, Pops, but—please.

They're winded, sweating. My father's eyes are dilated. Peter's bare chest is beaded with sweat. They see, however, that I'm not going to let them mix it up, so they go to neutral corners. I turn off the dragon, and we all walk off the court.

At home, Stefanie kisses me and asks how it went.

I'll tell you later, I say, reaching for the tequila.

I don't know when a margarita has ever tasted so good.

AFTER PLAYING WELL IN THE DAVIS CUP, I lose early in Scottsdale, a tournament I typically own. I play poorly in Atlanta and pull a hamstring. I lose in the third round in Rome and realize, reluctantly, that this can't go on. I can't play every tournament. Approaching thirty years old, I must choose my battles more carefully.

Every other interview now is about the end. I tell reporters that my best tennis is ahead of me, and they smile, wincingly, as if they hope I'm kidding. I've never been more serious.

When the time comes to defend at the 2000 French Open, I walk into Roland Garros expecting to feel waves of nostalgia. But it's all different—the place has been renovated. They've added more seats. They've redone the locker rooms. I don't like it. Not one bit. I wanted Roland Garros to stay the same forever. I want everything to stay the same. I hoped to walk on center court every year and conjure up 1999—when life changed. At the news conference after my win against Medvedev I told reporters that I could now leave tennis with no regrets. But one year later I realize that I was wrong. I will always have one regret—that I can't go back and relive the 1999 French Open again and again.

In the second round I face Kucera. He always has my number. The mere sight of me fills him with a quart of adrenaline. Even when I see him in the locker room before our match, he looks as if he's just been reminiscing about the time he beat me at the 1998 U.S. Open. He comes out playing superbly, running me ragged, and though I'm keeping pace, I develop blisters all over my right foot. I limp to the side and ask for an injury timeout. A trainer re-tapes my foot, but the real blister is on my brain. I don't win another game from that point on.

I look up at my box. Stefanie has her head down. She's never seen me lose like this.

Later I tell her that I don't understand why I sometimes come apart—still. She gives me insights from her experience. Stop thinking, she says. Feeling is the thing. *Feeling.*

It's nothing I haven't heard before. It sounds like a sweeter, softer version of my father. But when Stefanie says it, the words go in deeper.

We talk for days about thinking versus feeling. She says it's one thing not to think, but you can't then decide to feel. You can't *try* to feel. You have to let yourself feel.

Other times, Stefanie knows there is nothing to be said. She touches my cheek and tilts her head and I see that she gets it—that she's been there—and that's enough. That's exactly what I need.

We go to the 2000 Wimbledon. I take great pleasure in watching Stefanie explore London. At last, she says, she can actually see this beautiful city, because she's not looking at it through a haze of pressure and injuries. Tennis players travel as much as any athletes, but the stress and rigors of the game keep us from seeing. Now Stefanie gets to see everything. She walks everywhere, exploring all the shops and parks. She drops into a famous pancake restaurant she's always wanted to try. It serves 150 different kinds of pancake, and she samples just about every kind, without having to worry about feeling heavy-footed on the court.

True to form, I see nothing in London but my draw. With blinders on I fight my way to the semis. I face Rafter. He's putting together a beautiful career. Two-time U.S. Open champ. Former number one. Now they say he's trying to come back from shoulder surgery, though he's acing me left and right. When he's not acing me he's dancing in behind his serve, letting nothing past. I try lobbing him. I hit what feel like unreturnable shots as they leave my racket, but he always gets back in time. We play for three and a half hours, high-quality tennis, and it all comes down to the sixth game of the fifth set. Trying to put something extra on a second serve, I double-fault.

Break point.

I serve, he hits a crisp return, I net the ball.

I can't break him back. He's landing 74 percent of his first serves, and he first-serves his way into the final. He's earned the right to play Pete for the championship. I wanted to play Pete with Stefanie watching, but it's not to be. A year ago I beat Rafter here in the semis, when he felt the first twinges in his shoulder. Now he comes back and beats me in the semis with his shoulder fully healed. I like Rafter, and I like symmetry. I can't argue with that story line.

Stefanie and I fly home. I need rest. Then the bad news starts pouring in. My sister Tami has gotten a diagnosis of breast cancer. Days later, my mother gets the same diagnosis. I give up my spot on the Olympic team going to Sydney. I want to spend as much time as possible with my family. I need to shut down for the year, until January at least.

My mother won't hear of it.

Go, she says. Play. Do your job.

I try. I go to D.C., but play the way I always do when I can't concentrate. Against Corretja I break three rackets in anger and lose in two spiritless sets.

At the 2000 U.S. Open, I'm the number one seed. The favorite to win it. On the eve of the tournament, I sit with Gil at the Lowell Hotel, feeling not favored, but fucked. It should be a happy time. I could win this thing, I could shock the world. And I don't care.

Gil, why go on?

Maybe you shouldn't.

Why do I feel—*this* way—the old way—again?

It's a rhetorical question. Kacey is fully recovered, thriving, talking about college, but Gil never forgets what it's like to have someone you love lying in a hospital bed. He knows what I'm saying without my saying it: Why must the people we love suffer? Why can't life be perfect? Why, every day, somewhere on this earth, does someone have to lose?

You can't play, Gil says, unless you feel inspired. That's your nature. That's always been your nature, since you were nineteen years old. But you can't feel inspired unless the people around you are OK. I love you for that.

I'm letting people down if I don't play. I'm letting my family down if I do.

He nods.

Why do tennis and life always seem opposed?

He says nothing.

We've done it, haven't we? I mean, we've run the race—right? We're at the end of this bullshit, no?

I can't answer that, he says. I only know that there is still more inside you, and there is more inside me. If we walk away, fine. But we still have something left, and I think you promised yourself that you were going to see your game to the finish line.

On the first day of practice, hitting with Brad, I can't make a serve to save my life. I walk off the court, and Brad knows not to ask. I go back to the hotel and lie on the bed and stare at the ceiling for two hours, knowing I'm not going to be in New York for long.

In the first round I play a Stanford student, Alex Kim, who's sick with anxiety. I feel for him, but take him out in straight sets. In the second round I meet Clément. It's a hot day and we both have a full sweat going before the first point. I start fine, break him, go ahead 3–1. All's well. Then, suddenly, I've never played tennis before. In front of a packed house I disintegrate.

Again the sportswriters sound the old dirge. The end nears for Agassi. Gil tries to tell them what I'm going through. He says: Andre is fueled by his heart, emotions, and beliefs, and those he holds dearest to him. When all is not well you can see it in his actions.

On the way out of Arthur Ashe Stadium, a young girl says, I'm sorry you lost.

Oh honey, don't be too sorry.

She smiles.

I HURRY HOME TO VEGAS, to spend time with my mother. But she's untroubled, absorbed in her books and jigsaw puzzles, putting the rest of us to shame with her unshakable calm. I see that I've underestimated her through the years. I've mistaken her silence for weakness, acquiescence. I see that she is what my father made her, as we all are, and yet, beneath the surface, she's so much more.

I also see that, in this perilous moment of her life, she'd like a little credit. I've always taken it for granted that my mother *wanted* to be taken for granted, that she wanted to blend into the woodwork. But what she wants right now is to be noticed, appreciated. She wants me to know that she's stronger than I suspected. She's getting her treatments, not complaining, and if she takes pride in this, if she wants me to be proud, she also wants me to know I'm made of the same stuff. She survived my father, as did I. She'll survive this, and I will too.

Tami, getting treatment in Seattle, is also doing better. She's had surgery, and before she starts chemotherapy she comes to Vegas to spend time with the family. She tells me she's dreading the loss of her hair. I tell her I don't know why. Losing my hair was the best thing that ever happened to me. She laughs.

She says maybe it would be a good idea to get rid of her hair before the cancer takes it. An act of defiance, a seizing of control.

I like the sound of that, I say. I'll help.

We arrange a barbecue at my house, and before everyone arrives we shut ourselves into a bathroom. With only Philly and Stefanie as witnesses, we hold a formal head-shaving ceremony. Tami wants me to do the honors. She hands me the electric shearer. I set the blade at ooo, the tightest setting, and ask if she wants a mohawk first.

This might be your last chance to see how you look with one.

No, she says. Let's just go for broke.

I shave her fast and close. She smiles like Elvis on the day he went into the Army. As her hair cascades to the floor, I tell her everything's going to be great. You're free now, Tami. Free. Also, I tell her, at least *your* hair will grow back. With me and Philly—it's gone forever, baby. She laughs and laughs, and it feels good to make my sister laugh when every day does its best to make her cry.

BY NOVEMBER 2000 MY FAMILY is sufficiently on the mend that I'm ready to train again. In January we fly to Australia. I feel good when we land. I do love this place. I must have been an aborigine in another life. I always feel at home here. I always enjoy walking into Rod Laver Arena, playing under Laver's name.

I bet Brad that I'm going to win the whole thing. I can feel it. And when I do, he will have to jump in the Yarra River—a fetid, polluted tributary that wends through Melbourne. I batter my way to the semis and face Rafter again. We play three hours of hammer-and-tong tennis, filled with endless I-grunt-you-grunt rallies. He's ahead, two sets to one. Then he withers. The Australian heat. We're both drenched with sweat, but he's cramping. I win the next two sets.

In the final I face Clément, a grudge match four months after he knocked me out of the U.S. Open. I rarely leave the baseline. I make few mistakes, and those I do make, I put quickly behind me. While Clément is muttering to himself in French, I feel a serene calm. My mother's son. I beat him in straight sets.

It's my seventh slam, putting me tenth on the all-time list. I'm tied with McEnroe, Wilander, and others—one ahead of Becker and Edberg.

Wilander and I are the only ones to win three Australian Opens in the open era. At the moment, however, all I care about is seeing Brad do the backstroke in the Yarra, then getting home to Stefanie.

WE SPEND THE EARLY PART of 2001 nesting at Bachelor Pad II, converting it from bachelor pad to proper home. We shop for furniture that we both like. We give small dinner parties. We talk late into the night about the future. She buys me a kitchen chalkboard, for honey-do lists, but I convert it into an Appreciation Board. I hang the board on the kitchen wall and promise Stefanie that every evening I'll write something about my love for her—and the next evening I'll wipe the board clean and write something new. I also buy a crate of 1989 Beychevelle and we promise to share a bottle every year on the anniversary of our first date.

At Indian Wells I reach the final and face Pete. I beat him, and in the locker room after the match he tells me about his new life. He's recently married Bridgette Wilson, the actress.

I'm still allergic to actress, I say.

He laughs, but I'm not kidding.

He tells me he met her on the set of a movie—*Love Stinks*.

I laugh, but he's not kidding.

There is much I want to say to Pete, about marriage, about actresses, but I can't. Ours isn't that kind of relationship. There is much I'd like to ask him—about how he stays so focused, about whether or not he regrets devoting so much of his life to tennis. Our different personalities, our ongoing rivalry, precludes such intimacy. I realize that despite the effect we've had on each other, despite our quasi-friendship, we're strangers, and may always be. I wish him the best, and I mean it. To my mind, being with the right woman is true happiness. After all the time I've spent putting together my so-called team, the only thing I want now is to feel like a valued member of Stefanie's team. I hope he feels the same way about his bride. I hope he cares as much about his place in her heart as he seems to care about his place in history. I wish I could tell him so.

An hour after the tournament, Stefanie and I give a tennis lesson. Wayne Gretzky bought us at a charity auction, and he wants us to teach his kids. We have fun with the Gretzkys. Then, as darkness falls, we drive slowly back to Los Angeles. Along the way we talk about how cute the kids were. I think of the Costner kids.

Stefanie squints out the window, then at me. She says: I think I'm late.

What for?

Late.

Oh. You mean—*oh!*

We stop at several drugstores, buy every kind of pregnancy test on the shelves, then hole up at the Hotel Bel-Air. Stefanie goes into the bathroom, and when she comes out her expression is unreadable. She hands me the stick.

Blue.

What does blue mean?

I think it means—you know.

A boy?

I think it means I'm pregnant.

She does the test again. And again. Blue every time.

It's what we both wanted, and she's delighted, but frightened too. So many changes. What will happen to her body? We only have a few hours left together before I catch a red-eye to Miami and she flies to Germany. We go out to dinner, to Matsuhisa. We sit at the sushi bar, holding hands, telling each other it's going to be fantastic. I don't realize until later that this is the same restaurant where it all unraveled with Brooke. Just like tennis. The same court on which you suffer your bloodiest defeat can become the scene of your sweetest triumph.

After we're done eating and crying and celebrating, I say: I guess we should get married.

Her eyes widen. I guess so.

There will be no hoopla, we decide. No church. No cake. No dress. We'll do it on a free day during a lull in the tennis season.

I SIT DOWN FOR AN HOUR-LONG INTERVIEW with Charlie Rose, the genial TV host, during which I lie through my teeth.

I don't mean to lie, but each question Rose asks seems to come with an implied answer, an answer he's ready and eager to hear.

Did you love tennis at an early age?

Yes.

You loved the game.

I would sleep with a racket.

You look back on what your father did for you, do you say now: I'm glad that he gave me those early things that made me tough?

I'm definitely glad that I play tennis. I'm glad my dad started me in tennis.

I sound as though I've been hypnotized, or brainwashed, which isn't new. I say the same things I've said before, the same things I've mouthed during countless news conferences and interviews and cocktail-party conversations. Are they lies if I've come to partially believe them? Are they lies if, through sheer repetition, they've taken on a veneer of truth?

This time, however, the lies sound and feel different. They hang in the air, they have a bitter aftertaste. When the interview is over I feel a vague queasiness. Not guilt so much, but regret. A sense of missed opportunity. I wonder what would have happened, what Rose might have done or said, how much more we might have enjoyed the hour, if I'd leveled with him, and with myself. Actually, Charlie, I hate tennis.

The queasiness stays with me for days. It gets worse when the interview airs. I promise myself that one day I'll look an interviewer of Rose's stature right in the eye and tell him the unvarnished truth.

AT THE 2001 FRENCH OPEN, an invisible person is in my box. Stefanie is four months along, and the presence of our unborn child gives me the legs of a teenager. I reach the round of sixteen and play Squillari, with whom I have such history. It feels as we walk onto the court as if we have more history than France has with England. The sight of Squillari takes me straight back to 1999—one of the toughest matches of my career. One of the turning points. If he'd beaten me that day, two years ago, I don't know if I'd be here. I don't know if Stefanie would be here—and therefore our unborn child wouldn't be here.

Inspired by these thoughts, I'm locked in. As the match wears on, I grow fresher, more focused. My concentration is unbreakable. An unruly fan yells something obscene about me. I laugh. I take a nasty fall, twisting and cutting my knee. I shrug it off. Nothing can deter me—least of all Squillari. Gradually I lose all awareness of him. I'm out here by myself, more so than usual.

In the quarters I play Sébastien Grosjean, from France. I breeze through the first set, losing only one game, then Grosjean taps into some hidden reservoir of faith that he can win. Now our self-confidence is equal, but his shot-making is superior. He breaks me to go up 2–0, then breaks me again and wins the second set as easily as I won the first.

In the third set he breaks me right away, winning the game with a pretty lob. Then he holds, then breaks me again. I'm done for.

In the fourth set I have chances to break his serve, but I can't capitalize. I hit a backhand that's weak, unworthy of me, and as I watch it sail wide I know I'm running out of time. He's serving for the match, I'm holding on by my fingernails, and then I net a forehand. Match point. He closes me out with an ace.

Afterward, reporters ask if my concentration was broken by the arrival of President Bill Clinton. Of all the reasons I've ever heard, and offered, for losing a match, even I couldn't come up with one that lame. I didn't even know Clinton was there, I tell them. I had other things on my mind. Other invisible spectators.

I BRING STEFANIE TO GIL'S GYM, under the guise of a workout. She's beaming, because she knows why we're really here.

Gil asks Stefanie if she's feeling all right, if she'd like something to drink, if she'd like to sit. He guides her to an exercise cycle and she mounts sidesaddle. She studies the shelf Gil has built along one wall, to hold the trophies from my slams, including those I've had replaced since my post-*Friends* tantrum.

I fiddle with a stretching cord and then say: So, uhh, Gil, listen. We've picked out a name for our son.

Aw. What is it?

Jaden.

I like that, Gil says, smiling, nodding. Yes I do. I like that.

And—we also think we've got the perfect middle name.

What's that?

Gil.

He stares.

I say, Jaden Gil Agassi. If he grows up to be half the man you are, he'll be phenomenally successful, and if I can be half the father you've been to me, I'll have surpassed my own standards.

Stefanie is crying. My eyes are filled with tears. Gil is standing ten feet away, in front of the leg extension machine. He has his trademark pencil behind his ear, his glasses on the end of his nose, his da Vinci notebook open. He reaches me in three steps and folds me in his arms. I feel his necklace against my cheek. Father, Son, Holy Ghost.

I'M CLOSE TO BEATING RAFTER at the 2001 Wimbledon. Fifth set, serving for the match, two points from winning, I net a tentative forehand. On the next point I miss an easy backhand. He's broken back. Now it's he who thinks he's close to beating me.

I shout, *Motherfucker.*

336

A lineswoman promptly reports me to the umpire.

I get an obscenity warning.

Now I can think of nothing but this busybody lineswoman. I lose the set, 8–6, and the match. It feels disappointing and unimportant at the same time.

Along with Stefanie's health and our budding family, my thoughts are never far from my school, which is due to open this fall, with two hundred students, grades three through five—though we have plans to expand quickly to include kindergarten through twelfth grade. In two years we'll have the middle school built. In another two years, the high school.

I love our concepts, our designs, but I'm particularly proud of our commitment to putting money behind our ideas. Lots of money. Perry and I were horrified to learn that Nevada spends less than almost any other state on education—$6,800 per pupil, as compared with the national average of nearly $8,600. Thus, at my school we've vowed to make up the difference, and then some. Through a mix of state funding and private donors, we're going to invest heavily in kids and thereby prove that in education, as in all things, you get what you pay for.

We're also going to keep our kids in school more hours each day— eight instead of Nevada's customary six. If I've learned nothing else, it's that time and practice equal achievement. Further, we're going to insist that parents become intimately involved with the school. At least one parent per child will be required to spend twelve hours a month volunteering as a student aide in the classrooms or a monitor on school trips. We want parents to feel like shareholders. We want them fully committed and responsible for getting their children into college.

Many days, when I feel run-down or low, I drive to the neighborhood and watch the school take shape. Of all my contradictions, this is the most amazing, and the most amusing—a boy who despised and feared school becomes a man inspired and reenergized by the sight of his own school being built.

I can't be there on opening day, however. I'm playing in the 2001 U.S. Open. I'm playing *for* the school, therefore playing my best. I burn through four rounds and meet Pete in the quarters. From the moment we come out of the tunnel, we know this will be our fiercest battle yet. We just know. It's the thirty-second time we've played, he leads 17–14, and each of us wears an unusually grim game face. Right here, right now, this one will decide the rivalry. Winner take all.

Pete is supposed to be at half speed. He hasn't won a slam in fourteen months. He's been balky, and openly talking retirement. But all of that is irrelevant, because he's playing me. Still, I win the first set in a tiebreak, and now I feel good about my chances. I have a 49–1 record at this tournament when I win the first set.

Someone please remind Pete of the stats. He wins the second set in a tiebreak.

The third set also goes to a tiebreak. I make several foolish mistakes. Fatigue. He wins the third set.

In the fourth set we have several epic rallies. We go to still another tiebreak. We've played three hours, and neither of us has yet broken the other's serve. It's after midnight. The fans—23,000 plus—rise. They won't let us start the fourth tiebreak. Stomping and clapping, they're staging their own tiebreak. Before we press on they want to say thanks.

I'm moved. I see that Pete is moved. But I can't think about the fans. I can't let myself think about anything but reaching the sanctuary of a fifth set.

Pete knows that the advantage tips in my direction if this goes five sets. He knows that he needs to play a perfect tiebreak to prevent a fifth set. And so he does. A night of flawless tennis ends with my forehand in the net.

Pete screams.

I actually feel my pulse decrease. I don't feel bad. I try to feel bad, but I can't. I wonder if I'm growing accustomed to losing to Pete in big matches, or simply growing content with my career and life. Whatever the case, I put my hand on Pete's shoulder and wish him well, and though it doesn't feel like goodbye, it feels like a rehearsal for a goodbye that can't be far off.

IN OCTOBER 2001, three days before Stefanie is due to give birth, we invite our mothers and a Nevada judge to the house.

I love watching Stefanie with my mother. The two shy women in my life. Stefanie often brings her a couple of new jigsaw puzzles. And I adore Stefanie's mother, Heidi. She looks like Stefanie, so she had me at *guten tag.* Stefanie and I, barefoot and wearing jeans, stand before the judge in the courtyard. For wedding bands we use twists of old raffia Stefanie found in a drawer—the same stuff I used to decorate her first birthday card. Neither of us notices the coincidence until later.

My father insists he's not the least bit slighted by not getting an invite. He doesn't want an invite. The last thing he wants to do is attend a wedding. He doesn't like weddings. (He walked out in the middle of my first.) He doesn't care where or when or how I make Stefanie my wife, he says, so long as I do it. She's the greatest women's tennis player of all time, he says. What's not to like?

The judge runs through his legal rigmarole, and Stefanie and I are just about to say I do, when a team of landscapers arrive. I run outside and ask them to please turn off their lawnmowers and leaf blowers for five minutes so that we can get married. They apologize. One holds a finger over his lips.

By the power vested in me, the judge says, and at last, at long last, with two mothers and three landscapers looking on, Steffi Graf becomes Stefanie Agassi.

26

A SEASON OF BIRTH AND REBIRTH. Weeks after my school opens, my son arrives. In the delivery room, when the doctor hands me Jaden Gil, I feel bewildered. I love him so much that my heart splits open, like something overripe. I can't wait to get to know him, and yet, and yet. I also wonder, Just who is this beautiful intruder? Are Stefanie and I ready for a perfect stranger in the house? I'm a stranger to myself—what will I be to my son? Will he like me?

We bring Jaden home, and I spend hours staring at him. I ask him who he is, where he came from, what he'll be. I ask myself how I can be everything to him that I needed and never had. I want to retire, immediately, spend all my time with him. But now more than ever I need to play. For him, his future, and my other children at my school.

My first match as a father is a win against Rafter at the Tennis Masters Series tournament in Sydney. I tell reporters afterward that I doubt I'll be able to do this long enough that my new son will get to see me play, but it sure is a nice dream.

Then I pull out of the 2002 Australian Open. My wrist is throbbing, and I can't compete. Brad is frustrated. I wouldn't expect anything less. But this time he has trouble brushing aside his frustration. This time is different.

Days later he says we need to talk. We meet for coffee, and he lays it out.

We've had a great run, Andre, but we've gone as far as we can go. We're growing stagnant. Creatively. I've burned through my bag of tricks, buddy.

But—

We've had eight years, we could go on a few more, but you're thirty-two. You have a new family, new interests. It might not be such a bad idea to find a new voice for your home stretch. Someone to re-motivate you.

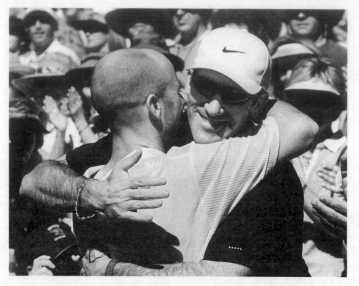

After beating Pete at Indian Wells, I celebrate with Brad, not knowing
it will be one of our last tournament victories together.

He pauses. He looks at me, then looks away. Bottom line, he says.
We're so close, my worst fear is that we get into an argument as the end
approaches, and it carries over.

I think: That could never happen, but better safe than sorry.

We hug.

As he walks out the door I feel the kind of melancholy you feel on a
Sunday night after an idyllic weekend. I know Brad does too. It might not
be the right way to end our journey, but it's the best way possible.

I CLOSE MY EYES and try to picture myself with someone new. The
first face I see is Darren Cahill. He's just finished a brilliant span coaching
Lleyton Hewitt, who's ranked number one, and among the best shot
selectors in the history of tennis, and a great deal of the credit must go to
Darren. Also, I recently bumped into Darren down in Sydney and we had
a long talk about fatherhood. It was a bonding moment. Darren, a fellow
new father, turned me on to a book about getting infants to sleep. He
swore by this book and said his son is known on tour as the baby who
sleeps like a drunkard.

I've always liked Darren. I like his easygoing style. I find his Aussie accent soothing. It almost puts *me* to sleep. I read the book he recommended and phoned Stefanie from Australia to read her passages. It worked. Now I dial him and tell him I've parted from Brad. I ask if he has any interest in the job.

He says he's flattered, but he's on the verge of signing to coach Safin. He'll think about it, though, and get back to me.

No problem, I say. Take your time.

I call him back in half an hour. I ask him, What the hell is there to think about? You can't coach Safin. He's a loose cannon. You've *got* to work with me. It feels right. I promise you, Darren, I have game left. I'm not done. I'm *focused*—I just need someone to help me keep the focus.

OK, he says, laughing. OK, mate.

He never once mentions money.

STEFANIE AND JADEN COME WITH ME to Key Biscayne. It's April 2002, days before my thirty-second birthday, and the tournament is crawling with players half my age, young Turks like Andy Roddick, the next *next* savior of American tennis, poor bastard. Also, there's a hot new wunderkind from Switzerland named Roger Federer.

I'd like to win this tournament for my wife and six-month-old son, and yet I don't worry about losing, don't care if I lose, *because* of them. Each night, within minutes of coming home from the courts, as I'm cradling Jaden and cuddling Stefanie, I can barely recall if I won or lost. Tennis fades as quickly as the daylight. I almost imagine that the calluses on my playing hand are disappearing, the inflamed nerves in my back cooling and mending. I'm a father first, a tennis player second, and this evolution happens without my being aware.

One morning Stefanie goes off to buy groceries and get in a fast workout. She dares to leave me alone with Jaden. My first time flying solo.

You two going to be OK? she asks.

Of course.

I sit Jaden on the bathroom counter, lean him against the mirror, let him play with my toothbrush while I get ready. He likes to suck on the toothbrush while watching me shave my head with the electric shearers.

I ask him, What do you think of your bald daddy?

He smiles.

You know, son, I was once like you: long hair flowing in every direction. You're not fooling anyone with that comb-over.

He smiles wider, no idea what I'm saying, of course.

I measure his hair with my fingers.

Actually, you look a little ratty there, buddy. You could use a clean-up.

I put a different attachment on the shearer, the attachment for trimming. When I run the shearer across Jaden's little head, however, it leaves a bright stripe of scalp down the middle, as white as a baseline.

Wrong attachment.

Stefanie will murder me. I need to even this boy's hair out before she gets home. But in my frantic attempt to even out the hair, I make it shorter. Before I know what's happened, my son is balder than I. He looks like Mini-Me.

When Stefanie comes through the door she stops in her tracks and stares, saucer-eyed. What the—? Andre, she says, what on earth is the matter with you? I leave you alone for forty-five minutes and *you shave the baby*?

Then she lets fly a burst of histrionic German.

I tell her it was an accident. The wrong attachment. I beg her forgiveness.

I know, I say, it looks like I did this on purpose. I know I'm always joking about wanting to *shave the world*. But honest, Stefanie, this was a mistake.

I try to remind her of that old wives' tale, that if you shave a child's head the hair will grow back faster and thicker, but she holds up a hand and starts laughing. She's bent over laughing. Now Jaden is laughing at Mommy laughing. Now we're all giggling, rubbing Jaden's head and mine, joking that the only one left is Stefanie, and she'd better sleep with one eye open. I'm laughing too hard to speak, and days later, in the final of Key Biscayne, I beat Federer. It's a good win. He's as hot as anyone on tour. He came into this tournament with twenty-three wins so far this year.

It's my fifty-first tournament victory, my seven hundredth victory overall. And yet I have no doubt I'll remember this tournament less for beating Federer than for that one belly laugh. I wonder if the laugh had something to do with the win. It's easier to be free and loose, to be yourself, after laughing with the ones you love. The right attachments.

I FALL INTO A NICE GROOVE with Darren in early 2002. We speak the same language, see the world in similar colors. Then he cements my trust, my unwavering confidence, by daring to fuss with my racket strings—and improving them.

I've always played with ProBlend, a string that's half Kevlar, half nylon. You can reel in an eight-hundred-pound marlin with ProBlend. It never breaks, never forgives, but also never generates spin. It's like hitting the ball with a garbage can lid. People talk about the game changing, about players growing more powerful, and rackets getting bigger, but the most dramatic change in recent years is the strings. The advent of a new elastic polyester string, which creates vicious topspin, has turned average players into greats, and greats into legends.

Still, I've always been reluctant to change. Now Darren urges me to try. We're in Italy, at the Italian Open. I've just played Nicolas Kiefer, from Germany, in the first round. I've beaten him, 6–3, 6–2, and I'm telling Darren that I should have lost. I played lousy. I have no confidence on this dirt, I tell him. The clay game has passed me by.

Give the new string a go, mate.

I frown. I'm skeptical. I tried changing my racket once. It wasn't pretty.

He puts the string on one of my rackets and says again, Just try.

In a practice session I don't miss a ball for two hours. Then I don't miss a ball for the rest of the tournament. I've never won the Italian Open before, but I win it now, because of Darren and his miracle string.

I SUDDENLY LOOK FORWARD TO the 2002 French Open. I'm excited, eager for the fight, and guardedly optimistic. I'm coming off a win, Jaden is sleeping a bit more, and I have a new weapon. In the fourth round I'm down two sets and a break to a wild card, a Frenchman named Paul-Henri Mathieu. He's twenty, but he's not in the shape I'm in. There's no clock in tennis, son. I can be out here all day.

Down comes the rain. I sit in the locker room and reminisce about Brad yelling at me in 1999. I hear his tirade, word for word. When we walk back onto the court I'm smiling. I'm up 40–love, and Mathieu breaks me. I don't care. I simply break back. In the fifth set he goes up, 3–1. Again I refuse to lose.

If it had been anyone but Agassi, Mathieu tells reporters afterward, I would have won.

Next I face Juan Carlos Ferrero, from Spain. Again it rains; this time I ask that the match be halted for the night. Ferrero is ahead, and he doesn't want to stop. He gets surly when officials grant my request and suspend the match. The next day he takes his surliness out on me. I have a small opportunity in the third set, but he quickly closes it. He wins the set, and I can see his confidence rising off him like steam as he closes me out.

I feel peaceful walking with Darren off the court. I like the way I played. I made mistakes, my game sprang leaks, but I know we'll work to patch them. My back is sore, but mostly from stooping to help Jaden walk. A wonderful soreness.

Weeks later we go to the 2002 Wimbledon, and my great new attitude abandons me, because my new string undoes me. On grass my newly augmented topspin makes the ball sit up like a helium balloon. In the second round I play Paradorn Srichaphan, from Thailand. He's good, but not this good. He's crushing everything I hit. He's ranked number sixty-seven, and I think it's impossible that he'll beat me, and then he breaks me in the first set.

I try everything to get back on track. Nothing works. My ball is a cream puff, and Srichaphan devours it. I've never seen an opponent's eyes grow quite so large as Srichaphan's when he tees up my forehand. He's swinging from his heels, and my only conscious, coherent thought is: I wish I could swing from my heels and be rewarded. How can I let everyone in this stadium know that this isn't me, this isn't my fault? It's the strings. In the second set I make adjustments, fight back, play well, but Srichaphan is supremely confident. He thinks it's his day, and when you think it's your day, it usually is. He hits a wild shot that magically catches a piece of the back line, then wins a tiebreak, going up two sets. In the third set I surrender peacefully.

It's cold comfort that, the same day, Pete loses.

Darren and I spend the next two days experimenting with different combinations of strings. I tell him I can't continue with his new polyester, and yet he's ruined me for the old string. If I have to go back to Pro-Blend, I say, I won't play tennis anymore.

He looks grim. After being my coach for six months, he's made one tiny adjustment to my strings, and he may have inadvertently hastened my retirement. He promises that he'll do everything in his power to find a combination of strings that's just right.

Find something, I tell him, that lets me swing from my heels and get rewarded. Like Srichaphan. Make me like Srichaphan.

Done, mate.

He works night and day and comes up with a combination he likes. We go to Los Angeles, and it's perfection. I win the Mercedes-Benz Cup.

We go to Cincinnati and I play well, just not well enough to win. Then in D.C. I beat Enqvist, always a tough matchup for me. I then face another kid who's supposed to be the next big thing—twenty-two-year-old James Blake. He plays pretty, graceful tennis, and I'm not in his league, not today. He's simply younger, faster, a better athlete. He also thinks enough of my history, my accomplishments, to bring his A game. I like that he comes out loaded for bear. It's flattering, even though it means I have no chance. The loss is nothing I can blame on my strings.

I go to the 2002 U.S. Open unsure what to expect from myself. I sail through the early rounds, and in the quarters I face Max Mirnyi, a Belarusian from Minsk. They call him the Beast, and it's an understatement. He's six foot five and hits a serve that's among the scariest I've ever faced. It has a burning yellow tail, like a comet, as it arcs high above the net and then swoops down upon you. I have no answer for that serve. He wins the first set with beastly ease.

In the second set, however, Mirnyi makes several unforced errors, giving me a boost, a bit of momentum. I start to see his first serve a little better. We play high-quality tennis all the way to the finish, and when his last forehand flies long, I can't believe it. I'm in the semis.

For my efforts I win a date with Hewitt, the number one seed, the winner of this year's Wimbledon. More germane, he's Darren's former pupil. That Darren coached Hewitt for years adds an extra level of intensity and pressure. Darren wants me to beat Hewitt; I want to beat Hewitt for Darren. But in the first set I quickly fall behind, 0–3. I have all this information in my head about Hewitt, data from Darren and from past experience, but it takes a while to sort through the data and solve him. When I do, everything quickly changes. I storm back and win the first set, 6–4. I see the pilot light in Hewitt's eyes go out. I win the second set. He rallies, wins the third. In the fourth set he suddenly can't make a first serve, and I'm able to pounce on his second. Jesus, I'm in the final.

Which means Pete. As always, Pete. We've played thirty-three times in our careers, four times in slam finals. He's got the overall edge, 19–14, and 3–1 in slam finals. He says I bring out the best in him, but I think he's brought out the worst in me. The night before the final I can't help but think of all the different times I thought I was going to beat Pete, knew I was going to beat Pete, needed to beat Pete, only to lose. And his success against me started right here, in New York, twelve years ago, when he stunned me in straight sets. I was the favorite then, as I am now.

Sipping Gil's magic water before bed, I tell myself that this time will be different. Pete hasn't won a slam in more than two years. He's nearing the end. I'm just starting over.

I climb under the covers and remember a time in Palm Springs, several years ago. Brad and I were eating at an Italian restaurant, Mama Gina's, and we saw Pete eating with friends on the other side of the dining room. He stopped by and said hello on his way out. Good luck tomorrow. You too. Then we watched him through the restaurant window, waiting for his car. We said nothing, each of us thinking of the difference he'd made in our lives. As Pete drove away I asked Brad how much he thought Pete tipped the valet.

Brad hooted. Five bucks, tops.

No way, I said. The guy's got millions. He's earned forty mil in prize money alone. He's got to be good for at least a ten spot.

Bet?

Bet.

We ate fast and rushed outside. Listen, I told the valet, give us the absolute truth: How much did Mr. Sampras tip you?

The kid looked at his feet. He didn't want to tell. He was weighing, wondering if he was on a hidden-camera show.

We told the kid we had a bet riding on this, so we absolutely were insisting he tell us. Finally he whispered: You really want to know?

Shoot.

He gave me a dollar.

Brad put a hand on his heart.

But that's not all, the kid said. He gave me a dollar—and he told me to be sure to give it to whichever kid actually brought his car around.

We could not be more different, Pete and I, and as I fall asleep the night before perhaps our *final* final, I vow that the world will see our differences tomorrow.

WE GET A LATE START, thanks to a New York Jets game that goes into overtime, delaying the TV broadcast, and this favors me. I'm in better shape, and I like that we're going to be out on the court until midnight. But I immediately fall behind two sets. Another drubbing at the hands of Pete—I cannot *believe* this is happening.

Then I notice Pete looking wrung out. And old. I win the third set by a mile, and the whole stadium can feel the momentum slide my way. The crowd is crazy. They don't care who wins, they just want to see an Agassi-Sampras five-setter. As the fourth set gets under way I know, deep in my heart, as I always know with Pete, that if I can get this thing to a fifth set, I'll win. I'm fresher. I'm playing better. We're the oldest players to meet in

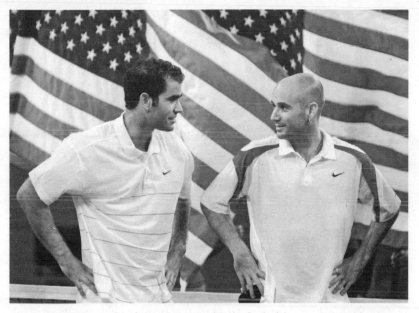

A private word with Pete Sampras after the final of the 2002 U.S. Open

the U.S. Open final in more than thirty years, but I'm feeling like one of the teenagers who have lately been kicking ass on tour. I feel like part of the new generation.

At 1–2, Pete is serving, and I have two break points. If I win this game I'll take the control of the set. So this is it, the game of the match. He locks in, saves the first, and on the second break point I hit a scorching return at his shoes. I think the ball is well behind him—I'm already celebrating—but somehow he turns and finds it and hits a half-volley that flops and dies on my side of the net. Deuce.

I'm spooked. Pete closes out the game, then goes on to break me.

Soon he's serving for the match, and when Pete serves for a match, he's a coldblooded killer. Everything happens very fast.

Ace. Blur. Backhand volley, no way to reach it.

Applause. Handshake at the net.

Pete gives me a friendly smile, a pat on the back, but the expression on his face is unmistakable. I've seen it before.

Here's a buck, kid. Bring my car around.

27

I OPEN MY EYES SLOWLY. I'm on the floor beside my bed. I sit up to say good morning to Stefanie, then realize she's in Vegas and I'm in St. Petersburg. No, wait—St. Petersburg was last week.

I'm in Paris.

No, Paris was after St. Petersburg.

I'm in Shanghai. Yes, that's right, China.

I go to the window, draw back the curtains. A skyline designed by someone on mushrooms. A skyline that looks like a sci-fi Vegas. Every building is crazily different, and all set against a hard blue sky. It doesn't matter where I am, strictly speaking, because parts of me are still in Russia and France and the last dozen places I've played. And the biggest part of me, as always, is home with Stefanie and Jaden.

No matter where I am, however, the tennis court is the same, and so is the goal—I want to be number one at the end of 2002. If I can put together a win here in Shanghai, one little win, I'll be the oldest year-end number one in men's tennis history, breaking Connors's record.

He's a punk—you're a legend!

I want this, I tell myself. I don't need it, but I do want it.

I order coffee from room service, then sit at the desk and write in my journal. It's not like me to keep a journal, but I've recently begun one, and it's quickly become a habit. I'm compelled to write. I'm obsessed with leaving a record, in part because I've developed a gnawing fear that I won't be around long enough for Jaden to know me. I live on airplanes, and with the world becoming more dangerous, more unpredictable, I fear that I won't be able to tell Jaden all that I've seen and learned. So every night, wherever I am, I jot a few lines to him. Random thoughts, impressions, lessons learned. Now, before going to the Shanghai stadium, I write:

Hey Buddy. You're in Vegas with Mom and I'm in Shanghai, missing you. I have a chance at finishing number one after this tournament. But I promise I can only think about getting home to you. I put a lot of pressure on myself with my tennis. But I'm strangely driven to continue. It took me a while to figure that out. I fought it for so long. Now I just work as hard as I can and let the rest fall where it may. It still doesn't feel great most of the time, but I push through it, for the sake of so much good. Good for the game, good for your future, good for many at my school. Always value others, Jaden. There is so much peace in taking care of people. I love you and am there for you always.

I close the journal, walk out of the room, and get clipped by Jiri Novak, from the Czech Republic. Humiliating. Worse, I can't leave the country and go home. I have to hang around an extra day to play a kind of consolation match.

Back at the hotel, choked with emotion, I write again to Jaden:

I just lost my match and I feel terrible. I don't want to go back out there tomorrow. So much so I was actually wishing for an injury. Picture that, not wanting to do something so much that you wish upon yourself injury. Jaden, if you ever feel overwhelmed with something like I was tonight, just keep your head down and keep working and keep trying. Face it at its worst and realize it's not so bad. That will be your chance for peace. I wanted to quit and leave and go home and see you. It's hard to stay and play, it's easy to go home and be with you. That's why I'm staying.

AT THE END OF THE YEAR, as expected, Hewitt is number one. I tell Gil we need to take it up a notch. He outlines a new regimen for the older me. He pulls ideas from his da Vinci notebooks, and we spend weeks working solely on my deteriorating lower body. Day in, day out, he stands over me as I build my legs, yelling, *Big thunder! Australia's calling!*

Weak legs command, Gil says. Strong legs obey.

By the time we board the Ambien Express, Vegas to Melbourne, I feel as if I could run or swim there. I'm the second seed in the 2003 Australian Open, and I come out growling, ferocious. I reach the semis and beat Ferreira in ninety minutes. In six matches I've dropped only one set.

In the final I face Rainer Schuettler, from Germany. I win three straight sets, losing only five games and tying the most lopsided victory ever at the Australian Open. My eighth slam, and it's my best performance ever. I tease Stefanie that it's like one of her matches, the closest I'll ever come to experiencing her kind of dominance.

As they hand me the trophy, I tell the crowd: There's not a single day that's guaranteed to us, and certainly days like this are very rare.

Someone says later that I sounded as if I'd had a near-death experience.

More like a near-life experience. It's how a person talks when he almost didn't live.

I'm the oldest player in thirty-one years to win a slam, and reporters won't let me hear the end of it. Again and again, before I leave Australia, reporters ask if I have a plan for retirement. I tell them I don't plan endings any more than I plan beginnings. I'm the last of a generation, they say. Last of the 1980s Mohicans. Chang announces he's retiring. Courier is already three years into his retirement. People treat me like a codger, because Stefanie is expecting again and it's well known that we tool around Vegas in a minivan. Still, I feel eternal.

Ironically, my lack of flexibility seems to be stretching out my career. It helps my durability. Since I can't turn well, I always keep the racket close to my body, always keep the ball out in front of me. Thus, I don't put unnecessary stress and torque on my frame. With such form, Gil says, my body might have another three years in it.

AFTER A SHORT BREATHER IN VEGAS, we fly to Key Biscayne. I've won this tournament two years in a row, five times overall, and nothing can stop me. I reach the final and beat Moyá, my old adversary from the French Open, who's ranked number five. Straight sets. My sixth win here, which tops Stefanie's record. Again, I tease her about finally doing something better than she did it. She's so competitive, however, I know not to tease her too much.

PLAYING IN THE U.S. MEN'S CLAY COURT CHAMPIONSHIPS, in Houston, I just need to reach the finals and I'll be ranked number one again. And I do. I beat Jürgen Melzer, 6–4, 6–1, and go out with Darren and Gil to celebrate. I throw down several vodka-cranberries. I don't care that I'm playing in the final against Roddick tomorrow—I'm already ranked number one.

Which is why I beat him. That perfect blend of caring and not caring, the best preparation.

Days before my thirty-third birthday, I'm the oldest player ever ranked number one. I fly to Rome, feeling like Ponce de León, and get off the plane feeling a geriatric twinge in my shoulder. In the first round I play poorly, but don't dwell on it, put it out of my mind. Weeks later, at the 2003 French Open, my shoulder is still sore, but my practices are crisp. Darren says I'm a force.

In the second round, I'm on the Suzanne Lenglen Court, a court filled with bad memories. Losing to Woodruff in 1996. Losing to Safin in 1998. I'm playing a kid from Croatia, Mario Ancic. I lose the first two sets and trail in the third. He's nineteen years old, six foot five, a serve-and-volleyer with no fear of me. The Lenglen court is supposed to be denser, slower, but today the ball is moving fast. I'm having an unusually hard time controlling it. I gather myself, however, and win the next two sets. In the fifth, exhausted, my shoulder falling off, I have match point four times, and lose them all. I double fault three of them. I beat the kid, at last, but only because he's slightly more afraid of losing than I am.

I'm in the quarters against Guillermo Coria, from Argentina, another youngster. He says publicly I'm his idol. Listen, I tell reporters, I'd rather not be his idol and play him on hard court than be his idol and play him on clay. How I hate this dirt. I lose four of the first five games. Then I win the set. How I love this dirt.

Coria shows no emotion, however. In the second set he jumps out to a 5–1 lead. He misses nothing. He's fast and getting faster. Was I ever that fast? I try to confuse him, rush the net—to no avail. He's just better than me today. He knocks me out of the tournament, and out of the number one slot.

In England, at a warm-up tournament before Wimbledon, I beat Peter Luczak, from Australia. It's the one thousandth match of my career. When someone tells me this, I feel an overpowering need to sit down. I have a glass of wine with Stefanie and try to run my mind over all one thousand matches. I remember every one of them, I tell her.

Of course, she says.

For Stefanie's birthday I take her to see Annie Lennox in London. She's one of Stefanie's favorites, but tonight she's my muse. Tonight she's

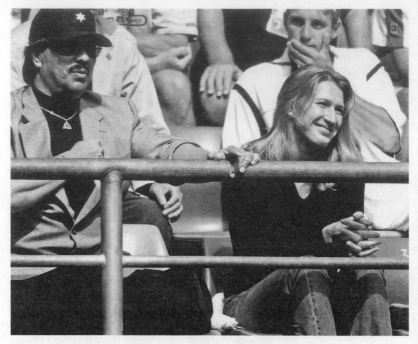

My two greatest sources of strength, Gil and Stefanie, sitting in my box
at the 2003 Australian Open

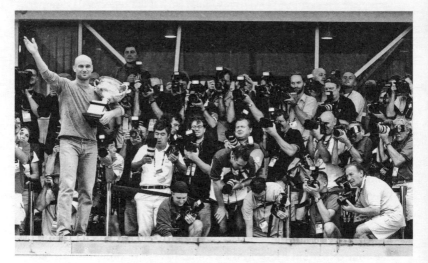

Shortly after winning the 2003 Australian Open

singing, speaking, directly to me. In fact I make a point to tell Gil that we'll need to include some Lennox on *Belly Cramps 2*. I might listen to her before every match.

> *This is the path I'll never tread*
> *These are the dreams I'll dream instead . . .*

I'M ONE OF THE FAVORITES at the 2003 Wimbledon. How? No father has won Wimbledon since the 1980s. Fathers don't win slams. In the third round I play Younes El Aynaoui, from Morocco. He's a new father too. I joke with reporters that I look forward to playing a man who gets as little sleep as I.

In his pre-match instructions Darren says: When you get this guy bled out to the backhand, early in the match, when you see him hit his slice, be sure to take it out of the air. That way you'll put him on notice that he can't get away with safe shots from a defensive position. He needs to hit something special. That's how you'll send him a message early and force him into errors later in the match.

Good advice. I quickly grab a lead, two sets to one, but El Aynaoui won't cave. He pours it on in the fourth, gets three set points. I don't want this thing going five. I refuse to let it go five. The final points of the fourth set are grueling, and I do everything required, everything Darren advised. When it's over, when I've won the set and match, I'm wiped out. I have a day off, but I know it's not nearly enough.

In the fourth round I face Mark Philippoussis, an Australian kid with tons of talent and a reputation for squandering it. His serve is big, infamously big, and never bigger than today. He's topping out at 140 miles an hour. He aces me forty-six times. Still, the match goes where we both know it's going, a fifth set. At 3–4, he's serving, and somehow I have break point. He misses the first serve. I taste the victory. He unloads a 138-mile-per-hour second serve, straight up the middle. Obscene speed, but that's right where I thought he'd hit it. I put the racket out, reflex the ball back to him, and he can only stand and watch. He almost gets whiplash. And yet it lands a half inch behind the baseline. Out.

Had it fallen in, I'd have had the break, the momentum, and I'd be serving for the match. But it's not to be. Now, believing he can win, Philippoussis stands a little taller, and breaks me. It's all gone in a blink. One minute, I'm almost serving for the match, the next minute he's raising his arms in conquest. Tennis.

In the locker room my body feels different. Grass has become an ordeal, and a five-setter on grass leaves me physically shattered. Also, the courts at Wimbledon are playing truer this year, which has meant longer rallies, more movement, more lunging and bending. My back is suddenly an issue. It's never been good, but now it's actively, troublingly bad. Pain runs from my back, down my butt, circumvents my knee, then reconnects with my shin and shoots down to my ankle. I'm grateful that I haven't beaten Philippoussis, that I haven't advanced in the tournament, because I'd have to forfeit the next match.

AS THE 2003 U.S. OPEN GETS UNDER WAY, Pete announces his retirement. He stops several times during his news conference to collect himself. I find myself deeply affected as well. Our rivalry has been one of the lodestars of my career. Losing to Pete has caused me enormous pain, but in the long run it's also made me more resilient. If I'd beaten Pete more often, or if he'd come along in a different generation, I'd have a better record, and I might go down as a better player, but I'd be less.

For hours after Pete's news conference I feel a sharp loneliness. I'm the last one standing. I'm the last American slam winner still playing. I tell reporters: You sort of expect to leave the dance with the ones you came with. Then I realize this is the wrong analogy, because I'm not leaving the dance—they are. I'm still dancing.

I reach the quarters. I face Coria, who knocked me out of the French Open. I'm itching to lace them up, get out there, but we're delayed for days by rain. Holed up in the hotel, there is nothing to do but wait and read. I watch raindrops slide down the window, each one as gray as the hairs of my stubble. Each raindrop seems like a minute forever melting away.

Gil forces me to drink Gil Water and rest. He says it's going to be good, but he knows. Time is running out. Finally the clouds part and we're on the court and Coria isn't the same guy I saw in Paris. He has a leg injury, which I exploit. I run him, merciless, grind him down to dust, and win the first two sets.

In the third set I have four match points—and lose them all. I look to the box and see Gil, squirming. In my entire career he's never once taken a bathroom break during one of my matches. Never. Not once. He says he doesn't want to take the chance that I'll look to my box and not see him there and panic. He deserves better than this. I refocus. I click the lens left, then right, and serve out the match.

There is no time to rest. All the rain has shrunk the tournament schedule. I have to play the semifinal the next day, against Ferrero, who just won the French Open. He has so much confidence, it's shooting from his pores. He's a hundred years younger than I am, and it shows. He puts me away in four sets.

I bow to all four corners, blow kisses to the crowd, and I think they know I've given them everything. I see Jaden and Stefanie waiting outside the locker room, Stefanie eight months pregnant with our second child, and the disappointment of the loss slides away like a raindrop.

OUR DAUGHTER IS BORN OCTOBER 3, 2003, another beautiful intruder. We name her Jaz Elle—and, as we did with our son, we secretly vow she won't play tennis. (We don't even have a tennis court in our backyard.) But there is something else that Jaz Agassi won't do—sleep. She makes her brother seem like a narcoleptic. Thus, I leave for the 2004 Australian Open looking like a vampire. Every other player, meanwhile, looks as if he's had twelve hours of sack time. They're all bright-eyed— and muscular. They seem bulkier than in years past, as if they all have their own Gils.

My legs stay fresh until the semis, when I run into Safin, who plays like a dingo. He missed most of last year with a wrist injury. Now, fully healed and rested, he's unstoppable. Side to side, back and forth, our rallies take forever. Each of us refuses to miss, to make an un- forced error, and after four hours neither of us wants the win any less. In fact, we each want it a little more. The difference is Safin's serve. He takes the fifth set, and I wonder if I've just had my last hurrah in Australia.

Is this the end? I've heard this question every other day for months, years, but this is the first time I'm the one asking.

REST IS YOUR FRIEND, Gil says. You need more rest between tour- naments, and you need to choose your battles ever more carefully. Rome and Hamburg? Pass. Davis Cup? Sorry, can't do it. You need to save up your sap for the big ones, and the next big one is the French Open.

As a result, when we arrive in Paris, I feel years younger. Darren looks over my draw and projects a clear path to the semis.

In the first round I play Jérôme Haehnel, a twenty-three-year-old from Alsace, ranked number 271, who doesn't even have a coach. No problem, Darren says.

Big problem. I come out flat. Every backhand finds the net. I scream at myself, You're *better* than this! It's not over yet! Don't let it end like this! Gil, sitting in the front row, purses his lips.

It's not just age, and it's not just the clay. I'm not hitting the ball cleanly. I'm rested, but rusty from the time off.

Newspapers call it the worst loss of my career. Haehnel tells reporters that his friends pumped him up before the match by assuring him that he was going to win, because I'd recently lost to a player just like him. Asked what he meant by a player just like him, he says: Bad.

We're down the homestretch, Gil tells reporters—all I can ask is that we don't limp across the finish line.

Come June, I pull out of Wimbledon. I've lost four straight matches—my worst losing streak since 1997—and my bones feel like china. Gil sits me down and says he doesn't know how much longer he can watch me go on like this. I need to think long and hard, for both our sakes, about the end.

I tell him I'll think about my retirement, but first I need to think about Stefanie's. She's been voted into the International Tennis Hall of Fame, of course: she has more slams than anyone in the history of tennis besides Margaret Court. She wants me to introduce her at the induction ceremony. We fly to Newport, Rhode Island. A big day. The first time we've ever left the children with someone else overnight, and the first time I've ever seen Stefanie truly, rigidly nervous. She dreads the ceremony. She doesn't want the attention. She worries that she'll say the wrong thing or forget to thank someone. She's shaking.

I'm not all that loose myself. I've obsessed for weeks about my speech. It's the first time I've ever spoken in public about Stefanie, and it's like writing something on the kitchen Appreciation Board for the world to read. J.P. helps me work through various drafts. I'm overprepared, and as I walk to the dais, I'm breathing hard. Then, the moment I start speaking, I relax, because the subject is my favorite and I consider myself an expert. Every man should have the chance to introduce his wife at her Hall of Fame induction ceremony.

I look out over the crowd, the fans, the faces of former champions, and I want to tell them about Stefanie. I want them to know what I know.

I compare her to the artisans and craftsmen who built the great medieval cathedrals: they didn't curtail their perfectionism when building the roof or the cellar or other unseen parts of the cathedrals. They were perfectionists about every crevice and invisible corner—and that's Stefanie. And yet also she's a cathedral, a monument to perfection. I spend five minutes extolling her work ethic, her dignity, her legacy, her strength, her grace. In closing, I utter the truest thing I've ever said about her.

Ladies and gentleman, I introduce you to the greatest person I have ever known.

28

EVERYONE AROUND ME TALKS INCESSANTLY OF RETIREMENT. Stefanie's retirement, Pete's retirement, mine. Meanwhile, I do nothing but play and keep my eye on the next slam. In Cincinnati, to everyone's surprise, I beat Roddick in the semis, which propels me to my first ATP final since last November. Then I beat Hewitt, making me the oldest winner of an ATP event since Connors.

The next month, at the 2004 U.S. Open, I tell reporters that I think I have a shot at winning this whole thing. They smile as if I'm demented.

Stefanie and I rent a house outside the city, in Westchester. It's roomier than a hotel, and we don't have to worry about pushing the stroller across busy Manhattan streets. Best of all, the house has a basement playroom, which is my bedroom the night before a match. In the basement I can move from the bed to the floor when my back wakes me, without disturbing Stefanie. Since fathers don't win slams, Stefanie likes to say, you can go to the basement and feel as single as you need to feel.

I see my life wearing on her. I'm a distracted husband, a tired father. She needs to carry more of the load with the children. Still, she never complains. She understands. Her mission, her passion every day, is to create an atmosphere in which I can think solely about tennis. She remembers how vital that was when she played. For instance, driving to the stadium, Stefanie knows exactly which Elmo songs on the car stereo will keep Jaden and Jaz quiet, so Darren and I can talk strategy. Also, she's like Gil about food: she never forgets that when you eat is as important as what you eat. After a match, driving home with Darren and Gil, I know that as we walk through the door there will be hot lasagna piled on a plate, the cheese still bubbling.

I also know Darren's kids and Jaden and Jaz will be fed and clean and tucked away for the night.

Because of Stefanie, I make it to the quarters, where I face the number one seed, Federer. He's not the man I beat in Key Biscayne. He's growing before my eyes into one of the game's all-time greats. He methodically builds a lead, two sets to one, and I can't help but stand back and admire his immense skills, his magnificent composure. He's the most regal player I've ever witnessed. Before he can finish me off, however, play is halted due to rain.

Driving back to Westchester, I stare out the window and tell myself: Don't think about tomorrow. Also, don't even think about dinner, because the match was cut short and I'm coming home hours earlier than expected. But of course Stefanie has a source with the weather service. Someone gave her a heads-up about the storm as it was swooping down from Albany, and she jumped into the car and rushed home and got everything ready. Now, as we walk through the door, she kisses us all and hands us plates in a single motion, fluid as her serve. I want to invite a judge to the house and renew our vows.

THE NEXT DAY howling winds come. Gusts of forty miles an hour. I fight through the winds, and through Federer's hurricane-force skills, and tie the match at two sets apiece. Federer glances at his feet, which is how he registers shock.

Then he adjusts better than I do. I have a sense he can adjust to anything, on the fly. He pulls out a tough fifth set, and I tell anyone who'll listen that he's on his way to becoming the best ever.

Before the winds settle down, retirement talk swirls again. Reporters want to know why I keep going. I explain that this is what I do for a living. I have a family and a school to support. Many people benefit from every tennis ball I hit. (One month after the U.S. Open, Stefanie and I host the ninth annual Grand Slam for Children, which collects $6 million. All told, we've raised $40 million for my foundation.)

Also, I tell reporters, I have game left. I don't know how much, but some. I still think I can win.

Again they stare.

Maybe they're confused because I don't tell them the full story, don't explain my full motivation. I can't, since I'm only slowly becoming aware of it myself. I play and keep playing because I *choose* to play. Even if it's not your ideal life, you can always choose it. No matter what your life is, choosing it changes everything.

. . .

AT THE 2005 AUSTRALIAN OPEN I beat Taylor Dent in three sets, advancing to the fourth round, and outside the locker room I stop for a very engaging TV commentator—Courier. It's odd to see him in this new role. I can't stop seeing him as a great champion. And yet TV suits him. He does it well and seems happy. I feel a good deal of respect for him, and I hope he feels some for me. Our differences feel long ago and juvenile.

He puts the microphone in front of my mouth and asks: How long before Jaden Agassi plays Pete's son?

I look into the camera and say: My biggest hope for my child is that he's focused on something.

Then I add: Hopefully he'll choose tennis, because I love it so much.

The old, old lie. But now it's even more shameful, because I've attached it to my son. The lie threatens to become my legacy. Stefanie and I are more resolved than ever that we don't want this crazy life for Jaden or Jaz, so what made me say it? As always, I suppose it was what I knew people wanted to hear. Also, flush from a win, I felt that tennis is a beautiful sport, which has treated me well, and I wanted to honor it. And maybe, standing before a champion I respected, I felt guilty for hating it. The lie may have been my way of hiding my guilt, or atoning for it.

IN THE LAST FEW MONTHS Gil has given a few hard twists to my training. He's had me eating like a Spartan warrior, and the new diet has honed me to a fine edge.

Also, I've had a cortisone shot, my third in the last year. Four is the maximum annual number recommended. There are risks, the doctors say. We simply don't know cortisone's long-term consequences for the spine and liver. But I don't care. So long as my back behaves.

And it does. I reach the quarters, where again I face Federer. I can't win a set. He dismisses me like a teacher with a dense pupil. He, more than any of the young guns taking control of the game, makes me feel my age. When I look at him, with his suave agility, his shot-making prowess and puma-like smoothness, I remember that I've been around since the days of wooden rackets. My brother-in-law, after all, was Pancho Gonzalez, a champion during the Berlin airlift, a rival of Fred Perry, and Federer was born the year I met my *friend* Perry.

. . .

I TURN THIRTY-FIVE just before Rome. Stefanie and the children come with me to Italy. I want to get out with Stefanie, see the Colosseum, the Pantheon, but I can't. When I came here as a boy, and as a young man, I was too consumed by inner torments and shyness to leave the hotel. Now, though I'd love to see the sights, my back won't permit it. The doctor says one long walk on pavement can mean the difference between the cortisone lasting three months or one.

I win my first four matches. Then I lose to Coria. Disgusted with myself, I feel guilty about getting a standing ovation. Again, reporters press the question of retirement.

I say: I only think about it fourteen times a year, because that's how many tournaments I play each year.

In other words: That's how many times I'm forced to sit through these news conferences.

In the first round of the 2005 French Open, I play Jarkko Nieminen, from Finland. Simply by stepping on the court, I set a record. My fifty-eighth slam. One more than Chang, Connors, Lendl, Ferreira. More than anyone in the open era. My back, however, is in no mood to commemorate the occasion. The cortisone has worn off. Serving is painful, standing is painful. Breathing is work. I think about walking to the net and forfeiting. But this is Roland Garros. I can't walk off this court, not *this* one. They'll have to carry me off this court atop my racket.

I swallow eight Advils. Eight. During the changeover I cover my face with a towel while biting on another towel to quell the pain. In the third set Gil knows something is terribly wrong. After hitting the ball, I don't sprint back to the center of the court. In all these years he's never seen me fail to sprint back to the center of the court. It's unthinkable, tantamount to him taking a men's-room break during one of my matches. Afterward, walking with Gil to a restaurant, I'm bent over like a giant shrimp. He says: We can't keep taking and taking from your body.

We pull out of Wimbledon, try to get ready for the summer hard courts. It's necessary, but feels like a gamble. Now I'll devote all my time and do all my work for fewer tournaments, which means the margin of error will be narrower, the pressure greater. The losses will hurt more.

Gil buries himself in his da Vinci notebooks. He's proud that I've never injured myself in his gym, and now I can see that, as my body ages, he's tense. His streak is on the line.

Some lifts you just can't do anymore, he says. Others you'll need to do twice as much.

We spend hours and hours in the weight room, discussing my core. From here until the finish line, Gil says, it's all about your core.

BECAUSE I'VE PULLED OUT OF WIMBLEDON, newspapers and magazines print a fresh batch of eulogies. *At an age when most tennis players—*

I swear off newspapers and magazines.

In late summer I play the Mercedes-Benz Cup and I win. Jaden is now old enough to watch me play, and during the trophy ceremony he comes running onto the court, thinking the trophy is his. Which it is.

I go to Montreal and scratch and claw my way to the final against a Spanish kid everyone is talking about. Rafael Nadal. I can't beat him. I can't fathom him. I've never seen anyone move like that on a tennis court.

At the 2005 U.S. Open I'm a novelty, a sideshow, a thirty-five-year-old playing in a slam. It's my twentieth year in a row at this tournament— many of this year's players haven't been alive twenty years. I remember playing Connors and knocking him out of his twentieth U.S. Open. I'm not the type to ask, Where did the years go? I know exactly where they went. I can feel every set in my spine.

I play Razvan Sabau, from Romania, in the first round. I've had my fourth and final cortisone shot of the year, so my back feels numb. I'm able to hit my meat-and-potatoes shot, which gives Sabau problems. When your basic shot hurts someone, when they're falling behind on the shot you can make a hundred out of a hundred times, you know the day is going to be fine. It's as though your jab is leaving marks on a guy's jaw, and you still haven't thrown your haymaker. I beat him in sixty-nine minutes.

Reporters say it was a massacre. They ask if I feel bad about beating him.

I say: I would never want to deprive anybody of the learning experience of losing.

They laugh.

I'm serious.

In the second round I play Ivo Karlovic, from Croatia. They list him as six foot ten, but he must have been standing in a ditch when they measured. He's a totem pole, a telephone pole, which gives his serve a sick trajectory. When Karlovic serves, the box technically becomes twice as large.

The net becomes a foot lower. I've never played anyone so big. I don't know how to prepare for an opponent his size.

In the locker room I introduce myself to Karlovic. He's sweet, fresh-faced, starry-eyed about being in the U.S. Open. I ask him to raise his serving arm as high as he can, then I call Darren over. We crane our necks, looking up, trying to see the tips of Karlovic's fingers. We can't.

Now, I say to Darren, try to imagine a racket in that arm. And now imagine him jumping. And *now*—imagine where the face of the racket would be and imagine the ball zinging off that racket. It's like he's serving from the freaking blimp.

Darren laughs. Karlovic laughs. He says, I would trade you my reach for your return game.

Fortunately, I know Karlovic's height will also be a liability for him at times in the match. Low balls will be problematic. Lunging won't be easy. Also, Darren says Karlovic's movement is dodgy. I remind myself not to spend energy worrying about how many times he aces me. Just wait for the one or two times he misses a first serve, then pounce on that second. Those will decide the match. And though Karlovic knows this also, I need to make him know it more. I need to make him feel it, by applying pressure on the second serve, which means never missing.

I beat him in straight sets.

In the third round I play Tomas Berdych, a tennis player's player. I faced him before, nearly two years ago, in the second round of the Australian Open. Darren warned me: You're about to play an eighteen-year-old kid who has real game, and you'd better be on it. He can rip the ball up both sides, he has a bomb of a serve, and in a few years he's going to be top ten.

Darren wasn't overselling it. Berdych was one of the best tennis players I'd faced all year. I beat him in Australia, 6–0, 6–2, 6–4, and felt fortunate. I thought: Good thing this is only best of five.

Now, surprisingly, Berdych hasn't improved much since then. His decision-making still needs work. He's like me before I met Brad: thinks he needs to win every point. He doesn't know the value of letting the other guy lose. When I beat him, when I shake his hand, I want to tell him to relax, it takes some people longer than others to learn. But I can't. It's not my place.

Next I play Xavier Malisse, from Belgium. He moves admirably well and has a slingshot of an arm. He features a meaty forehand and an acing serve, but he's not consistent. Also, his backhand is mediocre: it looks as if it should be great, because he's so comfortable hitting it, but he's more interested in the way it looks than actually executing it. He simply cannot hit a backhand up the line, and if you can't do that, you can't beat me. I control the court too well. If you can't hit a backhand up the line, I'll dictate every point. An opponent has to move me, stretch me off the mark, put me in a position where I'm dealing with him, or else he'll have to play on my terms. And my terms are harsh. Especially as I get older.

The night before the match, I have a drink with Courier at the hotel. He warns me that Malisse is playing well.

Maybe, I say, but I'm actually looking forward to it. You won't hear me saying this often, but this is going to be fun.

The match *is* fun, like a puppet show. I feel as if I'm holding a string and each time I pull it, Malisse jumps. I'm astonished, yet again, by the connection between two players on a tennis court. The net, which supposedly separates you, actually links you like a web. After two bruising hours you're convinced that you're locked in a cage with your opponent. You could swear that his sweat is spraying you, his breath is fogging your eyes.

I'm up two sets to none, dominating. Malisse has no faith in himself. He doesn't believe he belongs out here. But as the third set starts Malisse finally gets tired of being pulled from side to side. Such is life. He gets mad, plays with passion, and soon he's doing things that surprise even himself. He's hitting that backhand up the line, crisply, consistently. I glare at him with an expression that says, I'll believe that if you keep doing it.

He keeps doing it.

I see relief in his face and body language. He still doesn't think he's going to win, but he does think he's going to make a good show, and that's enough. He takes the third set in a tiebreak. Now I'm livid. I have better things to do than stand out here with you for another hour. Just for that, I'm going to make you cramp.

But Malisse isn't taking orders from me anymore. One set, one little set, has completely changed his demeanor, restored his confidence. He's no longer afraid. He only wanted to make a good show, and he has, so now he's playing with house money. In the fourth set our roles reverse, and he dictates the pace. He wins the set and ties the match.

In the fifth set, however, he's spent, whereas I'm just beginning to draw on funds long deposited in the Bank of Gil. It isn't close. Coming to the net, he smiles, accords me tremendous respect. I'm old, and he's made me older, but he knows that I've made him work, that I've forced him to dig deep and learn about himself.

In the locker room, Courier finds me, punches my shoulder.

He says, You called your shot. You told me you were going to have fun—you looked like you were having fun.

Fun. If I had fun, why do I feel as if I got hit by a truck?

I'M READY FOR A MONTH IN A HOT TUB, but my next match looms, and my opponent is playing like a man possessed. Blake. He smoked me the last time we met, in D.C., by getting and staying aggressive. Everyone says he's grown steadily better since that day.

My only hope is that he doesn't play aggressive this time out. Especially since it's cooler. In cool weather the court in New York plays slower, which favors a guy like Blake, who's so damned fast. On a slow court Blake can get to everything, and you can't, and thus he can make you press. You feel a need to do more than you normally do, and from there everything goes haywire.

The moment we step onto the court, my worst nightmare comes true. Blake is Mr. Aggressive, standing inside the baseline on my second serves, taking full cuts off both wings, making me feel urgency right from the opening minute. He smothers me in the first set, 6–3. In the second set he gives me a second helping of the same: 6–3.

Early in the third set the match takes on shades of Malisse. Except I'm Malisse. I can't beat this guy, I know I can't, so I may as well just try to give a good show. Freed from thoughts of winning, I instantly play better. I stop thinking, start feeling. My shots become a half-second quicker, my decisions become the product of instinct rather than logic. I see Blake take a step back and register the change. *What just happened?* He's been beating my brains in for seven straight rounds, and at the end of the eighth I land one sneaky punch, wobbling him just as the bell rings. Now he's walking to his corner, unable to believe that his hobbled, demoralized opponent still has life.

Blake has a huge following in New York, and they're all here tonight. Nike, which no longer endorses me, gives his supporters T-shirts and urges them to cheer. When I outplay Blake in the third, they stop cheering. When I win the set, they fall silent.

Throughout the fourth set, Blake's panicking, no longer being aggressive. I can see him thinking, can almost *hear* him thinking: Damn, I can't do anything right.

I win the fourth set.

Now that Blake has seen the benefits of my not thinking, he decides he's going to try it. As the fifth set unfolds, he turns off his brain. At last, after nearly three hours, we meet on equal terms. We're both on fire, and his on-fire is slightly better than my on-fire. In the tenth game he has a chance to serve out the match.

Then he starts thinking again. The contrarian brain. He presses, I hit three first-class returns, break him, and the crowd changes its mind. They chant, *An*-dre, *An*-dre.

I serve. I hold.

During the changeover the stadium sounds like a rock concert. My ears are ringing. My temples are pounding. It's so loud that I wrap my head in a towel.

He serves. He holds. We're going to a tiebreak.

I've heard old-timers say that the fifth set has nothing to do with tennis. It's true. The fifth set is about emotion and conditioning. Slowly I leave my body. Nice knowing you, body. I've had several out-of-body experiences over my career, but this one is healthy. I trust my skill, and I step out of its way. I remove myself from the equation. At match point, 6–5, I hit a solid serve. He returns to my forehand. I hit a quality ball to his backhand. He's moving around it, and I know—*mistake.* If he's running around my quality ball, that means he's pressing. He's not thinking clearly. He's putting himself out of position, letting the ball play him. He's not giving himself an opportunity to hit the best possible shot. Thus I know that one of two things is about to happen. He's going to be handcuffed by my ball and hit it weakly. Or he's going to be forced into an error.

Either way, I have a pretty good idea the ball is coming right here. I look at the spot where it's sure to land. Blake wheels, throws his lower torso out of the way and coldcocks the ball. It lands ten feet from where I expected. Winner.

I was completely wrong.

I do the only thing I can do. Walk back. Prepare for the next point.

At six–all we have a murderous rally, backhand to backhand, and I'm a big loose bag of rattling nerves. In a ten-stroke backhand rally, you know somebody's going to raise the stakes at any moment, and you're always sure it's going to be your opponent. I wait. And wait. But with each stroke, Blake doesn't raise the stakes. So it falls to me. I step in as if I'm going to cane the ball and instead I hit a backhand drop shot. I'm all in.

There are times in a match when you want to put just a solid, service-able swing on the ball, but your blood is so full of adrenaline that you hit it big. This happens often to Blake, not with his swing but his speed. He runs faster than he means to run. He feels so much urgency that he sprints to a ball and gets there sooner than he anticipated. This is what happens now. Sprinting all-out for my backhand drop, he has the racket gripped in such a way that he's going to have to dig, but instead he gets there so fast he doesn't need to dig. Meaning, the ball is on him and he has the wrong grip. Instead of crushing the ball, as he should, he's forced by his grip to punch the ball. Then he holds ground at the net, and I lace a backhand up the line. It passes him by a fair margin.

Now he's serving at 6–7. I have match point again. He misses the first serve. I have a nanosecond to decide where he's coming with his second serve. Aggressive? Safe? I decide he's going to err on the side of safety. He's going to roll it to my backhand. So how aggressive do I want to be? Where do I want to station myself? Should I make an irrevocable decision, stand where I can kill the ball if I'm correct, but where I won't be able to reach it if I'm wrong? Or should I split the difference, stand in the middle ground, where I'll be able to hit a moderately good shot on most serves, and a perfect shot on none?

If there is to be a final decision in this match, one final decision on this night of 100,000 decisions, I want that final decision to be mine. I irrevocably commit. He serves, as expected, to my backhand. It hangs just where I thought it would hang, like a soap bubble. I feel all the hairs on my body rise. I feel the crowd rise. I tell myself: Quality cut, rip it, rip it, *rip it, you fuck*. As the ball leaves my racket I track every inch of its flight. I see the shadow of the ball converging with the ball itself. As they slowly become one, I'm saying aloud: Ball, please please find a hole.

It does.

When Blake hugs me at the net, we know we've done something spe-cial. But I know it better, because I've played eight hundred more matches than he has. And this match stands apart from the others. I've never been more intellectually aware, never felt the need to be more intellectually aware, and I take a certain intellectual pride in the finished product. I want to sign it.

After they cut the tape off my feet, after the news conference, Gil and Perry and Darren and Philly and I go to P. J. Clarke's for food and drinks. By the time I get back to the hotel it's four in the morning. Stefanie is asleep. As I come in she sits up in bed and smiles.

You're crazy, she says.

I laugh.

That was unbelievable, she says. You *went places* out there.

I did, baby. I went places.

I lie on the floor next to the bed, try to fall asleep, but I can't stop replaying the match.

I hear her voice in the darkness somewhere above me, like an angel.

How do you feel?

It was a pretty cool way to spend an evening.

IN THE SEMIS I'm due to play Robby Ginepri, a touted kid from Georgia. CBS wants mine to be the late match. I go to the tournament director on my knees. I tell him, If I'm lucky enough to get through this match, I'll have to come back tomorrow. Please don't make a thirty-five-year-old man get home later than his twenty-two-year-old opponent in the final.

He reschedules my match, makes it the early semi.

After two five-setters in a row, no one gives me a chance against Ginepri. He's fast, solid off both sides, playing the best tennis of his life—and young. And even before dealing with Ginepri, I know the first thing I'll have to do is chisel through a wall of my own fatigue. The last three sets against Blake are the best tennis I've ever played, and the most draining. I tell myself to come out against Ginepri and manufacture adrenaline, pretend I'm down two sets, try to relocate that mindless state I found against Blake.

It works. Feigning urgency, I win the first set. Now my goal is to conserve energy for tomorrow's final. I begin to play safe tennis, thinking about my next opponent, and of course that lets Ginepri swing freely, take chances. He wins the second set.

I banish from my mind all thought of the final. I give Ginepri my full attention. He's gassed after expending so much energy to tie the match, and I win the third.

But he wins the fourth.

I need to start the fifth with fury. I also need to acknowledge that I can't win every point. I can't run after everything, can't lunge for each dink and drop. I can't go full-speed against a kid who's still teething. He wants to be out here all night, but I have forty-five minutes of energy left, forty-five minutes of a functioning body. Or maybe just thirty-five.

I win the set. It's not possible, but I'm in the final of the U.S. Open at thirty-five years old. Darren, Gil, and Stefanie scoop me off the locker-room floor and go into triage mode. Darren grabs my rackets and runs

them to Roman, the stringer. Gil hands me my Gil Water. Stefanie helps
me to the car. We race back to the Four Seasons to watch Federer and
Hewitt fight for the privilege of playing the old cripple from Vegas.

It's the most relaxed you can be before a final, watching the other
semi. You tell yourself: Whatever I'm feeling at this moment, it's better
than what those guys are feeling. Then Federer wins, of course. I lean
back on the couch and he's all I'm thinking about, and I know somewhere out there I'm all he's thinking about. Between now and tomorrow
afternoon I need to do everything a little better than he does it, including
sleep.

But I have children. I used to sleep until eleven thirty in the morning
on the day of a match. Now I can't sleep later than seven thirty. Stefanie
keeps the children quiet, but something in my body knows they're up,
they want to see their father. More, their father wants to see them.

After breakfast I kiss them goodbye. Driving to the stadium with Gil,
I'm quiet. I know I have no chance. I'm ancient, I've played three five-
setters in a row. Let's be real. My only hope is if it goes three or four sets.
If it's a fast match, where conditioning doesn't come into play, I might get
lucky.

Federer comes onto the court looking like Cary Grant. I almost wonder if he's going to play in an ascot and a smoking jacket. He's permanently smooth, I'm constantly rattled, even when serving at 40–15. He's
also dangerous from so many different parts of the court, there's
nowhere to hide. I don't do well when there's nowhere to hide. Federer
wins the first set. I go into frantic mode, do anything I can to knock him
off balance. I get up a break in the second. I break again and win the set.

I think to myself: Mr. Grant *might* just have a problem today.

In the third set, I break him and go up 4–2. I'm serving with a breeze
at my back, and Federer is shanking balls. I'm about to go up 5–2, and for
a fleeting moment, he and I both think something remarkable is about to
happen here. We lock eyes. We share a moment. Then, at 30–love, I hit a
kick serve to his backhand, he takes a swing, shanks it. The ball sounds
sick as it leaves his racket, like one of my deliberate misfires as a kid. But
this sick, ugly misfire somehow wobbles over the net and lands in. Winner. He breaks me, and we're back on serve.

In the tiebreak, he goes to a place that I don't recognize. He finds a
gear that other players simply don't have. He wins 7–1.

Now the shit is rolling downhill and doesn't stop. My quads are
screaming. My back is closing the store for the night. My decisions
become poor. I'm reminded how slight the margin can be on a tennis

court, how narrow the space between greatness and mediocrity, fame and anonymity, happiness and despair. We were playing a tight match. We were dead even. Now, due to a tiebreak that made my jaw drop with admiration, the rout is on.

Walking to the net, I'm certain that I've lost to the better man, the Everest of the next generation. I pity the young players who will have to contend with him. I feel for the man who is fated to play Agassi to his Sampras. Though I don't mention Pete by name, I have him uppermost in my mind when I tell reporters: It's real simple. Most people have weaknesses. Federer has none.

29

I PULL OUT OF THE 2006 AUSTRALIAN OPEN, then pull out of the entire clay season. I hate to do it, but I need to save myself for the 2006 Wimbledon, which I quietly, privately decide will be my last. I'm saving myself for Wimbledon. I never thought I'd say such a thing. I never dreamed a proper, respectful goodbye to Wimbledon would feel so important.

But Wimbledon has become hallowed ground for me. It's where my wife shined. It's where I first suspected that I could win, and where I proved it to myself and the world. Wimbledon is where I learned to bow, to bend my knee, to do something I didn't want to do, wear what I didn't want to wear, and survive. Also, no matter how I feel about tennis, the game is my home. I hated home as a boy, and then I left, and I soon found myself homesick. In the final hours of my career I'm continually chastened by that memory.

I tell Darren this will be my last Wimbledon, and the coming U.S. Open will be my last tournament ever. We make the announcement just as Wimbledon gets under way. Immediately after, I'm startled by how differently my peers look at me. They no longer treat me as a rival, a threat. I'm retired. I'm irrelevant. A wall is let down.

Reporters ask, Why now? Why did you choose to retire now? I tell them I didn't. I simply can't play anymore. That's the finish line I've been seeking, the finish line with the inexorable pull. Can't play, as opposed to won't play. Unwittingly, I've been seeking that moment when I'd have no choice.

Bud Collins, the venerable tennis commentator and historian, the coauthor of Laver's autobiography, sums up my career by saying I've gone from punk to paragon. I cringe. To my thinking, Bud sacrificed the truth on the altar of alliteration. I was never a punk, any more than I'm now a paragon.

Also, several sportswriters muse about my transformation, and that word rankles. I think it misses the mark. Transformation is change from one thing to another, but I started as nothing. I didn't transform, I formed. When I broke into tennis, I was like most kids: I didn't know who I was, and I rebelled at being told by older people. I think older people make this mistake all the time with younger people, treating them as finished products when in fact they're in process. It's like judging a match before it's over, and I've come from behind too often, and had too many opponents come roaring back against me, to think that's a good idea.

What people see now, for better or worse, is my first formation, my first incarnation. I didn't alter my image, I discovered it. I didn't change my mind. I opened it. J.P. helps me work through this idea, to explain it to myself. He says people have been fooled by my changing looks, my clothes and hair, into thinking that I know who I am. People see my self-exploration as self-expression. He says that, for a man with so many fleeting identities, it's shocking, and symbolic, that my initials are A.K.A.

Sadly, in the early summer of 2006, despite the best efforts of J.P. and others, I can't yet explain this to reporters. Even if I could, the press room at the All England Club isn't the place.

I can't explain it to Stefanie either, but I don't need to. She knows all. In the days and hours leading up to Wimbledon, she stares into my eyes and pats my cheek. She talks to me about my career. She talks about hers. She tells me about her last Wimbledon. She didn't know it would be her last. She says it's better this way, to know, to go out on my own terms.

Wearing a necklace made for me by Jaden—a chain of block letters that spells out *Daddy Rocks*—I face Boris Pashanski, from Serbia, in the first round. As I step on the court, the applause is loud and long. On the first serve, I can't see the court, because my eyes are filled with tears. Despite feeling as if I'm playing in a suit of armor, with a back that will not loosen, I persist, endure. I win.

In the second round I beat Andreas Seppi, from Italy, in straight sets. I'm playing well, which gives me hope going into my third-round match, against Nadal. He's a brute, a freak, a force of nature, as strong and balletic a player as I've ever seen. But I feel—the delusional effects of winning—that I might be able to make inroads. I like my chances. I lose the first set, 7–6, but take hope from how close it was.

Then he annihilates me. The match takes seventy minutes. My window of opportunity is fifty-five. That's when I start to feel my back. Late in the match, with Nadal serving, I can no longer stand still. I need to move around, stomp my foot, get the blood flowing. The stiffness is so severe, the pain so great, returning is the last thing on my mind. I'm thinking only of remaining vertical.

After, in a moment dripping with irony, Wimbledon officials break with tradition to hold an on-court interview with Nadal and me. They never hold on-court interviews. I tell Gil: Sooner or later, I knew I'd get Wimbledon to break with tradition.

Gil isn't laughing. He never laughs while a fight is still going on.

It's almost over, I tell him.

I go to Washington, D.C., and play an Italian qualifier named Andrea Stoppini. He beats me as if I'm the qualifier, and I feel ashamed. I thought I needed a tune-up for the U.S. Open, but this tune-up has left me shaken. I tell reporters that I'm struggling with the end more than I expected. I tell them that the best way I can explain it is this: Many of you, I'm sure, don't like your jobs. But imagine if someone told you right now that your story about me would be your last. After this, you'll never be able to write another word for as long as you live. How would you feel?

EVERYONE TRAVELS TO NEW YORK. The whole team. Stefanie, the children, my parents, Perry, Gil, Darren, Philly. We invade the Four Seasons and colonize Campagnola. The children smile to hear the applause as we walk in. To my ear, the applause sounds different this time. It has a different timbre. It has a subtext. They know this isn't about me, it's about all of us finishing something special together.

Frankie seats us at the corner table. He makes a big fuss over Stefanie and the children. I watch him serve Jaden all my favorite foods, and I watch Jaden enjoy them. I watch Jaz enjoy the food too, though she insists that each entrée remain separate. They mustn't touch. A variation of the blueberry muffin imperative. I watch Stefanie watching the kids, smiling, and I think of the four of us, four distinct personalities. Four different surfaces. And yet a matching set. Complete. On the eve of my final tournament, I enjoy that sense we all seek, that knowledge we get only a few times in life, that the themes of our life are connected, the seeds of our ending were there in the beginning, and vice versa.

In the first round I play Andrei Pavel, from Romania. My back seizes up midway through the match, but despite standing stick straight I manage to tough out a win. I ask Darren to arrange a cortisone shot for the next day. Even with the shot, I don't know if I'll be able to play my next match.

I certainly won't be able to win. Not against Marcos Baghdatis. He's ranked number eight in the world. He's a big strong kid from Cyprus, in the midst of a great year. He's reached the final of the Australian Open and the semis of Wimbledon.

And then somehow I beat him. Afterward I'm barely able to stagger up the tunnel and into the locker room before my back gives out. Darren and Gil lift me like a bag of laundry onto the training table, while Baghdatis's people hoist him onto the table beside me. He's cramping badly. Stefanie appears, kisses me. Gil forces me to drink something. A trainer says the doctors are on the way. He turns on the TV above the table and everyone clears out, leaving just me and Baghdatis, both of us writhing and groaning in pain.

The TV shows highlights from our match. SportsCenter.

In my peripheral vision I detect slight movement. I turn to see Baghdatis extending his hand. His face says, We *did* that. I reach out, take his hand, and we remain this way, holding hands, as the TV flickers with scenes of our savage battle.

We relive the match, and then I relive my life.

Finally the doctors arrive. It takes them and the trainers half an hour to get Baghdatis and me on our feet. Baghdatis leaves the locker room first, gingerly, leaning against his coach. Then Gil and Darren lead me out to the parking lot, enticing me forward a few more steps with the thought of a cheeseburger and a martini at P. J. Clarke's. It's two in the morning.

Christ, Darren says, as we emerge into the parking lot. The car is all the way over there, mate.

We squint at the lone car in the middle of the empty parking lot. It's several hundred yards away. I tell him I can't make it.

No, of course not, he says. Wait here and I'll bring it around.

He runs off.

I tell Gil that I can't stay upright. I need to lie down while we wait. He sets my tennis bag on the cement and I sit, then lie back, using the bag as a pillow.

I look up at Gil. I see nothing but his smile and his shoulders. I look just beyond his shoulders at the stars. So many stars. I look at the light stanchions that rim the stadium. They seem like bigger, closer stars.

Suddenly, an explosion. A sound like a giant can of tennis balls being opened. One stanchion goes out. Then another, and another.

I close my eyes. It's over.

No. Hell no. It will never really be over.

· · ·

I'M HOBBLING THROUGH THE LOBBY of the Four Seasons the next morning when a man steps out of the shadows. He grabs my arm.

Quit, he says.

What?

It's my father—or a ghost of my father. He looks ashen. He looks as if he hasn't slept in weeks.

Pops? What are you talking about?

Just quit. Go home. You did it. It's over.

He says he prays for me to retire. He says he can't wait for me to be done, so he won't have to watch me suffer anymore. He won't have to sit through my matches with his heart in his mouth. He won't have to stay up until two in the morning to catch a match from the other side of the world, so he can scout some new wonderboy I might soon have to face. He's sick of the whole miserable thing. He sounds as if—is it possible?

Yes, I see it in his eyes.

I know that look.

He hates tennis.

He says, Don't put yourself through this anymore! After last night, you have nothing left to prove. I can't see you like this. It's too painful.

I reach out and touch his shoulder. I'm sorry, Pops. I can't quit. This can't end with me quitting.

THIRTY MINUTES BEFORE THE MATCH, I get an anti-inflammatory injection, but it's different from the cortisone. Less effective. Against my third-round opponent, Benjamin Becker, I'm barely able to remain standing.

I look at the scoreboard. I shake my head. I ask myself over and over, How is it possible that my final opponent is a guy named B. Becker? I told Darren earlier this year that I wanted to go out against somebody I like and respect, or else against somebody I don't know.

And so I get the latter.

Becker takes me out in four sets. I can feel the tape of the finish line snap cleanly across my chest.

U.S. Open officials let me say a few words to the fans in the stands and at home before heading into the locker room. I know exactly what I want to say.

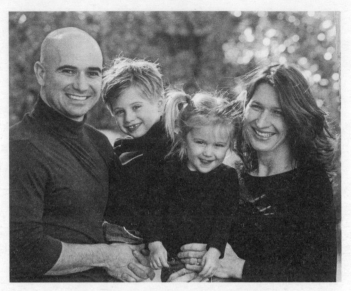

With Stefanie, Jaden, and Jaz in the fall of 2006

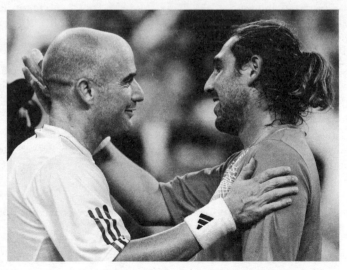

Marcos Baghdatis congratulates me after the second round
of the 2006 U.S. Open

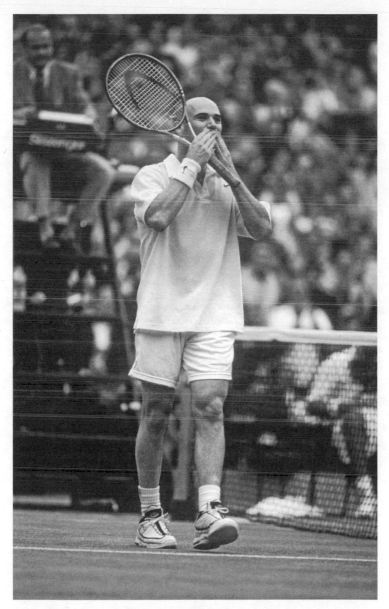

Centre Court, Wimbledon, 2000

I've known for years. But is still takes me a few moments to find my voice.

The scoreboard said I lost today, but what the scoreboard doesn't say is what it is I have found. Over the last twenty-one years I have found loyalty: You have pulled for me on the court, and also in life. I have found inspiration: You have willed me to succeed, sometimes even in my lowest moments. And I have found generosity: You have given me your shoulders to stand on, to reach for my dreams—dreams I could have never reached without you. Over the last twenty-one years I have found you, and I will take you and the memory of you with me for the rest of my life.

It's the highest compliment I know how to pay them. I've compared them to Gil.

In the locker room it's deathly quiet. I've noticed through the years that every locker room is the same when you lose. You walk in the door—which slams open, because you've pushed it harder than you needed to—and the guys always scatter from the TV, where they've been watching you get your ass kicked. They always pretend they haven't been watching, haven't been discussing you. This time, however, they remain gathered around the TV. No one moves. No one pretends. Then, slowly, everyone comes toward me. They clap and whistle, along with trainers and office workers and James the security guard.

Only one man remains apart, refusing to applaud. I see him in the corner of my eye. He's leaning against a far wall with a blank look on his face and his arms tightly folded.

Connors.

He's now coaching Roddick. Poor Andy.

It makes me laugh. I can only admire that Connors is who he is, still, that he never changes. We should all be so true to ourselves, so consistent.

I tell the players: You'll hear a lot of applause in your life, fellas, but none will mean more to you than that applause—from your peers. I hope each of you hears that at the end.

Thank you all. Goodbye. And take care of each other.

THE BEGINNING

RAIN HAS BEEN FALLING OFF AND ON ALL DAY.

Stefanie peers at the sky and says, What do you think?

Come on, I say—let's try. I'm willing if you are.

Willing. She frowns. She's always willing, but she can't speak for her calf, which has been giving her problems since she retired. Especially lately. She looks down. Darned calf. She has a charity match in Tokyo next week. She's playing to raise money for a kindergarten she's opened in Eritrea, and even though it's only an exhibition she wants to do well. She feels the old pressure to do well. Also, she can't help but wonder how much game she has left.

I wonder the same thing about myself. It's been a year since I walked off the court for the last time at the U.S. Open. It's autumn, 2007.

So we've been planning all week to get out there, hit with each other, but now the day has come and it's the one rainy day all year in Vegas.

We can't build a fire in the rain.

Stefanie looks again at the overcast sky. Then at the clock. Busy day, she says. She has to pick up Jaden at school. We only have this small window.

IF THE RAIN DOESN'T LET UP, if we don't hit, I might go down to my school, because that's where I go whenever I have time. I can't believe how it's grown: a 26,000-square-foot education complex with 500 students and a waiting list of eight hundred.

The $40 million campus features everything the kids could want. A high-tech TV production studio. A computer room with dozens of PCs along the walls and a big, white, fluffy couch. A topflight exercise room with machines as fancy as those at the most exclusive clubs in Vegas. There's a weight room, a lecture hall, and bathrooms as modern and clean as the ones in the city's finest hotels. Best of all, the place is still freshly painted and pristine, just as sparkling as it was on opening day. Students, parents, the neighborhood, everyone respects the school because everyone owns it. The area hasn't completely rebounded since we arrived. While I was giving a tour recently, someone was shot across the street. And yet in eight years not one window has been broken, not one wall has been sprayed with graffiti.

Everywhere you look are little touches, subtle details that signify this school is different, this place is about excellence, through and through. On the front window is etched one large word, our unofficial school motto: BELIEVE. Every classroom is flooded with soft natural daylight. Indirect, southern, bounced from skylights to high-tech reflectors, it's a diffuse glow that's ideal for reading and concentrating. Teachers never need to flick a light switch, which saves energy and money, but also spares students the headaches and general gloom caused by standard fluorescents, which I remember all too well.

Our grounds are designed like a college campus, with intimate quads and welcoming common areas. The walls are stone—muted purple and pale salmon quartzite from local quarries—and the walkways are lined with delicate plum trees, leading to one beautiful holly oak, a symbolic Tree of Hope, which we planted even before the groundbreaking. First things first, our architects figured, so they planted the Tree of Hope, then asked construction workers to keep the tree watered and lighted while they built the school around it.

The land on which the school sits is narrow, only eight acres, but the lack of space actually suited the architects' overall scheme. They wanted the flow of the campus to symbolize a short, serpentine journey. Like life. Wherever students stand, they can turn one way and see a glimpse of where they've been, or turn the other and see a hint of where they're headed. Kindergarteners and elementary schoolers can gaze at the tall high school buildings, waiting for them—though they can't hear the voices of the older kids. We don't want to scare them. High schoolers can glance back at the primary classrooms from which they set out—though they can't hear the high-pitched screaming on the playground. We don't want to disturb them.

The architects, local guys named Mike Del Gatto and Rob Gurdison, threw themselves into this project. They spent months researching the history of the neighborhood, examining charter schools throughout the nation, experimenting with ideas. Then they stayed up night after night, brainstorming around a ping-pong table in Mike's basement. They built the first cardboard-plywood model of the school on that ping-pong table, unaware of any coincidence or irony.

It was their idea to have the buildings teach, to tell stories. We told them the stories we wanted told. In the middle school we wanted enormous photos of Martin Luther King Jr., Mahatma Gandhi, and, of course, Mandela, with their inspirational words painted on raised glass beneath their portraits. Since most of our students are African American, we asked Mike and Rob to embed bricks of marbled glass in one wall, depicting the Big Dipper, and to the right one single brick of glass, representing the North Star. The Big Dipper and the North Star were beacons for runaway slaves, pointing them to freedom.

My small contribution to the aesthetics of the school: in the common area of the high school building I wanted a gleaming black Steinway. When I delivered the piano, all the students gathered around and I shocked them by playing Lean on Me. What delighted me most was that the students didn't know who I was. And when their teachers told them, they weren't all that impressed.

I dreamed of a school with the fewest possible dry routines, a place that fostered serendipity. A place where serendipity was the norm. And it's happened. On any given day something cool is likely to happen at Agassi Prep. President Bill Clinton might drop by and take a turn teaching history. Shaquille O'Neal might be the substitute in physical education. You might bump into Lance Armstrong walking the halls, or Muhammad Ali wearing a visitor badge, shadow-boxing a freshman. You might look up at any moment and see Janet Jackson or Elton John standing in the door of a classroom, or members of Earth, Wind & Fire auditing. More serendipity: When we dedicate the gymnasium, the NBA All-Star Game will be taking place in Vegas. We'll invite the rookie and sophomore All-Stars to play their traditional pickup game on our floor— the first game ever played at Agassi Prep. The kids will love that.

Our educators are the best, plain and simple. The goal in hiring them was to find sharp, passionate, inspired men and women who were willing to lay it on the line, to get personally involved. We ask one thing of every teacher: to believe that every student can learn. It sounds like a painfully obvious concept, self-evident, but nowadays it's not.

Of course, because Agassi Prep has a longer day and a longer year than other schools, our staff might earn less per hour than staffs elsewhere. But they have more resources at their fingertips, and so they enjoy greater freedom to excel and make a difference in children's lives.

We thought it important that students wear uniforms. Tennis shirt with khaki pants, shorts, or skirt, in official school colors—burgundy and navy. We think it creates less peer pressure, and we know it saves our parents money in the long run. Every time I walk into the school I'm struck by the irony: I'm now the enforcer of a uniform policy. I look forward to the day when some Wimbledon official happens to be in Vegas and asks for a tour. I can hardly wait to see the look on his or her face when I mention my school's strict dress code.

We have another code that might be my favorite feature of the school. The Code of Respect that begins each day. Whenever I'm down there I poke my head into a random classroom and ask the children to stand with me and recite.

> *The essence of good discipline is respect.*
> *Respect for authority and respect for others.*
> *Respect for self and respect for rules.*
> *It is an attitude that begins at home,*
> *Is reinforced at school,*
> *And is applied throughout life.*

I promise them that if they memorize that simple code, keep it close to their hearts, they will go very far.

Walking the halls, peering into the classrooms, I can see how the children value this place. I can hear it in their voices, discern it in their postures. From the teachers and staff I've heard their stories, and I know the many ways this school enriches their lives. Also, we ask them to write personal essays, which we excerpt in the program for the yearly fund-raiser. Not all the essays are about trials and hardships. Far from it. But those are the ones I remember. Like the girl living alone with her frail mother, who's been unable to work for years due to an incurable lung disease. They share a cockroach-infested apartment in a neighborhood ruled by gangs, so school is the girl's refuge. Her grades, she says with touching pride, are outstanding, *because I rationalized that if I did well in school no one would question what was going on at home, and I wouldn't have to tell my story. Now, at seventeen, despite being forced to watch my mother deteriorate, to have lived with The Bloods and cockroaches, to work to support my family, I am college bound.*

Another senior writes about her painful relationship with her father, who's spent much of her childhood in jail. Recently, when he got out, she went to meet him and found him painfully thin, living with a haggard woman *in a broken motor home that reeked of sewage and crystal meth.*

Desperate not to repeat the mistakes of her parents, the girl pushes herself to succeed at Agassi Prep. *I won't let myself down the way others have. It's up to me to change the course of my future and I will never give up.*

Not long ago, while walking through the high school, I was flagged down by a boy. He was fifteen, shy, with soulful eyes and chubby cheeks. He asked if he could speak to me privately.

Of course, I said.

We stepped into an alcove off the main hallway.

He didn't know where to start. I told him to start at the beginning.

My life changed a year ago, he said. My father died. He was killed. Murdered, you know.

I'm so sorry.

After that, I really lost my way. I didn't know what I was going to do.

His eyes grew cloudy with tears.

Then I came to this school, he said. And it gave me direction. It gave me hope. It gave me *a life.* So I've been keeping an eye out for you, Mr. Agassi, and when you came by, I had to introduce myself and tell you— you know. Thanks.

I hugged him. I told him that it was I who needed to thank him.

IN THE UPPER GRADES, the focus is squarely on college. The kids are told again and again that Agassi Prep is only a stepping-stone. Don't get comfortable, we tell them. College is the main goal. Should they happen to forget, reminders are everywhere. College banners line the walls. A main hallway is named College Street. A metal sky bridge between the two main buildings has never been used, and never will be used, until the first seniors receive their diplomas and embark for college in 2009. Walking across that bridge, the seniors will enter a secret room, sign their names in a ledger, and leave notes to the next class, and the next, and all senior classes to come. I can see myself addressing that first senior class. I'm already working with J.P. and Gil, obsessing over my speech.

My theme, I think, will be contradictions. A friend suggests I brush up on Walt Whitman.

Do I contradict myself? Very well, then, I contradict myself.

I never knew this was an acceptable point of view. Now I steer by it. Now it's my North Star. And that's what I'll tell the students. Life is a tennis match between polar opposites. Winning and losing, love and hate, open and closed. It helps to recognize that painful fact early. Then recognize the polar opposites within yourself, and if you can't embrace them,

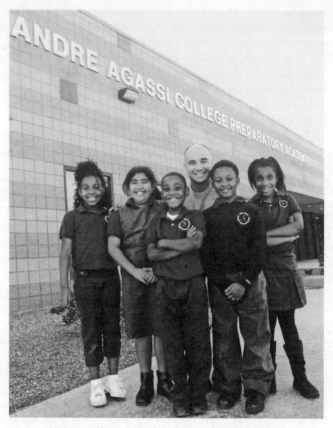

Visiting with a group of students at the Andre Agassi
College Preparatory Academy

or reconcile them, at least accept them and move on. The only thing you cannot do is ignore them.

What other message could I hope to deliver? What other message could they expect from a ninth-grade dropout whose proudest accomplishment is his school?

IT'S STOPPED RAINING, Stefanie says.

Come on, I say. Let's go!

She pulls on a tennis skirt. I throw on some shorts. We drive to the public court down the street. In the little pro shop, the teenage girl behind the counter is reading a gossip magazine. She looks up, and her chewing gum almost falls out.

Hello, I say.

Hi.

Are you open?

Yeah.

Could we rent a court for an hour?

Um. Yeah.

How much does it cost?

Fourteen dollars.

OK.

I hand her the money.

She says, You can have center court.

We walk downstairs to a mini amphitheater, where a blue tennis court is surrounded by metal bleachers. We set down our bags, side by side, then stretch and groan, teasing each other about how long it's been.

I rummage in my bag for wristbands, tape, gum.

Stefanie says, Which side do you want?

This one.

I knew it.

She hits a forehand softly. I creak like the Tin Man as I lumber toward it, then punch it back. We have a gentle, tentative rally, and suddenly Stefanie laces a backhand up the line that sounds like a freight train going by. I shoot her a look. It's going to be like that, is it?

She hits a Stefanie Slice to my backhand. I sit down on my legs and cane it, hard as I can. I yell to her, That shot has paid a lot of bills for us, baby!

She smiles and blows a lock of hair from her eyes.

Our shoulders loosen, our muscles warm. The pace quickens. I strike the ball clean, hard, and my wife does the same. We shift from hitting without purpose to playing crisp points. She hits a wicked forehand. I hit a screaming backhand—into the net.

First backhand crosscourt I've missed in twenty years. I stare at the ball, lying against the net. For a moment it bothers me. I tell her it bothers me. I feel myself getting irritated.

Then I laugh, and Stefanie laughs, and we begin again.

With every swing she's visibly happier. Her calf is feeling good. She thinks she'll be fine in Tokyo. Now that she's not worried about the injury, we can play, really play. Soon we're having so much fun that when the rain comes, we don't notice. When the first spectator arrives, we don't notice him either.

One by one, more arrive. Faces appear throughout the bleachers, as one person presumably phones another person, who phones two more people, to tell them we're out here, on a public court, playing for nothing but pride. Like Rocky Balboa and Apollo Creed after the lights are off and the gym is locked.

The rain falls harder. But we ain't stopping. We're going all-out. The people who show up now have cameras. Flashes go off. They seem unusually bright, reflected and magnified by the raindrops. I don't care, and Stefanie doesn't notice. We're not fully conscious of anything but the ball, the net, each other.

A long rally. Ten strokes. Fifteen. It ends with me missing. The court is strewn with balls. I scoop up three, put one in my pocket.

I yell to Stefanie, Let's both come back! What do you say?

She doesn't answer.

You and me, I say. We'll announce it this week!

Still no answer. Her concentration, as usual, puts mine to shame. In the same way that she wastes no movement on the court, she never wastes words. J.P. points out that the three most influential people in my life—my father, Gil, Stefanie—aren't native English speakers. And with all three, their most powerful mode of communication may be physical.

She's engrossed in each shot. Each shot is important. She never tires, never misses. It's a joy to watch her, but also a privilege. People ask what it's like, and I can never think of the perfect word, but that word comes close. A privilege.

I miss again. She squints, waits.

I serve. She returns, then gives the Stefanie wave, as if swatting a mosquito, meaning she's done. Time to pick up Jaden.

She walks off the court.

Not yet, I tell her.

What? She stops, looks at me. Then she laughs.

OK, she says, backpedaling to the baseline. It makes no sense, but it's who I am, and she understands. We have things to do, wonderful things. She can't wait to go and get started, and neither can I. But I also can't help it.

I want to play just a little while longer.

ACKNOWLEDGMENTS

THIS BOOK would not exist without my friend J. R. Moehringer.

It was J.R., before we even met, who first made me think seriously about putting my story on paper. During my final U.S. Open, in 2006, I spent all my free time reading J.R.'s staggering memoir, *The Tender Bar*. The book spoke to my heart. I loved it so much, in fact, that I found myself rationing it, limiting myself to a set number of pages each night. At first *The Tender Bar* was a crucial distraction from the difficult emotions at the end of my career, but gradually it added to the overall anxiety, because I feared the book would run out before the career did.

Just after my first-round match, I phoned J.R. and introduced myself. I told him how much I admired his work, and I invited him to Vegas for dinner. We hit it off right away, as I knew we would, and that first dinner led to many more. Eventually I asked J.R. if he'd consider working with me, helping me tackle my own memoir and give it shape. I asked him to show me my life through a Pulitzer Prize–winner's lens. To my surprise, he said yes.

J.R. moved to Las Vegas and we got right to it. We have the same work ethic, the same obsessive all-or-nothing approach to big goals. We met each day and developed a strict routine—after wolfing down a couple of burritos, we'd talk for hours into J.R.'s tape recorder. No topics were out of bounds, so our sessions were sometimes fun, sometimes painful. We didn't go chronologically or topically; we simply let the talk flow, prodded now and then by stacks of clippings collected by our superb, young, soon-to-be-famous researcher, Ben Cohen.

After many months J.R. and I had a crate of tape cassettes—for better or worse, the story of my life. The intrepid Kim Wells then turned those tapes into a transcript, which J.R. somehow transformed into a story. Jonathan Segal, our wise, wonderful editor at Knopf, and Sonny Mehta, the Rod Laver of publishing, helped J.R. and me polish that first draft into a second and a third, which was then excruciatingly fact-checked by

Eric Mercado, the second coming of Sherlock Holmes. I've never spent so much time reading and rereading, debating and discussing words and passages, dates and numbers. It's as close as I'll ever come, or want to come, to studying for final exams.

I asked J.R. many times to put his name on this book. He felt, however, that only one name belonged on the cover. Though proud of the work we did together, he said he couldn't see signing his name to another man's life. These are your stories, he said, your people, your battles. It was the kind of generosity I first saw on display in his memoir. I knew not to argue. Stubbornness is another quality we share. But I insisted on using this space to describe the extent of J.R.'s role and to publicly thank him.

I also want to mention the dedicated team of first readers to whom J.R. and I passed copies and excerpts of the manuscript. Each contributed in significant ways. Deepest thanks to Phillip and Marti Agassi, Sloan and Roger Barnett, Ivan Blumberg, Darren Cahill, Wendy Netkin Cohen, Brad Gilbert, David Gilmore, Chris and Varanda Handy, Bill Husted, McGraw Milhaven, Steve Miller, Dorothy Moehringer, John and Joni Parenti, Gil Reyes, Jaimee Rose, Gun Ruder, John Russell, Brooke Shields, Wendi Stewart Goodson, and Barbra Streisand.

A special thanks to Ron Boreta for being rock solid, for reading me as closely as he read this book, for giving me invaluable advice about everything from psychology to strategy, and for helping me rethink and revise my longstanding definition of the words *best friend*.

Above all, I want to thank Stefanie, Jaden, and Jaz Agassi. Forced to do without me on countless days, forced to share me for two years with this book, they never once complained, they only encouraged, which enabled me to finish. The steadfast love and support of Stefanie provided constant inspiration, and the daily smiles of Jaden and Jaz converted to energy as quickly as food turns to blood sugar.

One day, while I was working on the second draft, Jaden had a playmate over to the house. Manuscripts were piled high along the kitchen counter, and Jaden's friend asked: What's all that?

That's my Daddy's *book,* Jaden said in a voice I'd never heard him use for anything but Santa Claus and Guitar Hero.

I hope he and his sister feel that same pride in this book ten years from now, and thirty, and sixty. It was written for them, but also to them. I hope it helps them avoid some of the traps I walked right into. More, I hope it will be one of many books that give them comfort, guidance, pleasure. I was late in discovering the magic of books. Of all my many mistakes that I want my children to avoid, I put that one near the top of the list.

ILLUSTRATION CREDITS

Page

A NOTE ON THE TYPE

THIS BOOK was set in Minion, a typeface produced by the Adobe Corporation specifically for the Macintosh personal computer, and released in 1990. Designed by Robert Slimbach, Minion combines the classic characteristics of old style faces with the full complement of weights required for modern typesetting.

Composed by North Market Street Graphics,
Lancaster, Pennsylvania

Designed by Virginia Tan